Cancer Drug Discovery

Kyu-Won Kim • Jae Kyung Roh
Hee-Jun Wee • Chan Kim

Cancer Drug Discovery

Science and History

Springer

Kyu-Won Kim
College of Pharmacy
Seoul National University
Seoul
Korea (Republic of)

Hee-Jun Wee
College of Pharmacy
Seoul National University
Seoul
Korea (Republic of)

Jae Kyung Roh
Department of Internal Medicine
Yonsei University College of Medicine
Seoul
Korea (Republic of)

Chan Kim
Department of Internal Medicine
CHA Bundang Medical Center
Seongnam
Korea (Republic of)

Originally published by PanMun Education Co., Seoul, 2015
ISBN 978-94-024-0842-3 ISBN 978-94-024-0844-7 (eBook)
DOI 10.1007/978-94-024-0844-7

Library of Congress Control Number: 2016958571

Printed on acid-free paper

This Springer imprint is published by Springer Nature
The registered company is Springer Science+Business Media B.V. Dordrecht

Preface

This book was written with the aim to provide a comprehensive and multifaceted overview of the history of the development of anticancer drugs and to present future directions for the development of new anticancer drugs. First, this book examines the scientific progress in biological science periodically and the influence such progress had in cancer research. Furthermore, this book outlines the development process of anticancer drugs with a focus on the characteristic drug groups of each era, in relation with the advancements in the relevant fields of chemistry and biological science and also presents a brief mechanism of the drugs. After examining the side effects of each anticancer drug and the treatments for alleviating the effects, this book finally sums up the limitations of the current anticancer drugs and seeks new directions for the development of anticancer drugs.

During the last 60 years, research in biological science has centered on the cell, and cellular molecules, with an emphasis on the activities and functions of various genes. Accordingly, cancer research has also focused on cancer cells; the differences between normal cells and cancer cells, including their genetic variations, were discovered and corresponding molecule-targeted anticancer drugs developed.

The development process of anticancer drugs indicates that leukemia, which can be easily observed through the microscope, served as the model during the early days of cancer research and that the rapid proliferation of the leukemia cells was accepted as the general characteristic of cancer cells. As a result, development of anticancer drugs that have anti-proliferative effects began, starting with the alkylating agent in 1946, based on the unity assumption that all cancer cells characteristically grows abnormally. The search for a standard treatment for all cancers was launched through the development of such cytotoxic anticancer drugs.

Alkylating agents, which are one of the first types of anticancer drugs developed during this process, inhibit persistent cell proliferation, which is the representative feature of cancers, by causing DNA damage, and was developed especially during the 1940s to the early 1970s. The second type, antimetabolites, have been developed since the late 1940s and display structural mimicry with precursors of DNA synthesis, thus inhibiting cell proliferation by inhibiting activities of various enzymes contributing to DNA replication. In addition, as a result of a large-scale drug screening that began in 1954, plant alkaloids and anticancer antibiotics were developed from the 1960s and continued to be developed until the 1990s. Anticancer drug screenings on chemical molecules also proceeded at the same time, leading to the development of various chemical anticancer drugs from the mid-1960s which continued to be developed until the mid-2000s. These drugs form the third type of anticancer drugs. The fourth type of anticancer drugs, consisting of immunotherapy and miscellaneous anticancer drugs, were developed in the mid-1960s, proceeded to be developed from the 1980s to the 1990s and are still consistently being developed. Immunotherapy anticancer drugs, which activate the immune system to eliminate cancer cells, include cytokines such as interferons, humanized antibodies, and dendritic cells, while asparaginase and others were developed as miscellaneous type of anticancer drugs. Before the molecule-targeted anticancer drugs were developed, the fifth type of anticancer drugs, hormonal cancer drugs were developed for treating several cancers based on the understanding of the biological characteristics of cancers. Hormonal anticancer drugs for treating testosterone- or estrogen-dependent cancers such as diethylstilbestrol or tamoxifen were developed from the 1940s and are continued to be used today. Beginning from the 1990s, new types of molecule-targeted anticancer drugs were rapidly developed, forming the sixth type of anticancer drugs. Molecule-targeted anticancer drugs are products of in-depth biological research on cancers that was intensified from the 1980s. In other words, molecular mechanisms of tumorigenesis and malignancy were better understood by extensive research which used molecular biology as its major research technologies. In particular, various factors that play important roles in various types of cancers were discovered, facilitating the development of new drugs targeting the discovered factors. These molecule-targeted anticancer drugs are forming a major anticancer drug group starting from the 2000s.

Accordingly, this book presents an overview of the scientific discoveries and history of the development of anticancer drugs in the following order. Chapter 1 summarizes the characteristics of cancer in accordance to the development of science. This chapter describes the characteristics of the cancer cells based on the research that focused exclusively on cancer cells, similarly to biological science which mainly focuses on cells. Moreover, this chapter provided characteristics of cancer which interacts with its surrounding microenvironment. In particular, this chapter provides a systematic explanation of cancer in relation with the vascular system, lymphatic system, and immune system, which also relates to the new research prospects presented in the final chapter of this book. Chapter 2 examined the relation between the development of biological science since the advent of the cell theory in 1838 with the corresponding history of cancer research and development of anticancer drugs and summarized the relation through a chronological table. Chapter 3 provided images that explain a historical background of cancer chemotherapy and describe chronologically the developmental history of screening systems of anticancer drugs. Chapters 4–9 classified the characteristics and effects of approximately 160 anticancer drugs, which used the screening system described in Chapter 3 for development, into 6 groups and provided a comprehensive account of the development process and history of each group. Chapter 10 provided details on the side effects of the clinical use of the anticancer drugs introduced in Chapters 4–9, along with the drugs that can alleviate such side effects. Finally, in Chapter 11, this book provided new anticancer drugs that will be researched and developed, based on research focusing on the difference between cancer cells and normal cells which has been conducted since the 1980s. This book also suggested a cell network research for a next research methodology, based on the perspective that cancer is related with various systemic characteristics of the human body. In other words, this book emphasizes that the research on cell network of the tissue level is necessary.

This book, in short, is a review of the past and current research conducted on anticancer drugs and a proposal for a new direction of cancer research for the future. I would like to express my gratitude to Professor Jae Kyung Roh, Dr. Hee-Jun Wee, and Dr. Chan Kim for joining me as co-authors to write this book. I also thank my graduate students at the research center who helped me with the images and tables included in this book. I also extend my gratitude to Professor Seishi Murakami at the Cancer Research Institute of Kanazawa University, Japan, who has always been a source of advice and encouragement throughout the past 35 years of research on cancer. Lastly, I thank Dr. Jeong Hun Kim at Seoul National University Hospital who helped me throughout my personal ailment. This book would not have been published without their help.

Seoul, Korea
January, 2016

Kyu-Won Kim

Contents

Part I A Scientific Overview on Cancer

1 Advancements in Life Sciences and Characteristic Features of Cancer Cells 3
1.1 Characteristics of Cancer Cells 5
1.2 Characteristic Interactions of Cancer Cells with Neighboring Cells and the Tumor Microenvironment 9
1.2.1 Stromal Cells 9
1.2.2 Angiogenesis 16
1.2.3 Metastasis of Malignant Cancer 19
1.2.4 Avoidance of Immune Surveillance 21
1.2.5 Tumor-Promoting Inflammatory Responses 22
References 23

2 Advancement of the Science and History of Cancer and Anticancer Drugs 25
References 54

Part II Cancer Drug Discovery: Types and History

3 Chronology of Anticancer Drug Development 59
3.1 A Historical Background of Cancer Chemotherapy 59
3.2 Development of the Anticancer Drug Screening Systems 60
3.2.1 Transplantable Tumor Models in Animals 60
3.2.2 Chemical Tumor Induction and Anticancer Drug Screening Using Inbred Mice 61
3.2.3 Solid Tumor Animal Models and Xenograft Screening Methods 62
3.2.4 Anticancer Drug Screening Methods Based on Human Cancer Cell Lines 63
3.2.5 Mechanism-Based Anticancer Agent Screening Method 63

3.3 Chronology of the Anticancer Drug Development 64
3.4 Clinical Application of Anticancer Drugs 68
References 69

4 Alkylating Anticancer Drugs 71
4.1 Classical Alkylating Drugs 73
4.1.1 Bis Amine/Nitrogen Mustards 73
4.1.2 Alkyl Sulfonate: Busulfan 80
4.1.3 Aziridines (Ethylenimines) 81
4.1.4 Nitrosoureas 83
4.2 Nonclassical Alkylating Drugs 85
4.2.1 Hydrazine: Procarbazine 85
4.2.2 Triazenes 86
4.2.3 Altretamines 88
4.3 Alkylating-Like Agents: Platinum Compounds 88
4.3.1 Cisplatin 89
4.3.2 Carboplatin 90
4.3.3 Oxaliplatin 91
References 91

5 Antimetabolic Anticancer Drugs 95
5.1 Folic Acid Derivatives 95
5.1.1 Methotrexate 96
5.1.2 Pemetrexed 98
5.1.3 Pralatrexate 99
5.2 Purine Analogs 100
5.2.1 6-Mercaptopurine and 6-Thioguanine 100
5.2.2 Fludarabine 101
5.2.3 Pentostatin (2′-deoxycoformycin) 102
5.2.4 Cladribine 103
5.2.5 Clofarabine 104
5.2.6 Nelarabine 104
5.3 Pyrimidine Analogs 105
5.3.1 Fluoropyrimidines 105
5.3.2 Deoxycytidine 108
References 110

6 Natural Product Anticancer Drugs 113
6.1 Plant-Derived Anticancer Drugs 114
6.1.1 Vinca Alkaloids 114
6.1.2 Macrolide: Eribulin 116
6.1.3 Taxane 117
6.1.4 Ixabepilone 120
6.1.5 Podophyllotoxins: Topoisomerase II Inhibitors 120
6.1.6 Camptothecins: Topoisomerase I Inhibitors 122
6.1.7 Omacetaxine Mepesuccinate
(Homoharringtonine, HHT) 123

6.2 Anticancer Antibiotics . . . 125
6.2.1 Actinomycin D (Dactinomycin) . . . 126
6.2.2 Anthracycline . . . 126
6.2.3 Mithramycin (Plicamycin) . . . 130
6.2.4 Bleomycin . . . 130
References . . . 131

7 Immunotherapeutic Anticancer Drugs and Other Miscellaneous Anticancer Drugs . . . 135
7.1 Immunotherapeutic Anticancer Drugs . . . 135
7.1.1 Cytokines . . . 136
7.1.2 Denileukin Diftitox (DAB389IL2) . . . 138
7.1.3 Levamisole . . . 139
7.1.4 BCG (Bacillus Calmette-Guérin) . . . 140
7.1.5 Imiquimod . . . 141
7.1.6 Ipilimumab . . . 142
7.1.7 Sipuleucel-T . . . 143
7.1.8 Thalidomide . . . 144
7.1.9 Lenalidomide and Pomalidomide . . . 145
7.2 Other Miscellaneous Anticancer Drugs . . . 146
7.2.1 Mitotane (o,p-Dichlorodiphenyldichloroethane) . . . 146
7.2.2 Asparaginase . . . 146
7.2.3 Porfimer Sodium: Photodynamic Therapy (PDT) . . . 147
7.2.4 Arsenic Trioxide . . . 148
7.2.5 Hydroxyurea (Hydroxycarbamide) . . . 149
References . . . 150

8 Hormonal Anticancer Drugs . . . 155
8.1 Hormonal Anti-prostate-Cancer Drugs . . . 155
8.1.1 LHRH Agonists/Antagonists . . . 158
8.1.2 Anti-androgens . . . 159
8.1.3 CYP17A1 Inhibitor: Abiraterone . . . 161
8.2 Hormonal Anti-breast-Cancer Drugs . . . 162
8.2.1 Selective Estrogen Receptor Modulator (SERM) . . . 163
8.2.2 Anti-estrogen: Fulvestrant . . . 165
8.2.3 Aromatase (CYP29) Inhibitors . . . 167
8.3 Other Hormonal Anticancer Drugs . . . 169
8.3.1 Prednisone . . . 169
8.3.2 Testolactone . . . 169
8.3.3 Progestin . . . 170
8.3.4 Somatostatin . . . 170
References . . . 171

9 Molecular Targeted Anticancer Drugs . . . 175
9.1 Tretinoin (All-*Trans* Retinoic Acid, ATRA) . . . 179
9.2 Bcr-Abl Inhibitors . . . 180
9.2.1 First Generation Bcr-Abl Inhibitor: Imatinib . . . 181
9.2.2 Second Generation Bcr-Abl Inhibitors . . . 184

9.3 EGFR Inhibitors . . . 186
9.3.1 First Generation EGFR Inhibitors . . . 187
9.3.2 Afatinib: Second Generation EGFR Inhibitor . . . 189
9.3.3 Monoclonal Antibodies Against EGFR . . . 190
9.4 HER2 Inhibitors . . . 192
9.4.1 Monoclonal Antibodies Against HER2 . . . 193
9.4.2 HER2 Small Molecule Inhibitors . . . 195
9.5 Angiogenesis Inhibitors . . . 196
9.5.1 Bevacizumab . . . 196
9.5.2 Aflibercept . . . 198
9.5.3 Small Molecule VEGFR Inhibitors: Multi-targeted Kinase Inhibitors . . . 198
9.6 Other Kinase Inhibitors . . . 204
9.6.1 Ruxolitinib: JAK-1,2 Inhibitor . . . 204
9.6.2 Crizotinib: ALK and ROS1 Inhibitor . . . 206
9.6.3 B-Raf Kinase Inhibitors . . . 207
9.6.4 Trametinib: MEK Inhibitor . . . 208
9.6.5 Ibrutinib . . . 209
9.7 mTOR Inhibitors . . . 210
9.7.1 Temsirolimus . . . 211
9.7.2 Everolimus . . . 211
9.8 Other Targeted Anticancer Antibody Drugs . . . 212
9.8.1 Rituximab . . . 212
9.8.2 Ibritumomab Tiuxetan . . . 214
9.8.3 Tositumomab Iodine-131 . . . 214
9.8.4 Alemtuzumab . . . 215
9.8.5 Ofatumumab . . . 215
9.8.6 Brentuximab Vedotin . . . 215
9.8.7 Obinutuzumab . . . 217
9.9 Epigenetic Anticancer Drugs . . . 217
9.9.1 DNA Methylation Inhibitors: Azanucleosides . . . 217
9.9.2 Histone Deacetylase (HDAC) Inhibitors . . . 219
9.10 Proteasome Inhibitors . . . 222
9.10.1 Bortezomib . . . 222
9.10.2 Carfilzomib . . . 224
9.11 Vismodegib: Hedgehog Pathway Blocker . . . 224
References . . . 226

10 Complications of Anticancer Drugs and Their Management . . . 239
10.1 Chemotherapy-Induced Nausea and Vomiting (CINV) . . . 239
10.1.1 Emetogenic Risk of Anticancer Drugs . . . 240
10.1.2 Types of Anti-emetics . . . 240
10.1.3 Prevention and Treatment of Chemotherapy-Induced Nausea and Vomiting . . . 242
10.2 Myelotoxicity (Bone Marrow Toxicity) . . . 243
10.2.1 Neutropenia . . . 243
10.2.2 Anemia . . . 243

10.2.3 Thrombocytopenia . . . 244
10.3 Chemotherapy-Induced Diarrhea . . . 245
10.3.1 Cause of Diarrhea . . . 245
10.3.2 Treatment . . . 245
10.4 Chemotherapy-Induced Constipation . . . 245
10.4.1 Cause of Constipation . . . 245
10.4.2 Treatment . . . 246
10.5 Chemotherapy-Induced Urinary Toxicity . . . 246
10.5.1 Cisplatin-Induced Nephrotoxicity . . . 246
10.5.2 Hemorrhagic Cystitis . . . 246
10.5.3 Nephrotoxicity of Targeted Agents . . . 247
10.6 Chemotherapy-Induced Pulmonary Toxicity . . . 247
10.6.1 Bleomycin-Induced Pulmonary Fibrosis . . . 247
10.7 Chemotherapy-Induced Neurotoxicity . . . 248
10.7.1 Platinum-Induced Neurotoxicity . . . 248
10.7.2 Methotrexate-Induced Neurotoxicity . . . 248
10.7.3 Taxane-Induced Neurotoxicity . . . 248
10.8 Cardiotoxicity . . . 249
10.8.1 Chemotherapy-Induced Cardiotoxicity . . . 249
10.8.2 Anthracycline-Induced Cardiotoxicity . . . 249
10.9 Chemotherapy-Induced Oral Mucositis . . . 250
10.9.1 Pathogenesis and Clinical Features . . . 250
10.9.2 Prevention and Treatment . . . 250
10.10 Anorexia . . . 251
10.11 Tumor Lysis Syndrome . . . 251
10.12 Extravasation of Anticancer Drugs . . . 253
10.12.1 Skin Irritation from Extravasation of Anticancer Drugs . . 253
10.12.2 Treatment of Extravasation . . . 253
10.13 Chemotherapy-Induced Skin Toxicity . . . 254
10.13.1 Hyperpigmentation . . . 254
10.13.2 Nail Change . . . 255
10.13.3 Hand-Foot Syndrome (Palmar-Plantar Erythrodysesthesia) . . . 255
10.13.4 Acneiform Eruption . . . 255
References . . . 255

Part III A Paradigm Shift in Cancer Research

11 Advancements in Bioscience and New Cancer Drugs . . . 259
11.1 Development of Cancer Drugs According to Scientific Advancements . . . 259
11.2 New Anticancer Drugs . . . 261
11.2.1 Development of Novel Targeted Agents . . . 261
11.2.2 Future Research Prospects According to the Paradigm Shift . . . 264
References . . . 276

Contributors

Kyu-Won Kim

1976	College of Pharmacy, Seoul National University, Seoul, Korea B.S.
1985	University of Minnesota, Minneapolis, U.S.A. Ph.D.

Professional Training:

2000–Present	Professor College of Pharmacy, Seoul National University, Korea
2001–Present	Full member The Korean Academy of Science and Technology
2011–2012	Vice-chairman The Korean Cancer Association
1987–2000	Assistant Professor, Associate Professor, Professor Department of Molecular Biology Pusan National University, Korea
1985–1987	Postdoctoral Fellow Department of Cancer Genetics Dana-Farber Cancer Institute, Harvard Medical School, USA

Awards and Honors:

2005	Ho-Am Prize in medicine, Ho-Am Foundation
2003	The Highest Award for Korea Science, the President of Korea

Jae Kyung Roh

1973	Yonsei University, College of Medicine, Seoul, Korea M.D.
1990	Yonsei University, Graduate School, Seoul, Korea Ph.D.

Professional Training:

2014–Present	Professor Emeritus Yonsei Cancer Center, Yonsei University College of Medicine Honorary Director Cheil Hospital Women's Cancer Center, Seoul, Korea
1981–2014	Assistant Professor, Professor in Medicine Division of Medical Oncology, Yonsei Cancer Center
2008–2011	Chairman National Bioethics Committee, Korea
2006–2008	Chairman Board of Directors, The Korean Cancer Association
2005–2011	Vice President(Health Division) The Korean Federation of Science & Technology Societies(KOFST)
2000–2010	Director Cancer Metastasis Research Center, Yonsei University College of Medicine
1983–1986	Fellow in Medical Oncology Vincent T. Lombardi Cancer Research Center, Georgetown University, School of Medicine, Washington, D.C., USA

Awards and Honors:

2014	ROK Order of Service Merit (4th Class) Green Stripes

Hee-Jun Wee

1989	Pusan National University, Pusan, Korea B.S.
2003	Kyoto University, Kyoto, Japan Ph.D.

Professional Training:

2010–Present	Research Assistant Professor College of Pharmacy, Seoul National University, Korea
2006–2010	Research Assistant Professor Department of Biochemistry, School of Medicine, Chungbuk National University, South Korea
2003–2006	Research Fellow Institute of Molecular and Cell Biology, Singapore

Chan Kim

2005	Yonsei University College of Medicine, Seoul, Korea M.D.
2013	Korea Advanced Institute of Science and Technology (KAIST), Daejeon, Korea Ph.D.

Professional Training:

2015–Present	Assistant Professor Medical Oncology, CHA Bundang Medical Center, CHA University, Seongnam, Korea
2014–2015	Clinical Fellow Yonsei Cancer Center, Severance Hospital, Seoul, Korea
2013–2014	Postdoctoral Fellow Laboratory of Vascular Biology and Stem Cells, KAIST, Daejeon, Korea
2006–2010	Residency in Internal Medicine Severance Hospital, Seoul, Korea
2005–2006	Rotating Internship Severance Hospital, Seoul, Korea

Part I
A Scientific Overview on Cancer

Chapter 1
Advancements in Life Sciences and Characteristic Features of Cancer Cells

Advances in modern life sciences have primarily focused on cellular research because of the "Cell Theory" (Schleiden and Schwann 1838), which defines the cell as the basic unit of all organisms. Since cells are the common structural unit of a variety of organisms including animals and plants, it was hypothesized that complex life phenomena of multicellular organisms could be understood by studying individual cells. Molecular-level research began in 1953, when the double helix structure of DNA—the genetic material that transmits cellular characteristics to the next generation—was elucidated by Watson and Crick. Subsequently, advances in the understanding of the functions and mechanisms of cells were made rapidly.

As molecular-level research of DNA, RNA, and proteins uncovered the mysteries of life, Monod claimed that life phenomena at the molecular level were similar in all organisms.

> What is true for *E. coli* must also be true for elephants. – J. Monod (1954)

The aforementioned statement implies that studies on unicellular *E. coli* can aid our understanding of a larger and more complex organism such as an elephant. This rationale is based on the hypothesis that the cell is the basic unit of all life forms and hence, the life phenomena of a unicellular organism are identical to those of a multicellular organism. Therefore, it was thought that the complex life phenomena of the metaphorical elephant as well as humans, our main interest, could be understood by studying them at the cellular level. Furthermore, such research could improve our understanding of fatal human diseases and consequently therapies could be offered.

This argument has been the unwavering foundation of life science research for the last 60 years. Therefore, this viewpoint has also dominated cancer research, the most studied area in life sciences to date. Consequently, wide-ranging and complex molecular mechanisms underlying cancer have been well characterized. Herein, we briefly examine the characteristics of cancer as elucidated by this approach and describe the history of the development of anticancer drugs based on these characteristics. We also discuss whether the understanding of cancer at the molecular level should be our ultimate goal.

K.-W. Kim et al., *Cancer Drug Discovery*, DOI 10.1007/978-94-024-0844-7_1

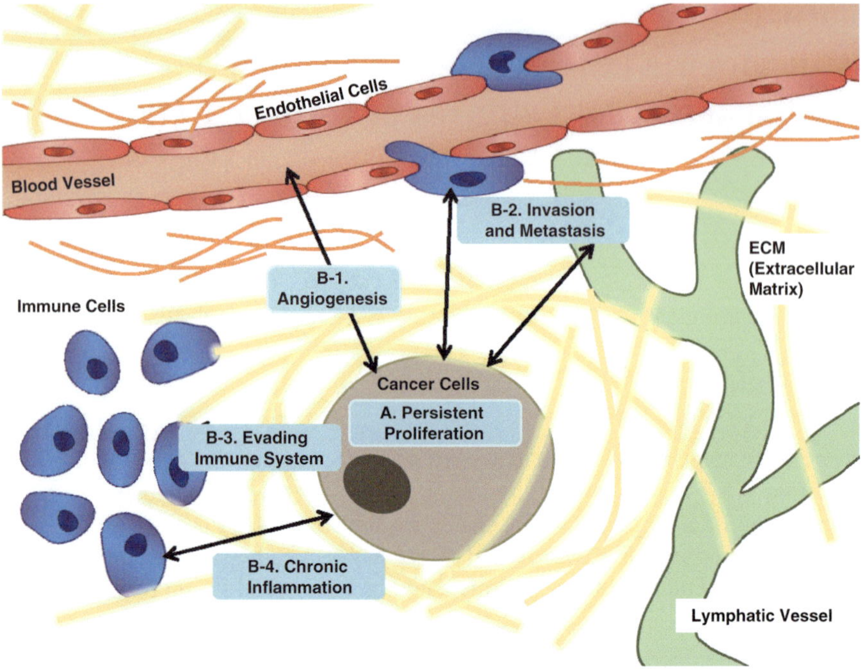

Fig. 1.1 Representative characteristics of malignant cancer. (**a**) Characteristics of cancer cells. (**b**) Properties of cancer cells are regulated by their interaction with surrounding stromal cells and a tumor microenvironment

Moreover, we discuss the characteristics of malignant cancer; these can be broadly classified into two categories, as presented in Fig. 1.1. The first category focuses on the characteristics of cancer cells, and is directly related to their continuous growth. The continuous proliferative capability of cancer cells is a result of changes perpetuated by genetic mutations in signal transduction pathways associated with cell division.

The second category of characteristics depends upon the interactions between cancer cells, neighboring cells, and the microenvironment. These characteristics include induction of angiogenesis by stimulating neighboring blood vessels, invasion of cancer cells into surrounding tissues, metastasis through the vascular and lymphatic systems, avoidance of immune cell-mediated cytotoxicity, and tumor-induced inflammatory reactions in the proximate immune cells.

Most of the currently available cytotoxic chemotherapeutics inhibit the continuous proliferation of cancer cells, and anticancer drugs with molecular targets that are under development focus on this particular feature of cancer cell. In the following section, we first briefly describe the results of research on cancer cell characteristics.

1.1 Characteristics of Cancer Cells

The representative characteristic of cancer cells is abnormal continuous growth. Among the ten hallmarks of cancer cells proposed by Hanahan and Weinberg in 2011 [1], sustained proliferative signaling, evasion of growth suppressors, resistance to cell death, and replicative immortality are directly related to the sustained proliferation of cancer cells. In addition, since "deregulating cellular energetics" and "genome instability and mutation" are also related to the continuous growth of cancer cells, six out of the ten hallmarks are associated with abnormal growth. Therefore, the ability of cancer cells to proliferate continuously is the defining characteristic of cancer, and drugs targeting this property can be used as anticancer drugs.

The results of all the research to date on the continuous growth of cancer cells have been summarized below. Unlike normal cells, cancer cells continuously proliferate due to growth factors responsible for the proliferation and persistent activation of cell surface receptors (particularly receptor tyrosine kinases). Cancer cells continuously produce growth factors, thereby stimulating themselves and neighboring normal cells. In addition, they enhance the responses of growth factor receptors by upregulating cancer cell surface receptors and allowing receptors to function without growth factors, resulting in persistent activation of proliferation-related signal transduction processes. Activation of a persistent proliferation signal is also induced by activating mutations in downstream mediators, such as B-Raf and phosphoinositide 3-kinase (PI3-kinase). Mutations in the phosphatase and tensin homolog (PTEN) phosphatase and mammalian target of rapamycin (mTOR) kinase, which are involved in feedback regulation of cell proliferation, also contribute to the persistent proliferation of cancer cells [2] (Fig. 1.2).

Another mechanism that perpetuates the proliferation of cancer cells is the inactivation of antiproliferative factors. Factors that inhibit cell proliferation are known as tumor suppressors and mainly include the retinoblastoma (Rb) and p53 proteins [3]. These proteins are responsible for initiating cell proliferation and activating senescence as well as apoptosis. Therefore, loss of function of these proteins causes persistent cell division (Fig. 1.3).

"Contact inhibition" is another mechanism that inhibits cell proliferation, which ordinarily involves the Merlin protein encoded by the neurofibromatosis type 2 (NF2) gene [4]. Cancer cells are thought to be resistant to this particular antiproliferative mechanism (Fig. 1.4).

Additionally, evasion of apoptosis can result in the continuous proliferation of cancer cells. Apoptosis is regulated by intracellular and extracellular mechanisms; the Fas ligand/Fas receptors initiate the extracellular mechanism, while caspase 8 and 9 are involved in the intracellular mechanism. The intracellular mechanism is involved more closely in the development of cancer. Apoptosis is regulated by interactions between antiapoptotic (e.g., Bcl-2, Bcl-XL) and proapoptotic (e.g., Bax, Bim, Puma) regulators [5]. The tumor suppressor p53 induces apoptosis when DNA

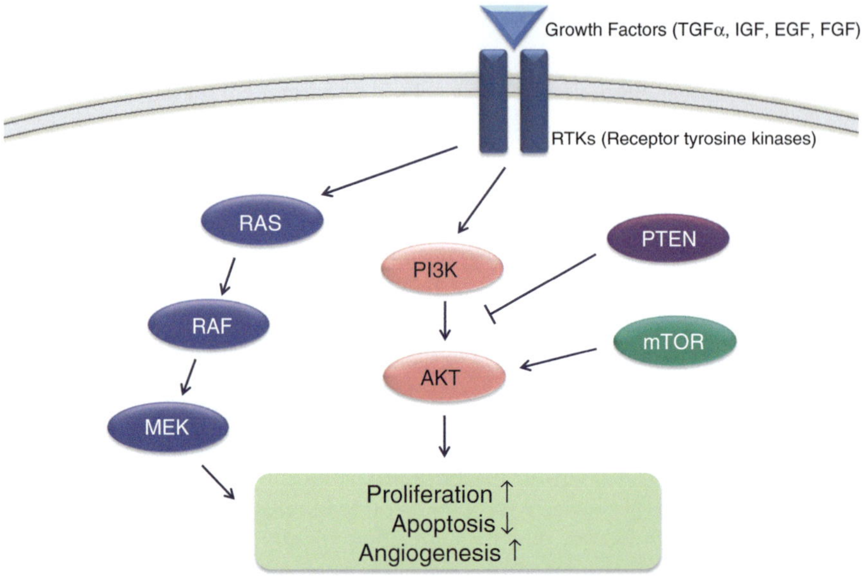

Fig. 1.2 Signal transduction pathways promote carcinogenesis. Two activated PI3K/AKT pathways in cancer cells prevent apoptosis and allow the cell cycle to progress without arresting at the G_0 restriction point, promoting cell division and proliferation. In addition, the RAS/RAF/MEK pathways are activated in cancer cells. This promotes carcinogenesis by activating cell division, preventing apoptosis, and inducing angiogenesis. Furthermore, the mTOR kinase in cancer cells activates AKT, promoting cell division and proliferation, while the PTEN phosphatase, which blocks the PI3K/AKT pathways, is suppressed. As a result, apoptosis is inhibited and abnormal cell proliferation occurs

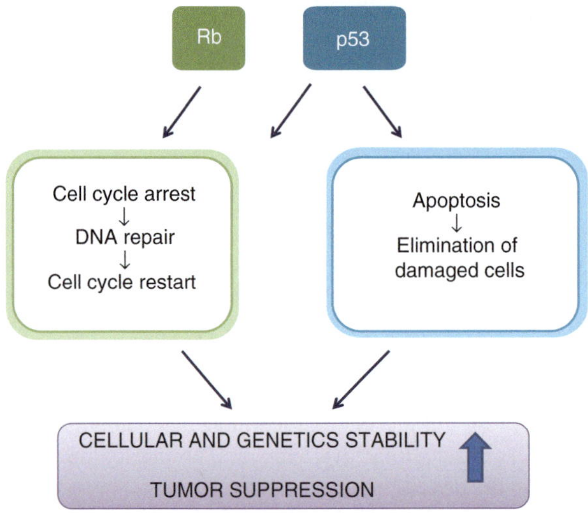

Fig. 1.3 Tumor suppression functions of Rb and p53. Rb is responsible for halting the cell cycle at the G_0 restriction point to prevent cell cycle progression in cells with DNA damage. Rb is phosphorylated when the damaged DNA is repaired, losing its ability to arrest the cell cycle, and the cell cycle resumes. p53 induces apoptosis in cells with DNA damage so that damaged cells are removed efficiently. Thus, Rb and p53 contribute to genetic stability by preventing mutations due to DNA damage and inhibiting the development of tumor cells

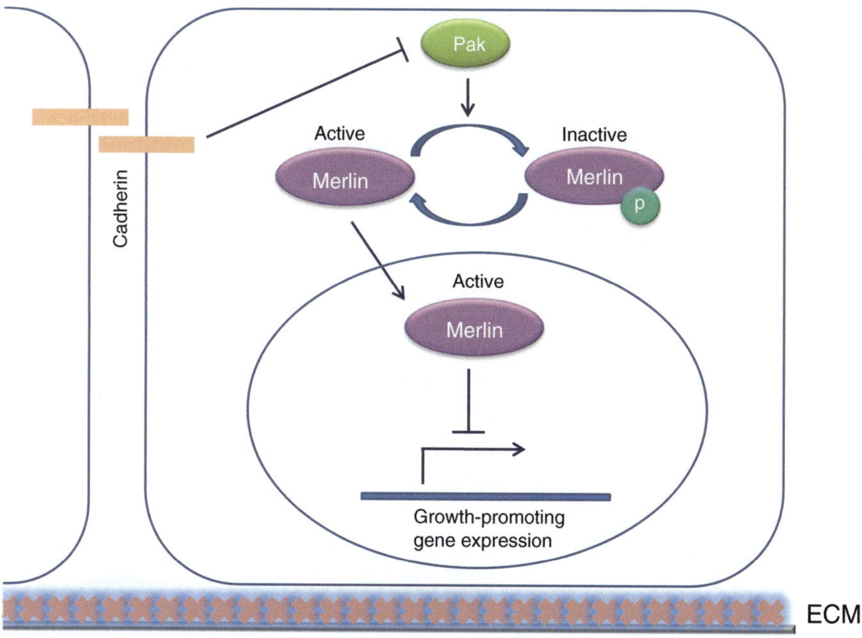

Fig. 1.4 Merlin is a tumor suppressor involved in "contact inhibition." Normal cells stop growing when they encounter neighboring cells, and cell division is inhibited. Merlin is responsible for this phenomenon called "contact inhibition." In normal cells, p21-activated kinase (PAK) activity is inhibited by cell contact, along with Merlin activation. Activated Merlin translocates to the nucleus and prevents cell division by suppressing the expression of mitogenic genes. However, abnormal proliferation can occur in cancer cells because they become resistant to contact inhibition

is damaged and an abnormal chromosome is formed. Therefore, resistance to or evasion of apoptosis in tumor cells is closely related to the dysfunction of the p53 protein, and an increase in antiapoptotic regulators (Bcl-2, Bcl-XL). Inversely, a decrease in proapoptotic regulators (Bax, Bim, Puma) can prevent apoptosis in tumor cells (Fig. 1.5).

For sustained proliferation, chromosomes have to replicate continuously and unlike normal cells, cancer cells are able to do this. Presumably, cancer cells obtain this capability through a "crisis phase" after overcoming senescence. Telomeres and telomerase activity that facilitates the addition of repeat sequences to telomeres are closely involved in this process. Increased telomerase activity or a special recombination mechanism allows cancer cells to maintain a telomere length sufficient for evading senescence or apoptosis [6]. Besides maintaining telomere length, telomerase influences cell proliferation by amplifying the Wnt pathway, and increasing DNA damage repair and RNA synthesis (Fig. 1.6).

For continuous cancer cell proliferation, abnormal expression of cell division genes is required. Abnormal expression can result from chromosomal instability and mutagenesis. Chromosomal instability is closely related to telomere damage and can cause the amplification or loss of a chromosome. An increase in mutational

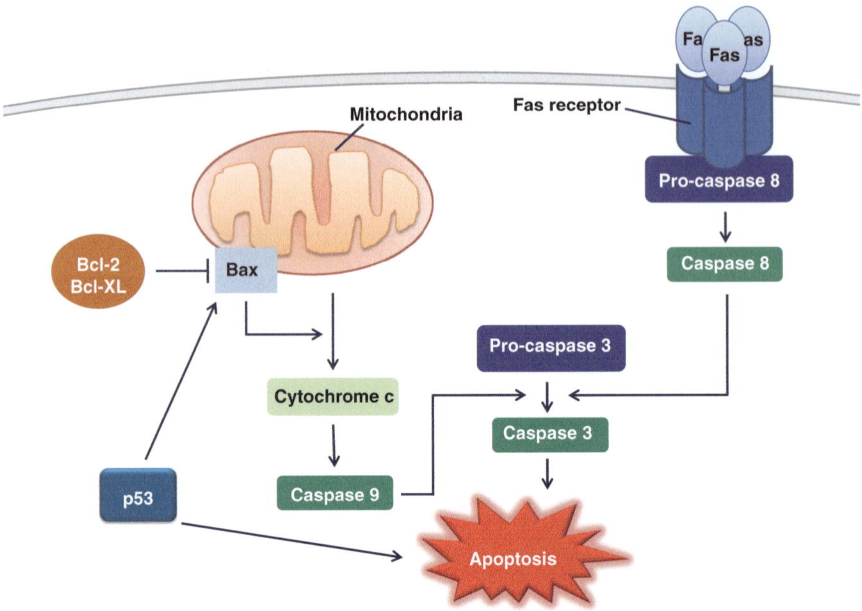

Fig. 1.5 Signal transduction in apoptosis. Apoptosis is induced by both extracellular and intracellular pathways. The Fas ligand/Fas receptor is involved in the extracellular pathway; procaspase 8 is activated to caspase 8 by Fas. The activated caspase 8 and caspase 9 which is activated by cytochrome c activate procaspase 3 to caspase 3. Activated caspase 3 in turn induces apoptosis. The intracellular mechanism is regulated by the interaction between antiapoptotic regulators and proapoptotic regulators. Apoptosis occurs as antiapoptotic regulators (Bcl-2, Bcl-XL) decrease and proapoptotic regulators (Bax, Bim, Puma, etc.) increase. Apoptosis is also induced by p53. However, the apoptosis pathways are inactivated in cancer cells, making continuous proliferation possible

load is associated with an increased sensitivity to mutagens, defective DNA repair mechanisms, or loss of the ability to remove cells harboring mutations. Chromosomal instability is increased by defective chromosome maintenance and repair, which results in frequent mutations [7]. This in turn, enables continuous cancer cell division and induces gene expression necessary for carcinogenesis (Fig. 1.7).

In addition, an energy mechanism known as the "Warburg effect" allows cancer cells to generate ATP by aerobic glycolysis even in the presence of oxygen. Because aerobic glycolysis has a very low ATP synthesis rate compared to normal mitochondrial oxidative phosphorylation, glucose uptake via the glucose transporter increases dramatically in cancer cells, allowing adequate ATP synthesis [8]. Aerobic glycolysis activates oncogenes such as RAS and MYC, which promote continuous cell division by supplying essential amino acids and nucleic acids, and enable the survival of cancer cells by increasing glycolysis in hypoxic conditions. Furthermore, aerobic glycolysis acidifies the microenvironment of cancer cells and promotes degradation of the extracellular matrix (ECM), making invasion and metastasis easier (Fig. 1.8).

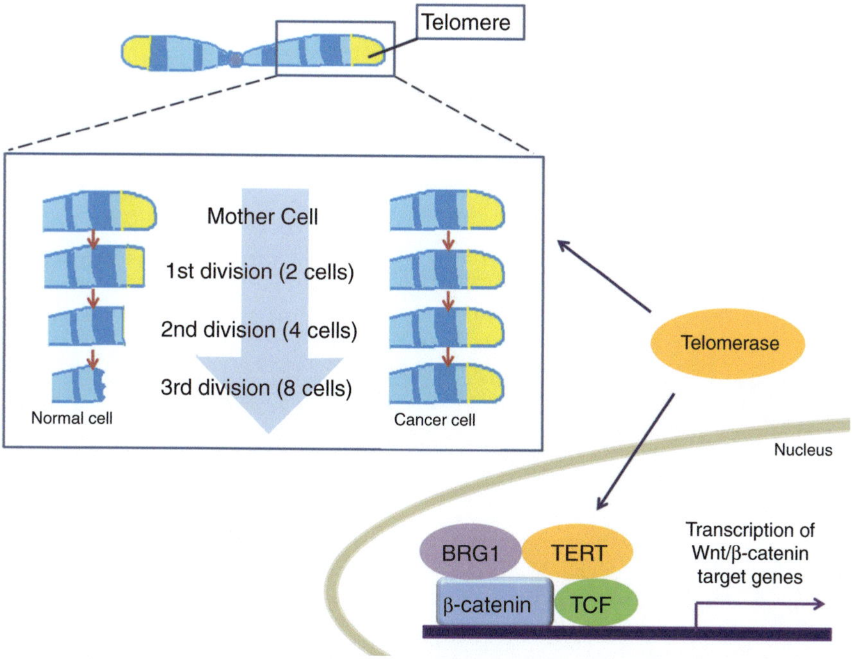

Fig. 1.6 Telomerase activation in cancer cells. Telomeres are the ends of chromosomes where the TTAGGG sequence is repeated. This sequence prevents chromosomal damage and recombination between chromosomes. Telomeres gradually shorten in each cell division and both chromosomes and telomeres are damaged after a certain number of cell division, eventually stopping cell division. All cells have the telomerase gene, which synthesizes telomeres. However, it is inactive in most normal cells and active in about 90 % of cancer cells. Because this enzyme maintains telomeres in cancer cells, they are immortal and have the ability to divide continuously. In addition, telomerase promotes cell proliferation by activating the Wnt pathway

1.2 Characteristic Interactions of Cancer Cells with Neighboring Cells and the Tumor Microenvironment

1.2.1 Stromal Cells

In the last 10 years, research has shown that cancer tissue is as complex as normal tissue, which includes a variety of cells. Thus, studying individual cancer cells according to the existing reductive viewpoint has limitations. As shown in Fig. 1.9, cancer cells manifest malignancy by interacting with not only diverse neighboring cell types, but also the ECM and due to various environmental factors such as O_2 and pH [9].

Among the ten hallmarks of cancer proposed by Hanahan and Weinberg in 2011 [1], apart from the six mentioned above, the remaining four hallmarks (inducing angiogenesis, activation of invasion & metastasis, avoidance of immune destruction,

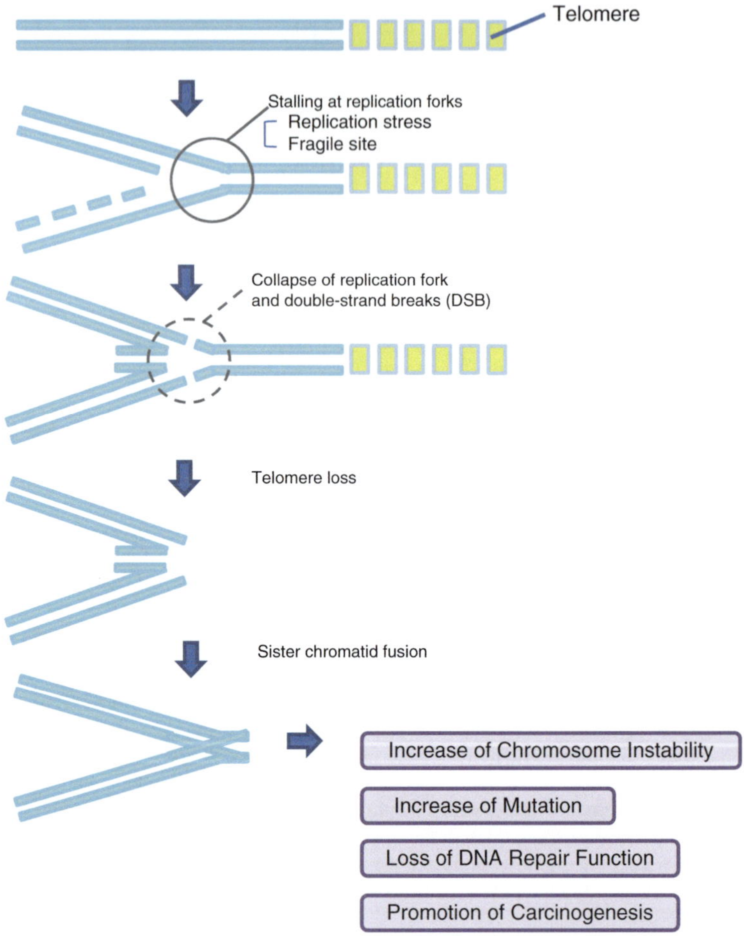

Fig. 1.7 Chromosomal instability increases due to telomere damage. In vigorously dividing cancer cells, double-strand breaks (DSBs) occur at fragile sites when the replication fork stalls and collapses due to replication stress. Distal ends are lost when broken strands are rejoined by non-homologous end joining (NHEJ). As telomeres are lost, chromosomal instability and the incidence of mutations increases. When chromosome repair ability is lost, carcinogenesis is promoted

and tumor-promoting inflammation) are manifested through interactions with neighboring cells and the tumor microenvironment.

Neighboring cells include endothelial cells and pericytes which are involved in angiogenesis. These cells create new blood vessels that transport oxygen and nutrients essential for cancer cell proliferation. Intratumoral blood vessels are formed by the "angiogenic switch," and endothelial cells constituting these tumor blood vessels are expected to be distinct from normal endothelial cells. This is because tumor blood vessels are different from normal blood vessels in many ways such as abnormal vessel structure and hyperpermeability [10] (Fig. 1.10).

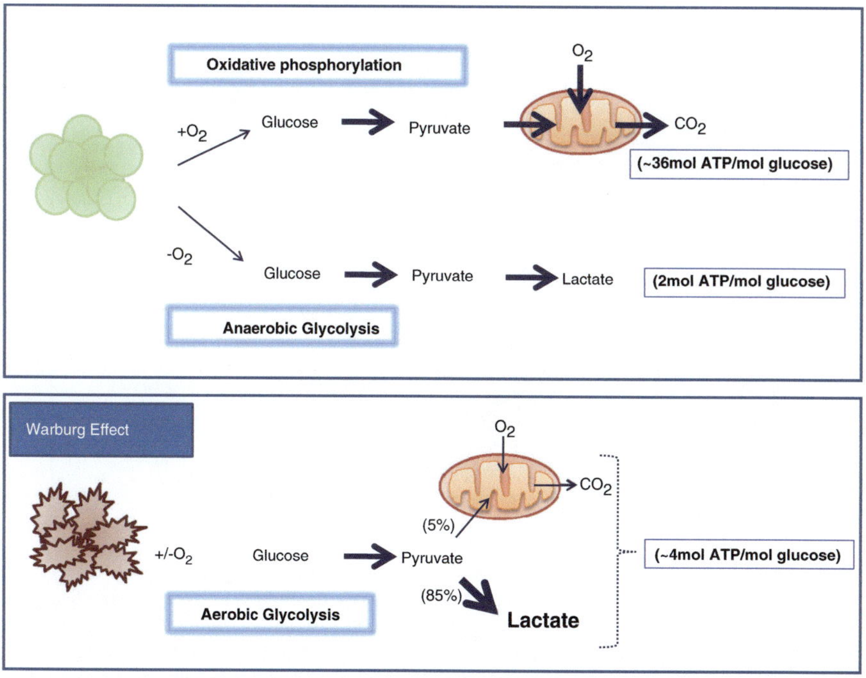

Fig. 1.8 The Warburg effect in cancer cells. In the presence of oxygen, differentiated normal cells convert glucose into pyruvate, after which a large amount of ATP is generated on complete oxidization by oxidative phosphorylation in the mitochondria. Oxygen is essential for this process because it acts as an electron donor in the glucose oxidization process. Under conditions of limited oxygen, cells produce lactate from pyruvate in a process other than oxidative phosphorylation. This process is called anaerobic glycolysis, resulting in the generation of only a small amount of ATP and the lactate produced this way goes through the glycolysis process. Warburg observed that cancer cells converted most of glucose into lactate even in the presence of oxygen. This phenomenon is called the "Warburg effect." Since this reaction takes place in the presence of oxygen, it is called aerobic glycolysis. Although only a small amount of ATP is produced, cancer cells can continuously produce the energy, amino acids, and nucleic acids needed for cell division through this reaction because the glucose uptake capability of cancer cells increases. In addition, cancer cells can continuously divide even under anaerobic or hypoxic conditions because glycolysis is constantly active due to the increased glucose uptake capability

Finger-shaped pericytes surrounding endothelial cells secrete angiopoietin-1 (Ang-1) or vascular endothelial growth factor (VEGF) to synthesize the basement membrane in collaboration with endothelial cells, playing an important role in angiogenesis and vessel maintenance. Therefore, if the pericytes do not cover the endothelial cells properly, intravasation of tumor cells occurs more readily.

Besides blood vessels, lymphatic vessels are also involved in metastasis. Although intratumoral lymphatic vessels are impaired and dysfunctional, functional lymphatic vessels grow in the periphery of tumors and may be involved in metastasis of cancerous cells to the lymph nodes [11] (Fig. 1.11).

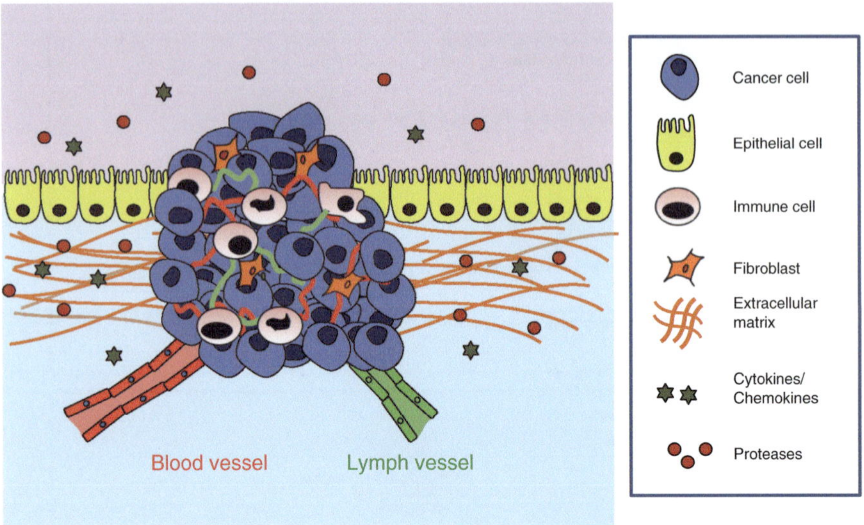

Fig. 1.9 Tumor microenvironment and diverse cell components. Tumor microenvironment refers to the diverse cellular environment of the tumor and consists of endothelial cells, pericytes, immune cells, ECM, fibroblasts, lymphatic vessels, other cell types, and signaling molecules. Through interactions with surrounding stromal cells and microenvironmental factors, tumor cells undergo carcinogenesis and eventually become metastatic. The characteristics properties of cancer cells including angiogenesis, invasion and metastasis, and tumor-promoting inflammation emerge from interactions with the tumor microenvironment as various signaling substances and enzymes are secreted from surrounding cells

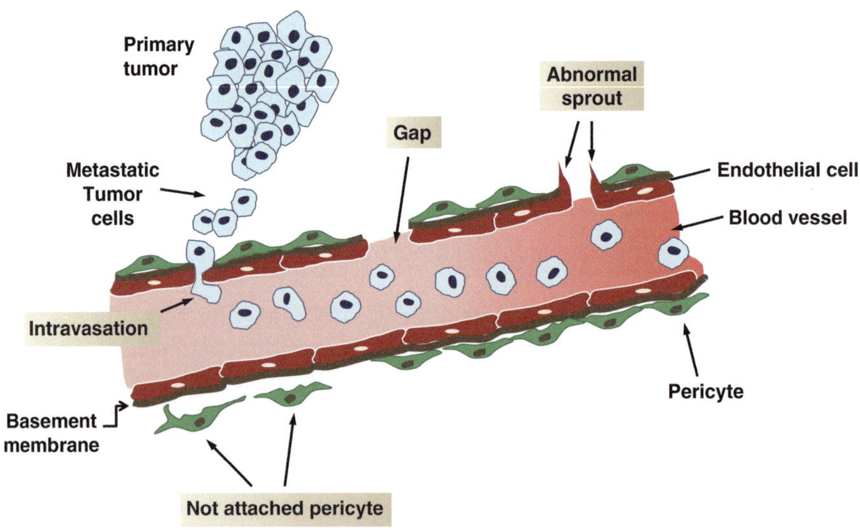

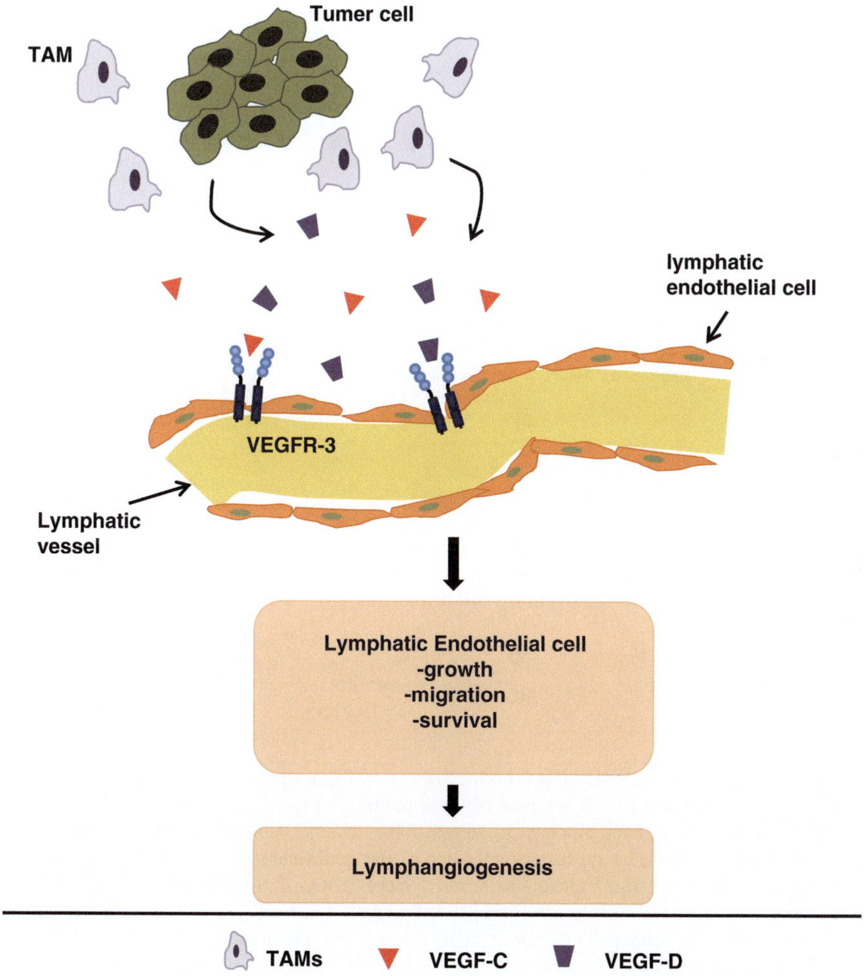

Fig. 1.11 Lymphangiogenesis and metastasis. New lymphatic vessels are generated around a tumor, through which cancer cells metastasize (lymphatic metastasis). Lymphangiogenesis requires lymphangiogenic factors such as VEGF-C and VEGF-D. Cancer cells and tumor-associated macrophages (TAMs) secrete VEGF-C and VEGF-D, which bind to VEGF receptor-3 (VEGFR-3), expressed on the surface of lymphatic vessels. As a result, the growth, migration, and survival of lymphatic endothelial cells increases and lymphangiogenesis is induced

Fig. 1.10 Endothelial cells and pericytes in tumors. Intratumoral blood vessels consisting of endothelial cells and pericytes surrounding endothelial cells are involved in angiogenesis. They supply oxygen and nutrients for the proliferation of cancer cells. Intratumoral blood vessels display abnormal structural and functional characteristics, differentiating them from normal blood vessels. That is, tumor blood vessels have irregular shapes and sizes, and are loosely connected. Furthermore, they are defective in the endothelial cell layer due to abnormal branching, which creates gaps between cells. As these tumor blood vessels are immature and hyperpermeable, their function is also disturbed. Therefore, cancer cells can easily intravasate through blood vessels and metastasize easily

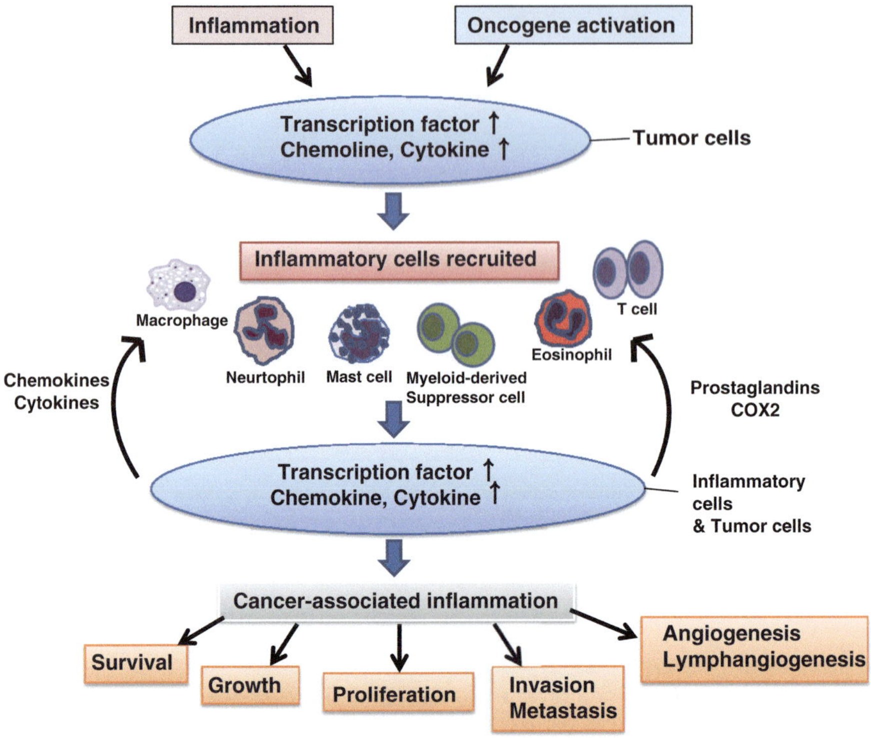

Fig. 1.12 Induction of inflammatory response in carcinogenesis. Transcription factors such as nuclear factor (NF)-kB, signal transducer and activator of transcription 3 (STAT3), and hypoxia-inducible factor-1α (HIF-1α) are activated in tumor cells by stimulation of external pathways such as inflammation and infection, or internal pathways such as activation of oncogenes and secretion of inflammation regulatory factors such as cytokines, chemokines, and cyclooxygenase 2 (COX2). These secretory factors recruit a variety of cells such as macrophages, neutrophils, mast cells, myeloid-derived suppressor cells, T cells, and eosinophils to cancer cells. When transcription factors such as NF-kB, STAT3, and HIF-1α are activated in immune and cancer cells, more cytokines, chemokines, and prostaglandins are produced, which in turn activates immune cells to induce carcinogenic processes such as cell survival, growth, proliferation, angiogenesis, lymphangiogenesis, and invasion and metastasis

Immune cells in the tumor microenvironment play a role in tumor-promoting inflammation. These include T lymphocytes, B lymphocytes, macrophages, mast cells, and neutrophils. These inflammatory cells amplify inflammatory responses by secreting growth factors like epidermal growth factor (EGF), VEGF, fibroblast growth factor 2 (FGF2), as well as chemokines and cytokines [12]. They also induce angiogenesis and upregulate production of ECM-degrading enzymes. Thus, they play an important role in tumorigenesis, invasion, and metastasis of tumor cells. These inflammatory cells include both terminally differentiated cells and undifferentiated progenitors (Fig. 1.12).

Other cells in the tumor microenvironment include fibroblasts, which have tumor-promoting functions such as the proliferation of cancer cells, angiogenesis, invasion, and metastasis [13] (Fig. 1.13).

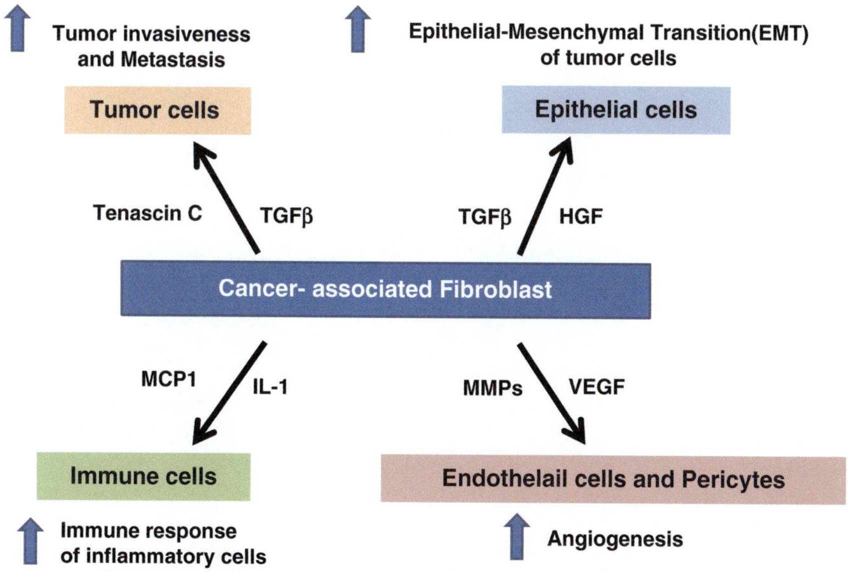

Fig. 1.13 Activated fibroblasts are involved in carcinogenesis. Fibroblasts surrounding tumor cells are frequently in an activated state and are called cancer-associated fibroblasts (CAFs). These fibroblasts secrete a variety of factors including growth factors and chemokines near tumor cells and affect tumor cells, immune cells, endothelial cells, pericytes, and epithelial cells, thereby playing an important role in carcinogenic processes such as progression and proliferation of cancer, angiogenesis, and metastasis. For example, tenascin C, an ECM protein secreted by fibroblasts, induces an ECM-like environment, which induces the invasion of tumor cells that secrete additional tumorigenic factors, eventually promoting tumor progression. By secreting cytokines and interleukins such as monocyte chemotactic protein 1 (MCP1) and interleukin-1, fibroblasts recruit immune cells to the inflammation site and induce immune cell-mediated inflammatory responses. Furthermore, by secreting matrix metalloproteinases (MMPs) and VEGF, fibroblasts assist endothelial cells and pericytes in inducing angiogenesis. By secreting potential tumor growth factors such as transforming growth factor-β (TGF-β) and hepatocyte growth factor (HGF) around epithelial cells, fibroblasts induce EMT in tumor cells and stimulate the proliferation and metastasis of tumor cells

In addition, myofibroblasts are found in wounds and chronically inflamed areas, and can induce fibrosis especially in the lung, kidney, and liver where chronic inflammation can occur.

Recently, cancer stem cells (CSCs) have been discovered in the tumor microenvironment. The origin of solid tumors from CSCs is not well understood. However, it is possible that CSCs develop due to mutations in normal stem cells and undifferentiated cells, or during EMT [14]. CSCs exhibit resistance to anticancer drugs and are activated when cancer relapses after a long latent period. They can also convert to fibroblasts or similar cells through EMT, or become endothelial-like cells through a differentiation process. Therefore, the diversity of tumor cells increases because of CSCs, producing a population of cells that vigorously promotes the progression of cancer (Fig. 1.14).

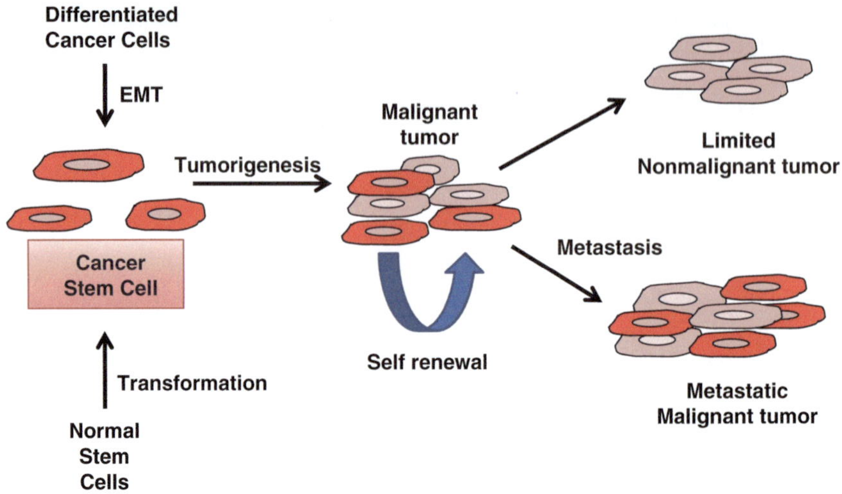

Fig. 1.14 Cancer Stem Cells (CSCs). CSCs are cancer cells with unlimited regenerative potential, and are defined as such when a tumor originating from these cells expresses the unique heterogeneity of the original tumor. They also possess differentiation, self-renewal, and tumorigenic capabilities. Depending on the tumor type, CSCs can be formed when either normal stem cells are transformed or cancer cells undergo epithelial-mesenchymal transition (EMT). CSCs form malignant tumors through carcinogenesis. These malignant tumors either differentiate into benign tumors or become metastatic tumors containing CSCs

1.2.2 Angiogenesis

As tumorigenesis progresses, tumor, unlike normal tissues, continuously generates new blood vessels necessary for the supply of oxygen and nutrients, and the removal of CO_2 and metabolic byproducts [15] (Fig. 1.15). Angiogenesis is regulated by a variety of factors; the representative proangiogenic factor is VEGF [16] (Fig. 1.16), whereas thrombospondin-1 (TSP-1) [17] (Fig. 1.17), angiostatin, and endostatin are the inhibitors. VEGF transmits a signal for angiogenesis via three types of receptors [vascular endothelial growth factor receptors (VEGFRs)-1 to 3], whose expression is regulated by oxygen levels and oncogenes.

Fig. 1.16 Angiogenesis induced by VEGF-A and VEGFR-2. VEGF-A is involved in angiogenesis in both normal and cancer cells, and exists in various isotypes (165,189,206,145,121 etc.). The most highly expressed isotype is VEGF-A165, which has a strong affinity to the receptor VEGFR-2. VEGFR-2 expression in endothelial cells increases under hypoxic conditions and induces a signal transduction pathway by binding to VEGF-A, which is secreted by cancer cells. That is, when VEGF-A binds to VEGFR-2, the signal transduction pathway is activated as the receptor is phosphorylated. As a result, angiogenesis is induced as proliferation, migration, differentiation, and survival of endothelial cells are promoted

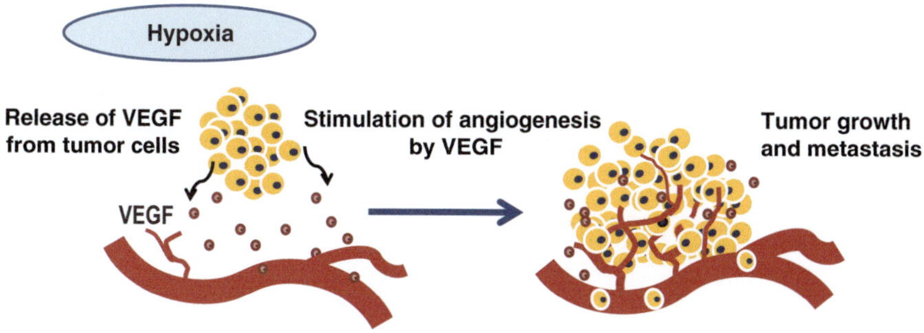

Fig. 1.15 Angiogenesis. To allow cancer cells to grow and metastasize to another organ, new blood vessels through which cancer cells receive a supply of oxygen and nutrients have to be generated. Under hypoxic conditions induced by active cancer cell proliferation, cancer cells facilitate angiogenesis from existing blood vessels by secreting proangiogenic factors, especially VEGF. Cancer cells rapidly proliferate after receiving oxygen and nutrients, and even metastasize through these new blood vessels

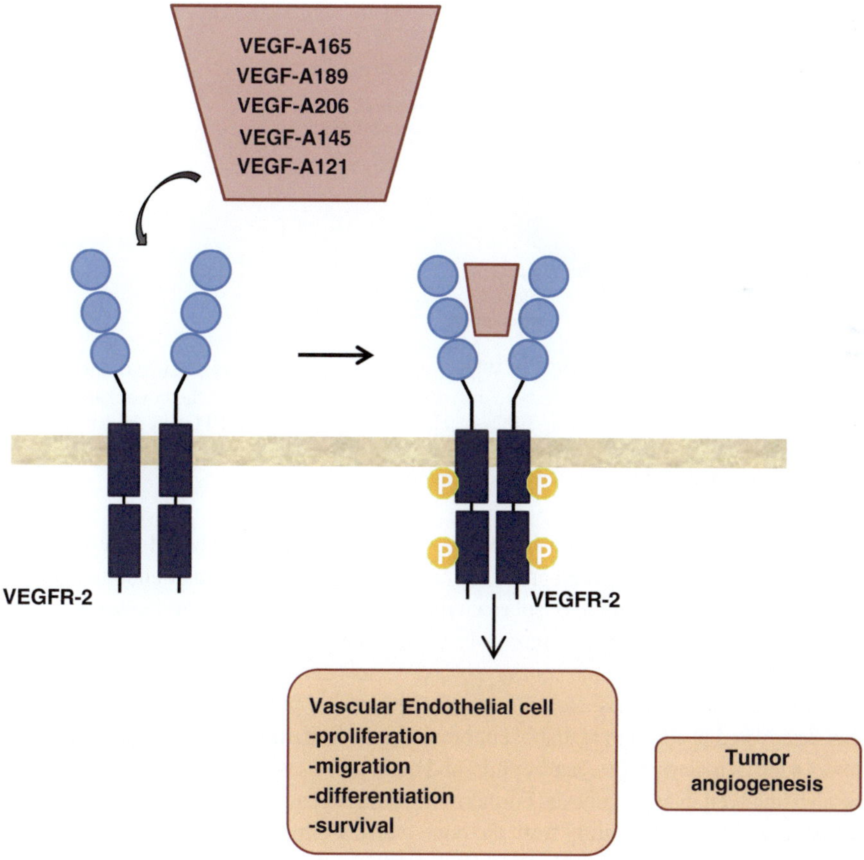

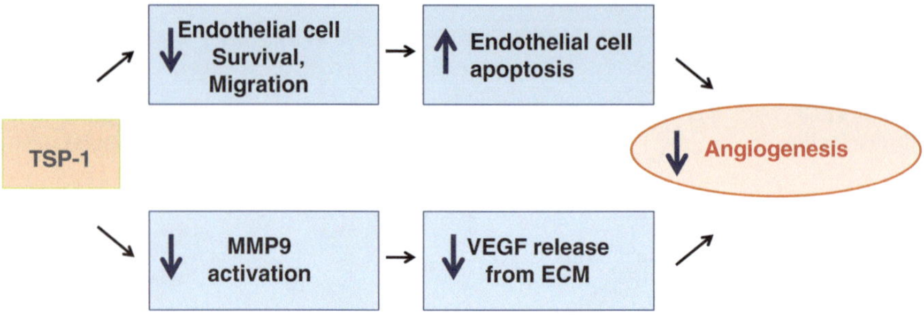

Fig. 1.17 Functions of TSP-1. TSP-1 is an anti-angiogenic factor produced by endothelial or immune cells, which decreases the density of blood vessels in normal tissues and suppresses the growth of cancer cells. TSP-1 suppresses angiogenesis by directly inhibiting proliferation, adhesion, and migration of endothelial cells. Alternatively, it suppresses VEGF-induced angiogenesis by decreasing the VEGF level

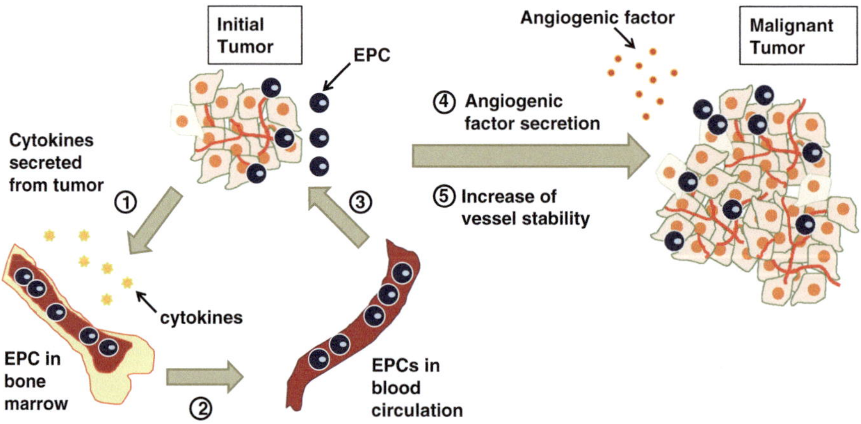

Fig. 1.18 Epithelial Progenitor Cells (EPCs). When a cancer cell secretes a bone marrow- stimulating cytokine, EPCs are generated in the bone marrow (*1*). EPCs generated in the bone marrow circulate in the blood (*2*), and circulating EPCs reach the cancer tissue (*3*). EPCs in the cancer tissue secrete proangiogenic factors that induce angiogenesis (*4*). In addition, EPCs also stabilize the blood vessel structure, and are thus, involved in angiogenesis (*5*)

Tumor blood vessels are immature, tortuous, dilated with disturbed blood flow, and exhibit microhemorrhage, abnormal proliferation, and apoptosis of vascular endothelial cells. Angiogenesis also occurs in dysplasia, which is an early stage of carcinogenesis, in situ carcinoma, and takes place vigorously in advanced vascular-rich tumors in the kidneys and glioblastomas. On the contrary, blood vessels decrease in cancers like pancreatic ductal adenocarcinomas. Recently, the importance of pericytes in angiogenesis has been discovered in addition to that of endothelial cells. Inflammatory cells surrounding tumors such as macrophages, neutrophils, and mast cells as well as myeloid progenitors are also involved in angiogenesis. Furthermore, it has been reported that endothelial progenitor cells (EPCs) originating from the bone marrow directly participate in angiogenesis in collaboration with pericytes [18] (Fig. 1.18).

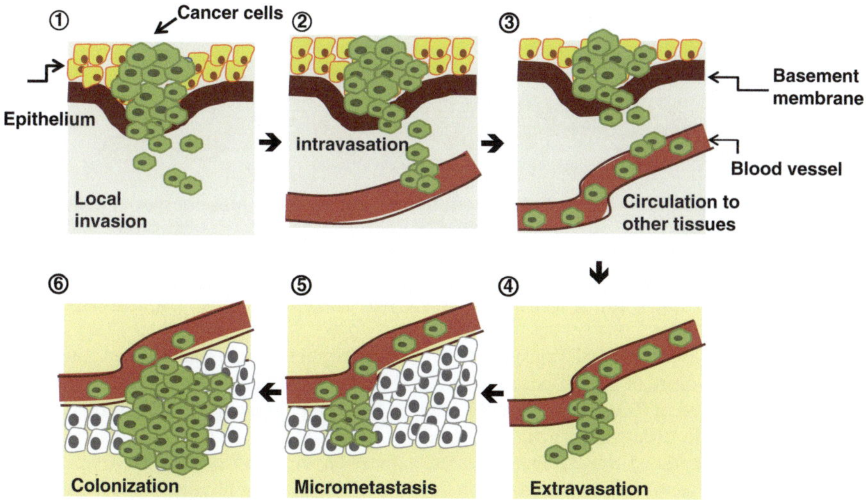

Fig. 1.19 Invasion-Metastasis cascade. (*1*) Invasion of the basal lamina after early cancer cell proliferation in the epithelial tissue. (*2*) intravasation of cancer cells into the tumor blood vessels. (*3*) Migration of cancer cells through systemic circulation (less than 1 in 1,000 cells survive to cause metastasis). (*4*) Extravasation of cancer cells from blood vessels after adhering to the blood vessel walls. (*5*) Micrometastasis in new tissue. (*6*) Colonization of metastatic cancer cells through continuous proliferation

1.2.3 Metastasis of Malignant Cancer

Metastasis of cancer is a multistep process, and generally, proliferating cancer cells go through the following steps: (1) local invasion, (2) intravasation into surrounding blood or lymphatic vessels, (3) migration through the vascular/lymphatic system, (4) extravasation, (5) micrometastasis, and (6) colonization [19] (Fig. 1.19).

EMT is expected to occur in the early stages of metastasis, wherein cancer cells transition from static epithelial cells to motile mesenchymal cells [20] (Fig. 1.20). In the EMT process, transcription regulators such as snail, slug, twist, and zeb1/2 are involved in the suppression of E-cadherin expression, loss of tight junctions, transition to fibroblasts, production of ECM-degrading enzymes, increase in motility, and resistance to apoptosis. Expression of these transcription regulators in cancer cells is regulated in a variety of ways depending on the stromal cells and tumor microenvironment. As a result, metastasis to distant organs involves a morphological change in cancer cells, and detachment from other cells and the ECM. Loss of function or mutations in E-cadherin, the prototypical cell-cell adhesion molecule, occur at the molecular level. Therefore, the interaction between cancer cells and surrounding stromal cells is very important in the process of metastasis. Mesenchymal stem cells (MSCs) in the adipose tissue stimulated by cancer cells secrete CCL5, which stimulates the metastatic function of cancer cells.

Furthermore, tumor-associated macrophages (TAMs) facilitate metastasis by secreting ECM-degrading enzymes such as metalloprotease and cathepsin

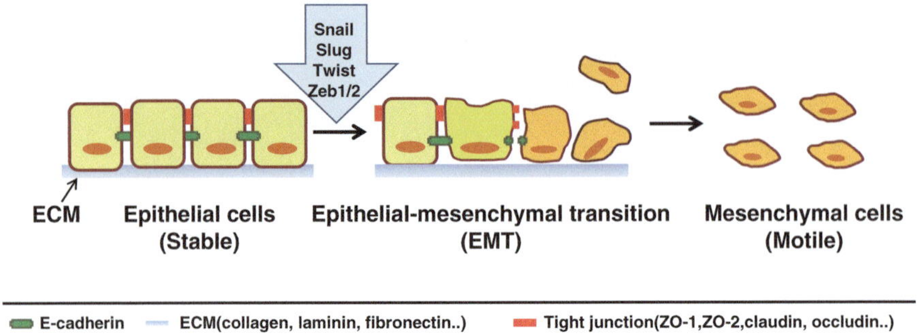

Fig. 1.20 Epithelial to Mesenchymal Transition (EMT). Transcription factors such as snail, slug, twist, and zeb1/2 are involved in EMT. Because of EMT, E-cadherin-mediated adhesion is lost and tight junctions (composed of ZO-1, ZO-2, claudin, and occludin) are disassembled. Transition to motile mesenchymal cells occurs when actin is reorganized and ECM proteins (collagen, laminin, fibronectin, etc.) are degraded due to the increased expression of ECM-degrading enzymes. Eventually, cell-cell contact is lost, and cells detach from the ECM, enabling migration and metastasis to other organs

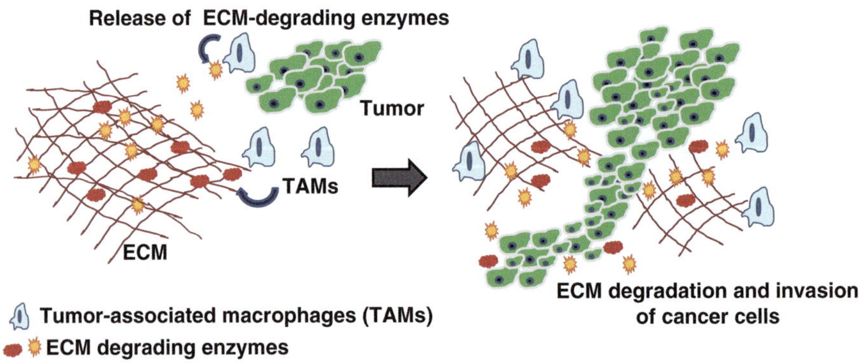

Fig. 1.21 Secretion of ECM-degrading enzymes by TAMs. ECM proteins are degraded by various ECM-degrading enzymes secreted by TAMs. Next, ECM-embedded growth factors and cytokines that increase migration and metastasis of cancer cells are activated, facilitating the invasion of cancer cells and metastasis to other organs

proteases [21]. In case of breast cancer, TAMs, which secrete EGF, and breast cancer cells, which produce colony stimulating factor-1, accelerate metastasis (Fig. 1.21). In the late stage of metastasis, when cancer cells settle in a new microenvironment, mesenchymal-epithelial transition (MET) occurs as opposed to EMT, and cancer cells halt migration and adapt to the new microenvironment forming a cancer mass. Because metastasis involves a variety of cell types in addition to cancer cells, and has several steps with complicated patterns, molecular-level research on metastasis is challenging and not feasible for the development of anticancer drugs.

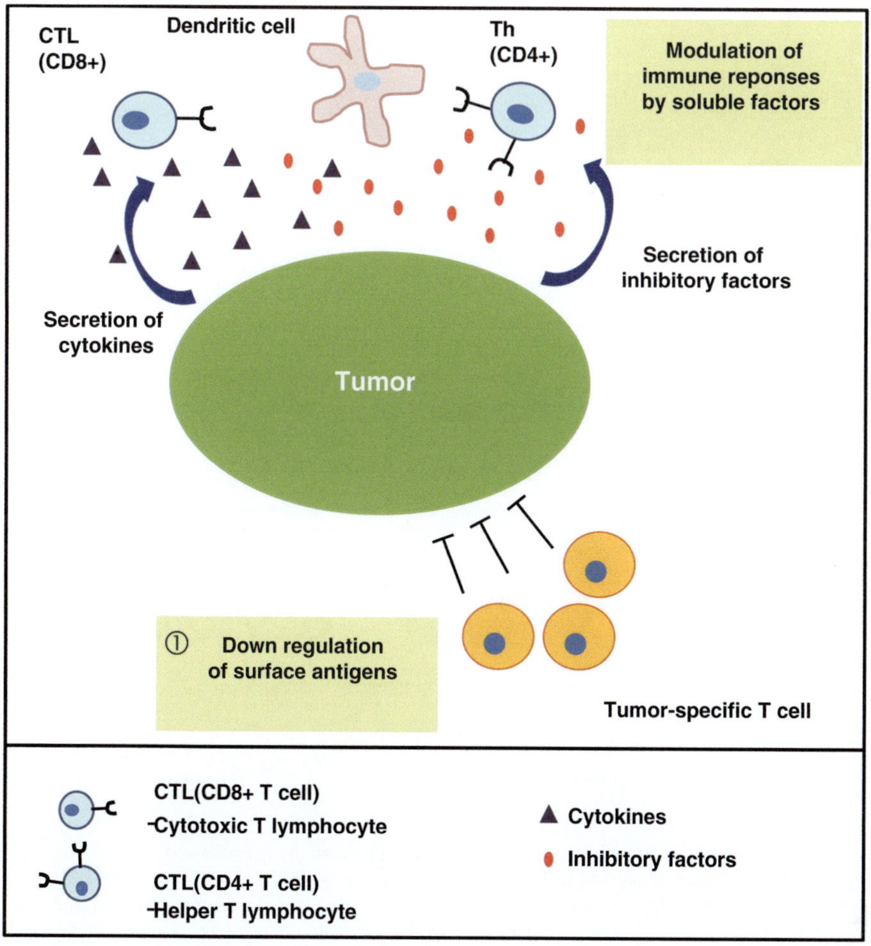

Fig. 1.22 Avoidance of immune surveillance. Cancer cells avoid the human immune system in a variety of ways. (*1*) Cancer cells avoid tumor-specific T cells by inhibiting the production of tumor-specific antigens. (*2*) Cancer cells regulate the immune response by secreting cytokines and immune response inhibiting factors, and expressing immune checkpoint molecules. This blocks the functions of immune cells such as CTLs, Th cells, and dendritic cells

1.2.4 Avoidance of Immune Surveillance

There is evidence to suggest that tumorigenesis can be prevented by the body's own immune cells. For instance, it has been reported that the incidence of tumors increased in mice that were deficient in cytotoxic T lymphocytes (CTLs), helper T cells, or natural killer (NK) cells. Inversely, prognosis of human colorectal and ovarian cancer patients improved after they were injected with a large number of CTLs and NK cells. Although further research of human cancers is needed, it is generally thought that malignant cancer cells have acquired the ability to avoid the human immune response [22] (Fig. 1.22).

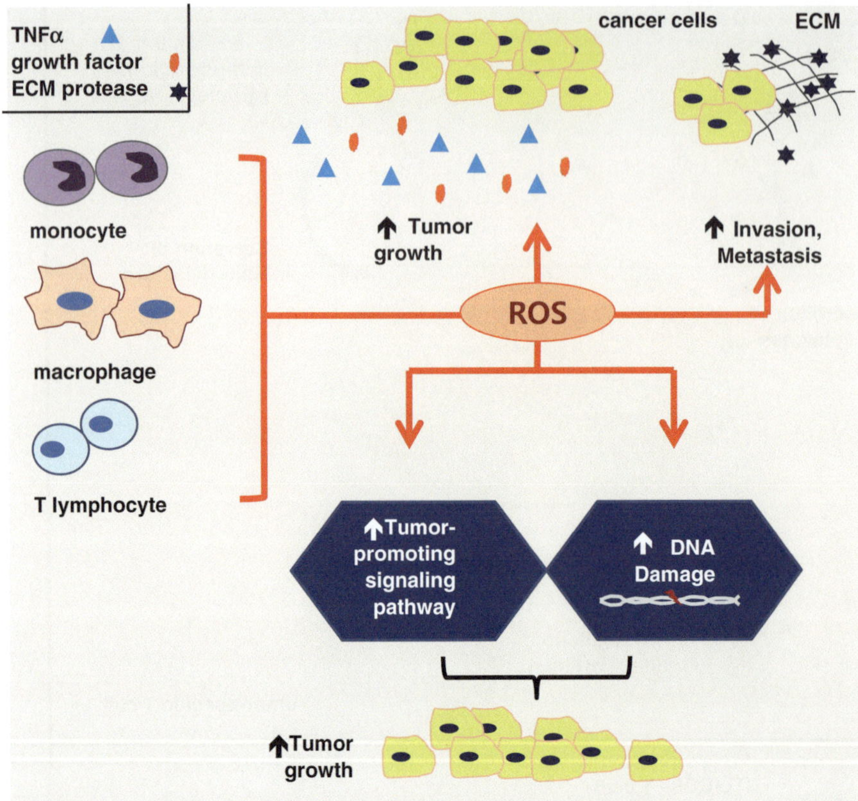

Fig. 1.23 Tumor-promoting inflammatory responses. ROS produced by immune cells (monocyte, macrophage etc.) activates signal transduction pathways that promote the growth of cancer cells and induce DNA damage that can cause cancer. In addition, they induce the proliferation and development of cancer cells by secreting tumor necrosis factor-α and various growth factors. They also enable cancer cells to migrate to other tissues through ECM and metastasize by secreting ECM-degrading enzymes

1.2.5 Tumor-Promoting Inflammatory Responses

Tumor cells continuously induce inflammatory responses through their interaction with neighboring immune cells, which are thought to play an important role in promoting carcinogenesis. That is, tumor-promoting inflammatory responses due to immune cells take place continuously from an early stage. These inflammatory responses are expected to be involved in carcinogenesis in a number of ways such as promoting the proliferation of cancer cells via secretion of growth factors and biologically active substances including reactive oxygen species (ROS), inhibiting cancer cell apoptosis, promoting angiogenesis, increasing invasion and metastasis through ECM-degrading enzymes, and inducing EMT etc. [23] (Fig. 1.23).

References

1. Hanahan D, Weinberg RA (2011) Hallmarks of cancer: the next generation. Cell 144:646–674
2. Luca AD, Maiello MR et al (2012) The RAS/RAF/MEK/ERK and the PI3K/AKT signalling pathways: role in cancer pathogenesis and implications for therapeutic approaches. Expert Opin Ther Targets 2:17–27
3. Kleinsmith LJ (2005) Principles of cancer biology. Pearson, San Francisco
4. Li W, Giancott FG (2010) Merlin's tumor suppression linked to inhibition of the E3 ubiquitin ligase CRL4(DCAF1). Cell Cycle 9:4433–4436
5. Kang MH, Reynolds CP (2009) Bcl-2 Inhibitors: targeting mitochondrial apoptotic pathways in cancer therapy. Clin Cancer Res 15:1126–1132
6. Mu J, Wei LX (2002) Telomere and telomerase in oncology. Cell Res 12:1–7
7. Murnane JP (2010) Telomere loss as a mechanism for chromosome instability in human cancer. Cancer Res 70:4255–4259
8. Vander Heiden MG, Cantley LC, Thompson CB (2010) Understanding the Warburg effect: the metabolic requirements of cell proliferation. Science 324:1029–1033
9. Balkwill FR, Capasso M, Hagemann T (2012) The tumor microenvironment at a glance. J Cell Sci 125:5591–5596
10. Dudley AC (2012) Tumor endothelial cells. Cold Spring Harb Perspect Med 2(3):a006536
11. Sundar SS, Ganesan TS (2007) Role of lymphangiogenesis in cancer. J Clin Oncol 25: 4298–4307
12. Mantovani A et al (2008) Cancer-related inflammation. Nature 454:436–444
13. Kalluri R, Zeisberg M (2006) Fibroblasts in cancer. Nat Rev Cancer 6:392–401
14. Pardal R, Clarke MF, Morrison SJ (2003) Applying the principles of stem-cell biology to cancer. Nat Rev Cancer 3:895–902
15. Weis SM, Cheresh DA (2011) Tumor angiogenesis: molecular pathways and therapeutic targets. Nat Med 17:1359–1370
16. Grothey A, Galanis E (2009) Targeting angiogenesis: progress with anti-VEGF treatment with large molecules. Nat Rev Clin Oncol 6:507–518
17. Zhang YW, Su Y, Volpert OV, Vande Woude GF (2003) Hepatocyte growth factor/scatter factor mediates angiogenesis through positive VEGF and negative thrombospondin-1 regulation. Proc Natl Acad Sci U S A 100:12718–12723
18. de la Puente P, Muz B, Azab F et al (2013) Cell trafficking of endothelial progenitor cells in tumor progression. Clin Cancer Res 19:3360–3368
19. Alberts B, Johnson A, Lewis J et al (2002) Molecular biology of the cell. 4th ed. Garland Science, New York
20. Kalluri R, Weinberg RA (2009) The basics of epithelial-mesenchymal transition. J Clin Invest 119:1420–1428
21. Pollard JW (2004) Tumour-educated macrophages promote tumour progression and metastasis. Nat Rev Cancer 4:71–78
22. Goldman B, DeFrancesco L (2009) The cancer vaccine roller coaster. Nat Biotechnol 27:129–139
23. Gyrd-Hansen M, Meier P (2010) IAPs: from caspase inhibitors to modulators of NF-kappa B, inflammation and cancer. Nat Rev Cancer 10:561–574

Chapter 2
Advancement of the Science and History of Cancer and Anticancer Drugs

Schleiden and Schwann first reported the Cell Theory in 1838, and Remak and R. C. Virchow advocated this theory for cancer in the mid-1850s. They named cancer "neoplasm," which was defined as a new mass of cells that emerges from abnormal proliferation of cells (Fig. 2.1). Thus, cancer was introduced into the field of science, was scientifically defined, and became an object of study.

In 1845, J. H. Bennett was the first to discover abnormal proliferation of leukocytes in blood. Later, in 1847, R. C. Virchow observed hazy pus-like characteristics in blood and named this disease "leukemia" (from the Greek word *leukos*, meaning "white").

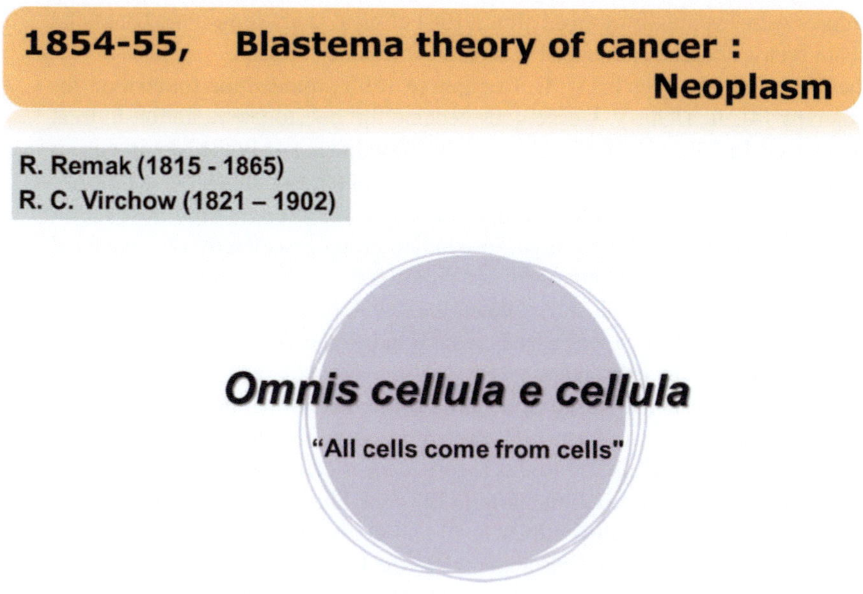

Fig. 2.1 Blastema theory of cancer: Neoplasm

K.-W. Kim et al., *Cancer Drug Discovery*, DOI 10.1007/978-94-024-0844-7_2

At this point in time, leukemia was the main focus of early cancer research and anticancer drug development. Solid cancers such as lung, colon, and liver cancers could not be properly studied because imaging techniques that could detect their occurrence and progression, such as MRI and CT, had not yet been developed. However, blood samples could be observed under a microscope to count the number of abnormal leukocytes, which made leukemia an adequate target of early cancer research. This allowed leukemia to become the basis for the development of anticancer drugs that suppressed proliferation of abnormal leukocytes. In 1860, M. A. Biermer reported the incidence of childhood leukemia, which became a major target of early anticancer drug development and treatment.

In 1889, S. Paget proposed the "seed and soil" theory as an explanation for metastasis, an important feature of malignant cancers [1]. This theory proposes the interaction between cancer cells and their surrounding tumor microenvironment, and is still widely accepted.

It was during this time that surgical therapy, one of the three major cancer treatments (along with radiotherapy and chemotherapy), began to be used, owing to the discovery of anesthetics and aseptic technique. In 1846, W. Morton performed the first surgical operation under ether anesthesia. In 1867, J. Lister became the first person to use aseptic technique during surgery [2]. These groundbreaking scientific advancements reduced the infection and pain associated with surgery; thus, surgical therapy was gradually introduced as a treatment for cancer.

In 1889, W. S. Halsted developed radical mastectomy, a typical surgical treatment for breast cancer [3]. During the 1950s and 1960s, radical mastectomy progressed to extreme limits, such as super-radical mastectomy and ultra-radical mastectomy, where surgical scopes were extended into the clavicles and ribs. These procedures were eventually stopped after a 1981 clinical study showed no beneficial effects in breast cancer treatment as compared with local surgery.

The discovery of x-rays by W. C. Rőntgen in 1895 provided the foundation for radiotherapy [4]. In 1896, V. Despeignes became the first to use radiation to treat gastric cancer. In 1902, E. H. Grubbe widely started using radiotherapy in cancer patients, and radiotherapy became increasingly popular [5]. In 1889, the Curiés discovered radium, which emitted stronger radiation, and brought high-dose radiotherapy to the forefront. Whereas high-dose radiotherapy was effective against local cancers, it triggered the development of secondary cancers due to radiation-induced mutation of normal cells. This necessitated the development of local radiotherapy for selective treatment of cancer tissues, which led to the development of various and precise radiotherapy equipment.

In 1890, D. P. Hansemann discovered chromosomal abnormalities in cancer cells [6]. Based on these abnormalities, T. H. Boveri proposed the carcinogenesis theory in 1914 (Fig. 2.2) [7]. According to this theory, cancer cells undergo constant division because of a chromosomal mutation in the cell. This definition simplified the characteristics of cancer at the cellular level and clarified the objective of cancer research by identification of the chromosome as the key substance of cell division.

The focus on the chromosomes of cancer cells in cancer research shared the direction of life science research in the early 1900s. During this time, life sciences

1914, Carcinogenesis theory by chromosome abnormality

T. H. Boveri (1862 – 1915)

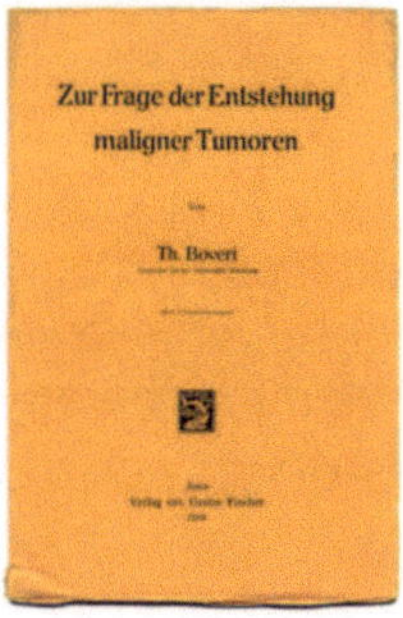

T. Boveri, "Zur Frage der Entstehung maligner Tumoren(On the problem of the origin of malignant tumors)", *Gustav Fisher (1914)*

" The origin of malignant tumors "

Fig. 2.2 Carcinogenesis theory by chromosome abnormality

were focused on the cell, but more specifically, on the genetic material inside the cell. In 1909, W. L. Johannsen named the mediator of genetic information the "gene" [8].

In 1915, T. H. Morgan, through his studies of Drosophila, proposed the theory that genes exist inside chromosomes [9]. There was much genetic research performed on the Drosophila chromosome, and in 1927, H. J. Müller discovered that x-rays could cause genetic mutation [10]. This discovery showed that radiation-(including x-rays) induced cancer lies in the genetic mutation of chromosomes in the cell.

Thereafter, the focus of life science and cancer research shifted from chromosomes to more essential material—genes. However, the true biological and chemical nature of this abstract concept called "gene" had yet to be determined. The importance of studying genes became widely acknowledged, and in 1938, W. Weaver named the research field that targets molecular substances in the cell, including genes, "molecular biology" [11].

Subsequently, the research areas of bioactive substances at the molecular level, including genes in the cell, were developed and defined. As the research target became clearer, O. T. Avery, C. M. MacLeod, and M. McCarty reported the results of their 1944 study that proved that DNA is the intracellular material of the gene. These results defined DNA as a molecule with genetic information, and made it the core target of molecular biology research [12].

Meanwhile, chemotherapy, one of the three major cancer treatments, commenced in the 1940s, nearly 100 years after cancer was named a "neoplasm" in the 1850s. Chemotherapy originated from N-mustard, which was used as a poisonous gas

1946, N-mustard as the first anticancer drug

L. S. Goodman (1906 – 2000) A. Gilman (1908 – 1984)

L. Goodman et al., Nitrogen Mustard Therapy, *J. A. M. A.*, 132, 126-132(1946)

··· Salutary results have been obtained particularly in Hodgkin's disease, lymphosarcoma and chronic leukemia. Indeed, in the first two disorders dramatic improvement has been observed. However, some patients fail to benefit from β-chloroethylamine therapy, and the cause of this failure is not known. ···

Fig. 2.3 N-mustard as the first anticancer drug

during the First and Second World Wars. The concept of chemotherapy emerged in 1909 when P. Ehrlich developed the syphilis medication Salvarsan 606; it was intended to be used to treat diseases with chemical substances.

N-mustard was the first chemical substance for anticancer chemotherapy, which was used as a poison gas during the Second World War. In 1943, a U.S. fleet anchored in Italy was bombed in an air raid by German Air Forces, killing 1,000 soldiers and residents. After reports that the deceased showed massive bone marrow damage, L. S. Goodman and A. Gilman used N-mustard to treat hematologic cancers such as leukemia in 1946 (Fig. 2.3) [13].

Anticancer chemotherapy was first proposed in 1948, when S. Farber used antifolate aminopterin in a child with leukemia (Fig. 2.4) [14]. The aminopterin temporarily alleviated the child's symptoms by inhibiting leukemic cell division, which indicated that cytotoxic chemical substances could treat cancer.

As previously mentioned, the target of early anticancer drug development was leukemia, of which cell proliferation was easily detected and measured. Therefore, early anticancer drugs were chemical substances that suppressed the rapid division of leukemic cells. S. Farber speculated that these chemical substances could also treat solid tumors with abnormally increased cell division, and proposed to use anticancer chemotherapy in solid tumors. In line with this proposal, G. B. Elion discovered the anticancer effect of 6-mercaptopurine in 1951, and clinical trials of this drug were performed to treat acute leukemia. In addition, in 1955 the American Cancer Chemotherapy National Service Center (CCNSC) conducted large-scale screening for chemotherapeutic agents, in which hundreds of thousands of synthetic chemical substances, fermentation products, and plant derivatives were used as candidate substances from 1955 to 1964. These efforts led to the development of various types of anticancer chemotherapy drugs such as 5-fluorouracil, which C. Heidelberger synthesized in 1957, and the plant derivative vincristine, developed in 1958 [15].

1948, Anticancer chemotherapy

S. Farber (1903 – 1973)

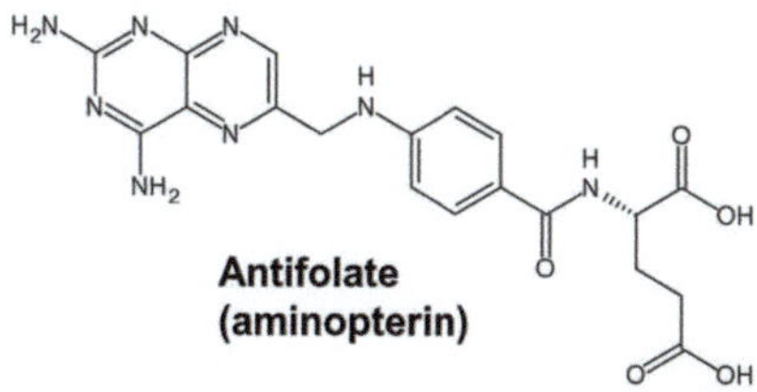

S. Farber et al., "Temporary Remissions in Acute Leukemia in Children Produced by Folic Acid Antagonist, 4-aminopteroyl-glutamic Acid(Aminopterin)", *The New England Journal of Medicine,* 238, 787-793(1948)

Fig. 2.4 Anticancer chemotherapy

Further investigation of these cytotoxic chemotherapy agents in clinical trials revealed that using a single type of anticancer drug caused cancer cells to become resistant to the drug and eventually caused cancer recurrence. In 1964, E. Frei and E. Freireich used multi-drug combination chemotherapy, in which existing anticancer drugs were combined and administered repetitively at high doses, and for the first time, they were used in children with leukemia.

The first high-dose combination chemotherapy was named "VAMP." It comprised vincristine, amethopterin (methotrexate), mercaptopurine, and prednisone (Fig. 2.5). However, this high-dose combination chemotherapy regimen had severe adverse effects; many clinical trials were conducted before the optimum dose of the anticancer drug was determined [16, 17]. The high-dose combination chemotherapy regimen was used in various protocols with different combinations, such as POMP in 1965 [18, 19] and MOPP in 1967 [20, 21].

In 1958, R. Hertz and M. C. Li used methotrexate to treat choriocarcinoma, which was the first attempt to treat a solid cancer in an adult patient using chemotherapy [22]. Actinomycin D, which S. A. Waksman discovered from actinomyces, was reported to have anticancer activity and was used for Wilm's tumor, another type of solid tumor, in 1959.

The therapeutic target of anticancer drugs shifted from hematologic tumors, such as leukemia, to solid tumors. However, the dominant hypothesis at the time was that all cancers had the same characteristic abnormal cell division. Based on this hypothesis, a "universal therapy" for cancer that could inhibit the abnormal proliferation of cancer cells using chemical substances was investigated in the 1960s (Fig. 2.6).

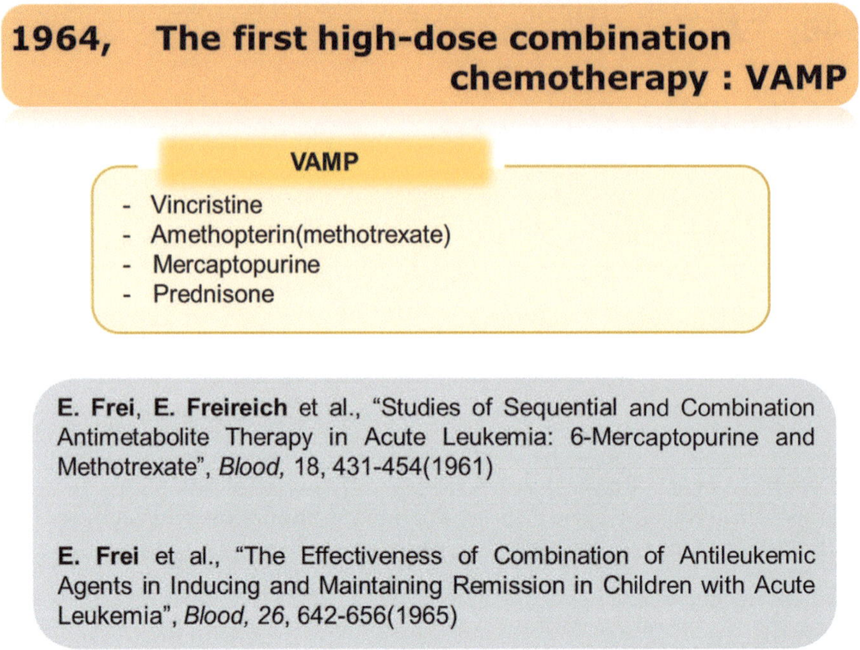

Fig. 2.5 The first high-dose combination chemotherapy: VAMP

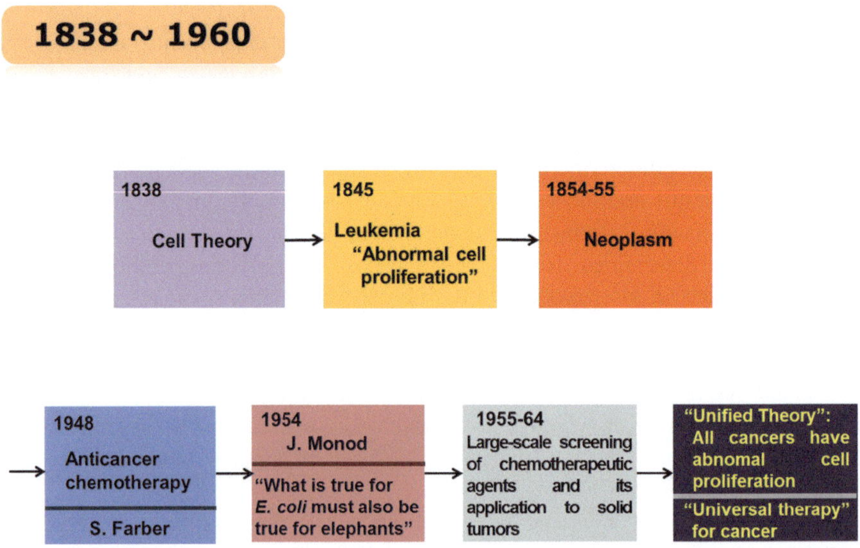

Fig. 2.6 Cancer research during 1838–1960s

In 1953, the molecular structure of DNA was discovered by J.D. Watson and F.H. Crick to be the double-helix structure. Soon after, in 1954, J. Monod proposed a theory that the life phenomenon at the molecular level is universal for all living organisms. Based on such hypotheses, molecular biological studies deciphered genetic codes and examined the molecular mechanisms of genetic information expressed as proteins through mRNA by focusing on the molecular targets of cell [23].

In the 1960s, it was incomprehensible to imagine the diversity and complexity of cancers at the molecular level; the development and application of anticancer drugs continued based on the assumption that all cancers have similarly abnormal cell proliferation. Etoposide (1966) and taxol (1967) were developed at this time and used as chemotherapeutic agents. Research achievements would be accumulated for decades after the 1960s to reveal the molecular mechanism of the abnormal proliferation of cancer cells and how this mechanism varies depending on the type of cancer.

In the bioscience field in the 1960s, S. Brenner, F. Jacob, and M. Meselson discovered mRNA, which mediates the transfer of genetic information from DNA to protein (1961) [24]. In the early 1960s, M. Nirenberg and H. G. Khorana deciphered the genetic code that explained the pathway of expression of the genetic information—the DNA-mRNA-protein chain [25, 26]. The revelation of the true nature of genetic information and the process of expression of this information to protein elucidated the relationship among genetic information and intracellular functions, various life phenomena, and carcinogenesis. Further, life science studies explained the correlation among storage (DNA), transfer (mRNA), and expression (protein) of the genetic information, and the DNA–mRNA–protein chain became the target of ardent efforts in the bioscience field to define biological activities and functions.

Meanwhile, in the United States, S. Farber of the Harvard Medical School and M. Lasker, who established the Lasker Awards, were urging the Congress and the President to enact the National Cancer Act through an extensive national campaign to cure cancer. After Apollo 11 successfully landed on the moon in 1969, M. Lasker, emboldened by the nation's confidence boost from its pioneering conquest of (outside) space, emphasized the need for national cancer research by describing it as conquering the "inner space" (cancer). In 1970, the National Program for the Conquest of Cancer was established and President Richard Nixon signed the National Cancer Act in 1971.

As a result of the National Cancer Act, nearly $1.5 billion was invested in cancer research in the U.S. between 1972 and 1974, which led to the rapid advancement of extensive anticancer treatment and cancer research nationwide. With the immense research funds, tremendous studies on anticancer drugs, clinical trials using these drugs in combination, and research on carcinogenesis were conducted. Correspondingly, numerous chemotherapeutic drugs, such as bleomycin (1973), adriamycin (1974), and cisplatin (1978), were developed in the 1970s and used for solid cancer treatment.

These anticancer drugs were used in high-dose combination chemotherapy regimens to induce a complete cure of solid cancers. In fact, it was predicted that in using these drugs, a generic treatment for all cancers would be developed. However, these cytotoxic anticancer drugs had several adverse effects, such as severe myelosuppression. Nevertheless, the high-dose combination chemotherapy regimen peaked in 1984–1985 and was widely used in the cancer therapy field, with nearly 6,000 relevant papers published in scientific journals during this time [27–29].

In 1982, a mega-dose combination chemotherapy was introduced to extreme levels above the lethal dose for bone marrow cells under the name of "STAMP" (Solid Tumor Autologous Marrow Program), using a combination of chemotherapy and autologous bone marrow transplantation that was developed by E. Frei [30]. However, this mega-dose combination chemotherapy was proven ineffective to the metastatic solid tumors during its final clinical trials in 2003, and was eventually discontinued.

Other advancements in bioscience in this period were the discovery of restriction enzymes by H. O. Smithies (1970) [31] and the synthesis of the first recombinant DNA by P. Berg using these restriction enzymes (1972) [32]. These advancements made possible the separation, manipulation, and recombination of genes, and led to a large-scale in vitro synthesis of proteins that could help treat diseases. These technologies stimulated industrialization in bioscience and eventually the biopharmaceutical industry emerged.

In 1975, G. Köhler and C. Milstein developed the monoclonal antibody technology that promoted in-depth studies on protein synthesis and function, which later greatly contributed to the development of anticancer drugs that inhibit the activity of certain proteins [33].

In 1977, W. Gilbert [34] and F. Sanger [35] invented the DNA-sequencing methods, which were crucial in deciphering genetic information. This breakthrough scientific discovery enabled decoding the genetic information of DNA and made possible to decipher the entire human genome. This discovery not only contributed to the understanding of the massive amount of human genetic information and normal human biological activities, but also helped to elucidate the pathological molecular pathways related to tumorigenesis. This research enabled the development of molecular targeted anticancer drugs, which was a new field of chemotherapy.

With the advancement of molecular biological technologies, such as defining the basic unit of a living organism as the cell, defining the gene, and defining the DNA that contained the genetic information, the objectives of bioscience research had become extremely sub-divided and detailed.

Advancements in molecular biology led to studies on the specific gene and carcinogenic processes of certain cancer cells. As a result, the hormone receptors that affect the proliferation of hormone-dependent cancers such as prostate, breast, and ovarian cancers were discovered. In 1977, an anti-estrogen hormone drug for estrogen-sensitive breast cancer named "tamoxifen" was developed. Tamoxifen suppressed the growth of cancer cells by binding to the estrogen receptor and blocking estrogen action. Such results implied the development of an anticancer drug that targeted a specific metabolic pathway of cancer cells, a mechanism quite different from the previous anticancer drugs that inhibited cell division.

In 1971, J. Folkman proposed angiogenesis as a main feature of malignant cancer [36]. This observation led to clinical, biochemical, and molecular biological studies of blood vessels around tumors and of angiogenesis, which is involved in the proliferation and metastasis of cancer; this promoted the development of anticancer drugs that inhibited angiogenesis. In 1975, a xenograft model of transplanted human cancer cells into an immune-deficient mouse was developed to study first-line anticancer drugs in a model simulating human cancer [37]. The resistance mechanism of anticancer drugs was reported in 1978 from the molecular biological studies of cancer cells, and was applied to the evaluation and new development of anticancer drugs [38, 39].

In the 1980s, hormone therapy and post-operative adjuvant chemotherapy were performed for breast and prostate cancers. In the 1970s and 1980s, cancers resistant to hormone therapy were reported and the molecular mechanism of anticancer drug resistance was gradually defined. However, as statistical research on cancer mortality in the 1980s showed that cancer mortality had not improved significantly until the mid-1980s, the importance of cancer prevention was noted, and subsequently, chemo-preventive research became routine. Smoking and asbestos were found to be related to carcinogenesis, therefore, not smoking and banning the use of asbestos became the main goals in cancer prevention. In 1973, B. Ames developed the Ames Test, which determined the carcinogenicity of chemical substances by measuring the degree of mutation of bacteria; [40] it was used to detect carcinogens.

In 1977, B. S. Blumberg [41, 42] identified the hepatitis B virus (HBV). The subsequent development of its vaccine in 1979 provided a treatment to prevent the progression of chronic hepatitis to liver cancer. In 1982, B. Marshall and R. Warren discovered *H. pylori*, a cause of gastritis [43]. The discovery that chronic gastritis caused by *H. pylori* could progress to gastric cancer led to the preventive treatment of some gastric cancers caused by bacterial infection.

The Pap smear method, which G. N. Papanicolaou devised [44, 45], and mammography could detect the precancerous stages of uterine cervical cancer and breast cancer, respectively, and therefore was used as preventive methods for these cancers.

Due to the extensive biochemical studies of carcinogenesis, not merely chemicals but other substances, such as hormones, viruses, and bacteria, were recognized to be carcinogens. Further research on these carcinogens and related types of cancer were performed, and their correlations were investigated in depth (Table 2.1).

As cancer prevention and early diagnosis became possible due to the aforementioned scientific discoveries, their importance became clearer. Since molecular mechanisms of carcinogenesis were not understood until the 1980s, it was still unclear in the 1960s and 1970s how HBV, *H. pylori*, and mutagenic chemicals individually caused tumorigenesis at the molecular level. Thus, the in-depth knowledge needed cancer treatment and prevention was limited. However, clinical studies during this time revealed that cancer had diverse characteristics with respect to their response to anticancer drugs as well as their invasion and metastatic abilities (Fig. 2.7).

Drosophila mutation was studied in 1910, and x-ray-induced mutation was studied in the 1920s, but no connection was revealed between the carcinogenic mechanism and genetic mutation.

Table 2.1 Carcinogens and related malignancies

Carcinogens	Related malignacies
Alkylating agents	AML, Bladder
Androgens	Prostate
Aromatic amines	Bladder
Arsenic	Lung, Skin
Asbestos	Lung, Mesothelioma, Peritoneum
Benzene	AML
Chromium	Lung
Epstein-Barr virus	Burkitt lymphoma, Nasal T cell lymphoma
Estrogens	Endometrium, Liver, Breast
Ethyl alcohol	Liver, Esophagus
Helicobacter pylori	Stomach, gastric MALT lymphoma
Hepatitis B or C virus	Liver
HIV virus	NHL, Kaposi sarcoma, Urologic malignancy, Squamouse cell carcinoma
Human papilloma virus	Cervis, Head & Neck
Immunosuppressive agents	NHL
Nitrogen mustard gas	Lung, Head & Neck
Nickel dust	Lung, Nasal cavity
Phenacetin	Kidney, Bladder
Polycyclic hydrocarbons	Lung, Skin
Schistosomiasis	Bladder (Squamous)
UV light	Skin (Squamous, Melanoma)
Tobacco	Lung, Head & Neck, Esophagus, Kidney, Bladder, Pancreas
Obesity	Colon, Breast, Esophagus, Endometrium, Kidney

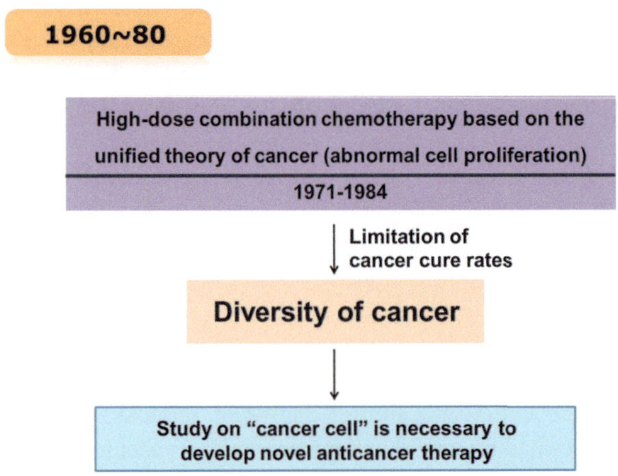

Fig. 2.7 Cancer research during 1960–1980s

After P. Rous discovered the Rous sarcoma virus in 1910 [46], D. P. Burkitt [47] discovered in 1958 that EBV causes Burkitt's lymphoma, and in 1983, it was reported that the human papilloma virus (HPV) [48] causes uterine cervical cancer. Based on these findings, it was proposed that viruses could cause cancer, as supported by the prevailing theory until the 1970s that the transformation of normal cells into cancer cells was caused by external factors.

In the 1950–1970s, x-ray, soot, tobacco smoke, and asbestos were thought to be the main causes of cancer. Other known causes were genetic factors, such as in the case of retinoblastoma and the Rous sarcoma virus, which causes sarcoma in chickens. Thus, cancer-inducing factors were shown to be genes, exogenous chemicals, and infectious agents such as viruses, but not one unified mechanism could integratively explain all these factors because they were so different from one another.

However, in 1970, D. Baltimore [49] and H. M. Temin [50] discovered the retrovirus, which revealed the process of reverse transcription from RNA to DNA and how insertion of the retrovirus into host chromosomes could induce mutation of genetic information. This discovery led to studies on the relationship between the retrovirus and human tumors.

In 1970, G. S. Martin, P. K. Vogt, and P. H. Duesberg [51] discovered the Src oncogene in RSV. This oncoprotein was revealed to have kinase activity and induced phosphorylation in other proteins. Such kinase could promote cell division, which explained the molecular pathway of carcinogenesis [52].

In 1976, J. M. Bishop and H. E. Varmus [53, 54] discovered that the Src oncogene existed not only in viruses but also in normal host cells. The oncogenes in the normal host cells were named "proto-oncogenes," and those in viruses were mutated. In 1981, based on this finding, it was suggested that proto-oncogenes in normal cells could be activated into oncogenes that cause abnormal cell division due to mutations caused by x-rays, exogenous chemicals, or viruses. This discovery was widely spread under the concept of "enemies within." [55]

Based on this discovery, a universal mechanism for tumorigenesis was proposed in the 1980s. The explanation that mutation factors (including x-rays, soot, tobacco smoke, and asbestos), genetic factors, and viruses induce genetic mutations, especially the activation of proto-oncogenes, eventually enabled integrated understanding of tumorigenesis at the genetic level.

In 1982, R. A. Weinberg, M. Barbacid, and M. Wigler reported the first Ras oncogene in humans [56–58]; in 1986, R. A. Weinberg again discovered the Rb (anti-oncogene or tumor suppressor gene) in humans [59, 60]. Thereafter, various mutations of Rb were discovered in different types of cancer, in addition to retinoblastoma. The Rb gene provided solid evidence that the inactivation of anti-oncogenes is involved in human tumor development.

In the 1980s, the dominant theory held was that tumors were caused by the activation of proto-oncogenes and the inactivation of tumor suppressor genes. Cancer was then widely believed to be induced by the abnormal regulation of gene expression from the mutation of normal genes in cells.

In the 1980s–1990s, many types of oncogenes and tumor suppressor genes were discovered in human tumors (Fig. 2.8), and their functions and mechanisms were discovered in vivo through transgenic mouse technology, which was developed in 1980 [61–63]. In 1983, K. Mullis invented PCR technology, which could amplify a

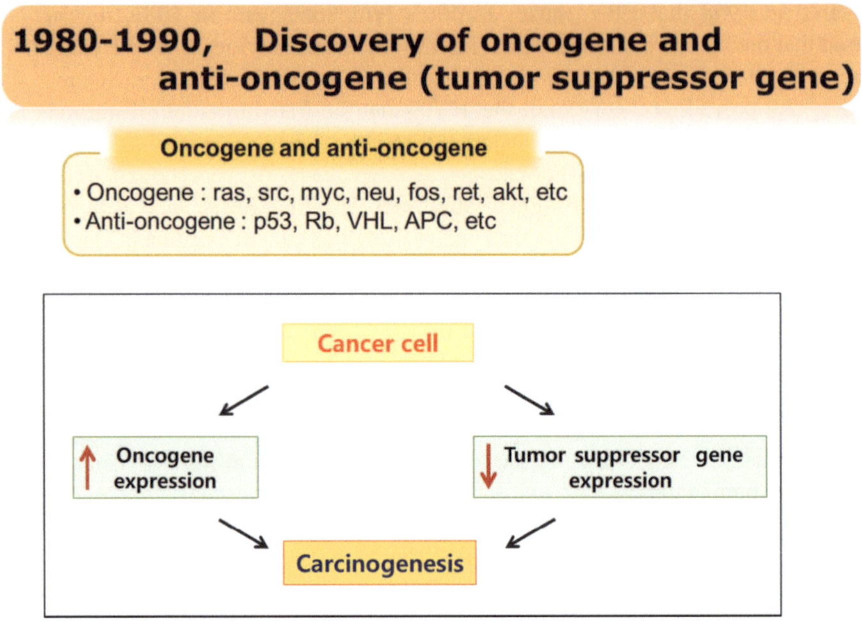

Fig. 2.8 Discovery of oncogene and anti-oncogene (tumor suppressor gene)

small amount of DNA. This invention led to a breakthrough progress in the identification of cancer genes and their functional studies during carcinogenesis. As a result, the correlation among various genes (i.e., the signal transduction process of the genes) was gradually understood.

According to epidemiologic studies on cancer mortality conducted in the U.S. between 1970 and 1994, the mortality rates of colon cancer decreased by nearly 30 %, and of cervical and uterine cancer, by nearly 20 %. The mortality rates of childhood cancer, Hodgkin's disease, and testicular cancer decreased as well [64]. Regarding lung cancer, its mortality rate in men decreased after it peaked in the 1980s, but its rate in women rapidly increased; its mortality rate in women over 55 years old greatly increased within a 30-year interval due to the increase in the female smoking rate in the 1950s.

As cancer occurrence caused by smoking increased, research of cancer prevention became routine. Epidemiologic, clinical, and biologic research findings also indicated that cancer is not a simple disease that could be overcome with a single therapy, but instead a complex genetic disease with various molecular characteristics. Therefore, basic research on the genetic characteristics of cancer was intensively conducted, and the research target was of course cancer cells. This was because the cancer cells were the most significant cells in cancer tissue. Hence, most studies focused on the genes of cancer cells, since cancer genes are responsible for the expression of the characteristics of cancer cells.

With this viewpoint, B. Vogelstein [65] proposed a theory in 1988 that cancer progresses through a multi-step process that involves the activation and inactivation of several genes. Related to this theory, the characteristics of malignant cancer such as abnormal cell proliferation, suppression of apoptosis, induction of angiogenesis, invasion, and metastasis, and their molecular mechanisms, were studied in detail at the genetic level.

As molecular changes in cancer cells during carcinogenesis were revealed, the characteristics of cancer cells were summarized by D. Hanahan and R. A. Weinberg, and they proposed the six hallmarks of cancer in 2000 [66] to be as follows: (1) it maintains a consistent proliferative signal; (2) it evades growth suppression; (3) it resists apoptosis; (4) it enables replicative immortality of chromosomes; (5) it induces angiogenesis; and (6) it activates invasion and metastasis abilities. These were further extended to ten hallmarks in 2011 [67]. Subsequently, attempts to treat cancer by targeting these characteristics developed rapidly. These attempts focused on the development of molecule-targeted anticancer drugs that target the genes related to the characteristics of cancer cells that differ from those of normal cells.

Throughout the 1980s–1990s, extensive basic research on cancer cells was carried out based on the understanding that the properties of cancer cells were crucial to the development of treatment of cancers. As a result, much information was accumulated on the many types of oncogenes and tumor suppressor genes involved in carcinogenesis, as well as on the signal transduction pathways in gene activation and their underlying mechanisms. These scientific advancements made possible the development of novel anticancer drugs.

Most of the anticancer drugs developed before the 1980s targeted the rapid cell division of cancer cells. Antifolates such as aminopterin, which was developed in the 1940s, inhibited cell division by blocking folic acid metabolism in the cell. N-mustard and cisplatin inhibited cell division by binding to DNA and blocking the gene replication needed for cell division [68]. Vincristine, developed in 1958, blocked cell division by suppressing the formation of cytoskeleton in the cell. However, these cytotoxic anticancer drugs suppressed not only the division of the cancer cells but also that of normal cells, which led to toxicities such as severe myelosuppression and epithelial cell damage of the skin and mucosa. Therefore, it was necessitated that new anticancer drugs should distinguish cancer cells from normal cells and attack only the cancer cells. The scientific evidence for such anticancer drugs was provided by basic research on cancer cells.

Based on such research, tamoxifen and trans-retinoic acid were developed as early molecular-targeted anticancer drugs. Tamoxifen was developed in 1977, based on the fact that specific breast cancers rely on estrogen signaling. In 1986, it was discovered that the PML-RARα fusion protein in acute promyelocytic leukemia (APL) was produced through chromosome translocation, and all-trans-retinoic acid (ATRA) showed an anticancer effect after combining with this protein.

As the various oncogenes and tumor suppressor genes discovered in previous studies acted as the core regulatory factors of cell division, anticancer drugs that targeted such factors began development. One example is trastuzumab (Herceptin), developed in 1990, an antibody that targeted the oncogene Her-2 of some breast cancers. Imatinib (Gleevec), which targeted the oncogene Bcr-Abl kinase of chronic myeloid leukemia (CML), was developed in 1996, and introduced the molecule-targeted therapy that inhibited only the activated oncogenes [69]. Next, molecular targeted agents that targeted the genetic mutations in cancer cells, the

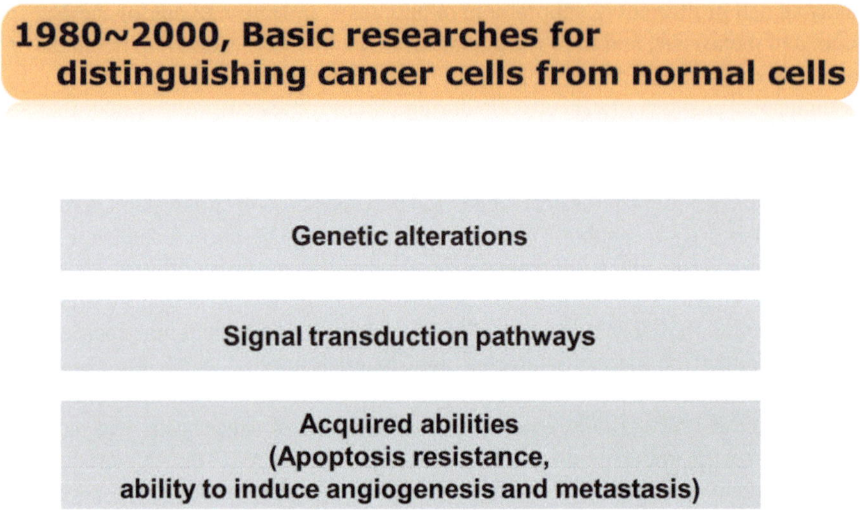

Fig. 2.9 Basic researches for distinguishing cancer cells from normal cells during 1980–2000

molecular differences in the signal transduction pathways, the apoptosis resistance of cancer cells, and the ability to induce angiogenesis and metastatic ability began development (Fig. 2.9). In 2005, a second generation CML drug named dasatinib (Sprycel) was developed for the mutated Bcr-Abl kinase of CML patients resistant to imatinib (Gleevec); the evolution of cancer and molecule-targeted agents began [70].

Since the introduction of Gleevec in 1996, hundreds of targeted agents for various cancers such as lung cancer, breast cancer, sarcoma, and melanoma are currently being developed.

Typical examples are bevacizumab (Avastin), which suppresses tumor angiogenesis; bortezomib (Velcade), which can treat multiple myeloma by blocking the degradation pathway of protein in cancer cells; olaparib (Lynpanza), developed in 2009 to treat breast cancers with BRCA gene mutation; and vemurafenib (Zelboraf), which was developed in 2011 to treat melanoma [71] (Fig. 2.10).

In 2001, the Human Genome Project (HGP) led by F. Collins and C. Venter [72, 73], considerably increased the possibility of the development of these molecule-targeted agents. The HGP could be one of the greatest scientific achievements of humankind. Following the formulation of the Cell Theory in 1838, the study objective of modern life sciences was focused on genes from chromosomes in the cell. HGP made possible the full interpretation of human genetic information, and would provide an opportunity to scientifically explain human biological activities, the study of which was previously considered to be beyond the limits of human ability. Many people believed that the HGP would make possible the discovery of the molecular mechanism and the treatment of various human diseases, including cancer. These expectations led to various studies on the gene mutations of human cancers using the rapid genomic DNA sequencing technology.

In 2004, a year after the discovery of the human genome sequence, B. Vogelstein [74] proposed the theory that cancer is in essence a genetic disease. The Cancer

1990-2010, Molecular targeted anticancer drugs: dozens of drugs are approved by FDA

Targeted anticancer drug

① **Avastin**: tumor angiogenesis inhibitor
② Bortezomib (Velcade)
: block protein degradation pathway, treatment of multiple myeloma

Avastin

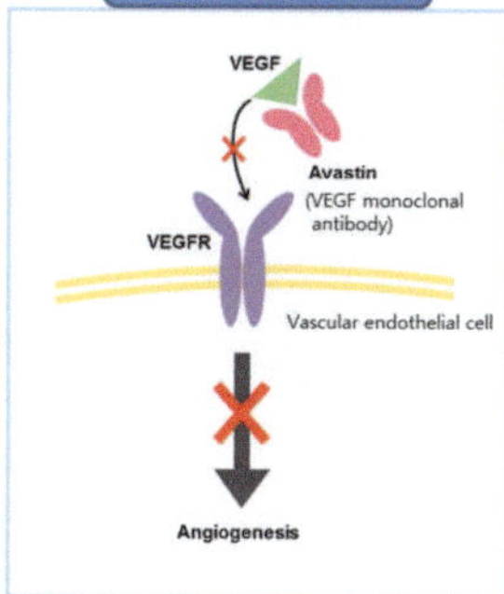

Bortezomib

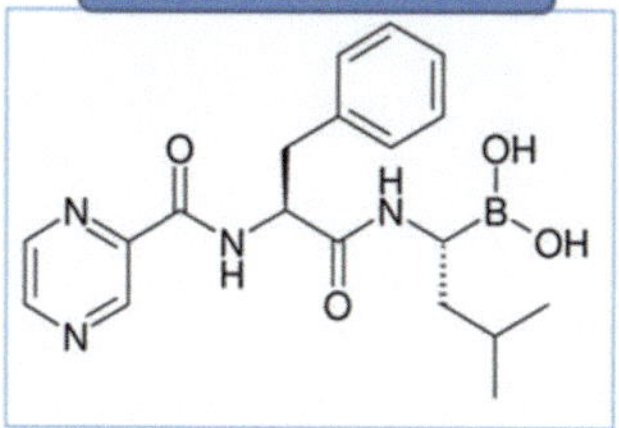

Fig. 2.10 Molecular targeted anticancer drugs

2004, "Cancer is, in essence, a genetic disease"

B. Vogelstein, **K. W. Kinzler**. "Cancer Genes and the Pathways They Control", *Nature Medicine*, 10, 789-799 (2004)

2005, The Cancer Genome Atlas

〈What is TCGA?〉

The Cancer Genome Atlas(TCGA) project
- A large-scale collaborative effort to characterize the genomic changes that occur in cancer
- Co-funded by NCI and the National Human Genome Research Institute (NHGRI)

〈Goal of TCGA〉

To improve ability to diagnose, treat and prevent cancer

Fig. 2.11 Cancer genome research

Table 2.2 Number of mutations in human cancers

Adult cancer	**No. of mutations**
Small cell lung cancer	163
Non-small cell lung cancer	147
Melanoma	135
Esophageal squamous cell carcinoma	79
Non-Hodgkin lymphoma	74
Head & neck cancer	66
Colorectal cancer	66
Esophageal adenocarcinoma	57
Gastric cancer	53
Endometrial cancer	49
Pancreatic cancer	45
Ovarian cancer	42
Prostate cancer	41
Hepatocellular cancer	39
Glioblastoma	35
Breast cancer	33
Chronic lymphocytic leukemia	12
Acute myeloid leukemia	8
Pediatric cancer	**No. of mutations**
Glioblastoma	14
Neuroblastoma	12
Acute lymphocytic leukemia	11
Medulloblastoma	8
Rhabdoid cancer	4

Genome Atlas (Fig. 2.11) for brain, lung, pancreatic, and ovarian cancers was promoted, and their entire genome was sequenced. As a result, dozens of mutated genes were discovered (Table 2.2), most of which were signal transduction factors such as serine/threonine kinases, tyrosine kinases, transcription factors, GTPases, and growth factors (Table 2.3) [74, 75].

In 2013, it was discovered that the number of mutations and the set of mutated genes differs from patient to patient, which gave rise to the concept of personalized therapy. These mutations could be divided into "driver mutations," which play an essential role in tumorigenesis, and "passenger mutations," which do not greatly affect tumorigenesis. The physiological function of these mutations in tumorigenesis and their connecting pathways were explained as well [75].

In the future, attempts will be made to understand the functions of these mutations and develop their targeted therapy agents. Such mutations closely related to increased cell division pathways (the cell cycle/death, RAS, and TGF-β signal transduction pathways), pathways related to the modulation of the cell fate (the Notch and chromatin-modified signal transduction pathways), and the genome-maintaining pathway through the DNA damage regulatory signal transduction pathway [75]. The

Table 2.3 Common genetic aberrations in human malignancies

Gene	Function	Genetic alterations	Associated tumors
AKT1	Serine/threonine kinase	Amplification	Stomach
AKT2	Serine/threonine kinase	Amplification	Ovary, Breast, Pancreas
BRAF	Serine/threonine kinase	Point mutation	Melanoma, Lung, Colon
CTNNB1	Signal transduction	Point mutation	Colon, Prostate, Melanoma
FOS	Transcription factor	Overexpression	Osteosarcoma
ERBB2	Receptor tyrosine kinase	Amplification, overexpresison	Breast, Stomach, Ovary, Brain
JUN	Transcription factor	Overexpression	Lung
MET	Receptor tyrosine kinase	Point mutation, rearrangement	Osteosarcoma, Kidney, Brain, Stomach
MYB	Transcription factor	Amplification	Leukemia, Colon, Melanoma
C-MYC	Transcription factor	Amplification	Breast, Colon, Stomach, Lung
L-MYC	Transcription factor	Amplification	Lung, Bladder
N-MYC	Transcription factor	Amplification	Lung, Brain
HRAS	GTPase	Point mutation	Colon, Lung, Pancreas
KRAS	GTPase	Point mutation	Melanoma, Colon, Leukemia
NRAS	GTPase	Point mutation	Various cancers
REL	Transcription factor	Point mutation, amplification	Lymphoma
WNT1	Growth factor	Amplification	Retinoblastoma

abnormally increased factors in these signal transduction pathways will be the target for future targeted anticancer drugs. Therefore, anticancer drugs that suppress or block such increased activity of cancer cells will be developed in the future.

Alternatively, there are attempts to develop targeted anticancer agents that focus on the loss-of-function of cancer cells, such as tumor suppressors, but this is not an easy task because protein functions are difficult to recover, and it will require a long time with abundant efforts. Meanwhile, the correlation between genetic diseases, their genetic abnormalities, and tumors has also been studied, and the relationships between various genetic diseases and the tumors that frequently accompany them have been summarized (Tables 2.4).

In the future, genetic mutations of individual patients will be analyzed, and it will become possible to provide each patient with individualized anticancer treatment by combining new targeted agents for such mutations with the previously developed cytotoxic anticancer drugs [76, 77].

In this chapter, the scientific discoveries and history of cancer and anticancer drugs following the Cell Theory in 1838 were briefly discussed. An overall chronological comparison regarding the scientific discoveries and history of cancer and anti-cancer drugs is summarized in Table 2.5.

Table 2.4 Genetic disorders and related malignancies

Syndrome	Gene	Chromosome	Inheritance	Associated tumors
Ataxia telangiectasia	ATM	11q22-q23	AR[a]	Breast
Autoimmune lymphoproliferative symdrome	FAS	10q24	AD[b]	Lymphoma
	FASL	1q23		
Bloom syndrome	BLM	15q26.1	AR	Various cancers
Cowden syndrome	PTEN	10q23	AD	Breast, Thyroid
Familial adenomatous polyposis	APC	5q21	AD	Colon
Familial melanoma	P16INK4	9p21	AD	Melanoma, Pancreas
Familial Wilms tumor	WT1	11p13	AD	Kidney
Hereditary breast/ovarian cancer	BRCA1	17q21	AD	Breast, Ovary, Colon, Thyroid
	BRCA2	13q12.3		
Hereditary diffuse gastric cancer	CDH1	16q22	AD	Stomach
Hereditary multiple exostoses	EXT1	8q24	AD	Chondrosarcoma
	EXT2	11p11-12		
Hereditary prostate cancer	HPC1	1q24-25	AD	Prostate
Hereditary retinoblastoma	RB1	13q14.2	AD	Retinoblastoma, Osteosarcoma
Hereditary nonpolyposis colon cancer (HNPCC)	MSH2	2p16	AD	Colon, Endometrium, Ovary, Stomach, Small bowel, Urothelial
	MLH1	3p21.3		
	MSH6	2p16		
	PMS2	7p22		
Hereditary papillary renal carcinoma	MET	7q31	AD	Kidney
Juvenile polyposis	SMAD4	18q21	AD	GIST, Pancreas
Li-Fraumeni	TP53	17p13.1	AD	Breast sarcoma
MEN type 1	MEN1	11q13	AD	Parathyroid, Endocrine, Pancreas, Hypothalamus
MEN type 2a	RET	10q11.2	AD	Medullary thyroid, Pheochromocytoma
Neurofibromatosis type 1	NF1	17q11.2	AD	Neurofibroma, Brain
Neurofibromatosis type 2	NF2	22q12.2	AD	Schwannoma, Meningioma, Spinal tumors
Nevoid basal cell carcinoma syndrome (Gorlin's syndrome)	PTCH	9q22.3	AD	Basal cell carcinoma, Medulloblastoma
Tuberous sclerosis	TSC1	9q34	AD	Angiofibroma, Angiomyolipoma
	TSC2	16p13.3		
Von Hippel-Lindau	VHL	3p25-26	AD	Kidney, Cerebellum, Pheochromocytoma

[a]*AR* autosomal recessive
[b]*AD* autosomal dominant

As shown in this table, current life sciences started with the definition of the basic unit of complex multicellular organisms, the Cell Theory, proposed in 1838. Subsequently, the majority of bioresearch was focused on cells, which became the research objective. This research objective became further subdivided by focusing on the gene and genetic information, among the various molecular substances in the cell. During this process, various scientific technologies and methodologies were developed to study cells, molecules and genes (DNA), and finally, the human genome was fully revealed and identified. In the past 40 years, along with the progress of scientific advancements, cancer research has also focused on cancer cells based on the definition of cancer as a "a new cell mass" ("neoplasm" in 1854–1855), and revealed various properties of cancer cells at the molecular and genetic level. As a result, anticancer drugs have been developed based on such research output from proliferation-inhibiting cytotoxic cancer drugs to molecular-targeted agents that target the abnormal genes of cancer cells. Therefore, the overall development of life sciences, cancer research, and anticancer drugs in the past 170 years was accomplished mainly at the molecular level by focusing on cells. Thus, anticancer drugs were developed based on the molecular properties of cancer cells.

Table 2.5 shows how past scientific developments led to the discovery of new anticancer drugs. For example, DNA-sequencing led to the discovery of the nature of the human oncogene and to the analysis of the genome of human cancer cells, which provided great opportunities to develop new molecular-targeted anticancer agents. The PCR and transgenic mouse technologies also led to an understanding of the functions and signal transduction pathways of oncogenes and tumor-suppressor genes, which eventually contributed to the development of new anticancer agents. In addition, monoclonal antibody technology provided the decisive technical basis for the development of various antibody-based cancer drugs that target specific proteins of cancer cells.

In Chaps. 4 to 9, the six classified cancer drugs and the developmental history of each drug are described. In Chap. 10, the adverse effects of anticancer drugs are summarized. In Chap. 11, the effectiveness of these drugs in cancer treatment is

Table 2.5 Advancement of science, history of cancer, and cancer drug development

Advancement of science		History of cancer		Cancer drug development	
[1801–1900]					
1838	"Cell Theory" *M. Schleiden* *T. Schwann*	1845	Discovery of leukemia *J.H. Bennett*		
1846	Discovery of anesthesia *W. Morton*	1847	Introduction of the name "leukemia" *R.C. Virchow*		
		1854–1855	Blastema theory of cancer—Neoplasm *R. Remak* *R.C. Virchow*		
1866	Discovery of the principles of heredity *G. Mendel*	1860	First known case of childhood leukemia *M.A. Biermer*		
1867	Use of an antiseptic *J. Lister*				
1879	Discovery of chromosomal duplication *W. Flemming*	1889	"Seed & Soil" hypothesis - organ-preference patterns of tumor metastasis *S. Paget*		
1890	Observation of chromosomal abnormalities in cancer *D.P. Hansemann*	1889	Invention of the radical mastectomy *W.S. Halsted*		
1895	Discovery of X-rays *W.C. Röntgen*				
1898	Discovery of radium *P. Curie & M. Curie*				
[1901–1930]					

1909	Discovery of Salvarsan, an antisyphilitic drug *P. Ehrlich*	1902	Radiation therapy for breast cancer treatment *E. Grubbe*		
1909	Introduction of the term "Gene" (plant) *W.L. Johannsen*	1910	Discovery of Rous Sarcoma Virus *P. Rous*		
1915	Genes are located on chromosoms *T.H. Morgan*	1912	Transplantable tumors *P. Rous*		
1927	Induction of mutation using X-rays *H.J. Müller*	1914	Carcinogenesis theory by chromosome abnormality (chromosomal theory of cancer) *T.H. Boveri*		
1928	Discovery of penicillin, an antibiotic *A. Fleming*				
[1931–1950]					
		1935	Discovery of tumor-causing papilloma virus *P. Rous*		
1938	Introduction of the term "molecular biology" *W. Weaver*	1937	Establishment of the National Cancer Institute (NCI)		
1940	Purification of actinomycin D *S. Waksman*				

(continued)

Table 2.5 (continued)

Advancement of science		History of cancer		Cancer drug development	
1943	Purification of streptomycin, an antituberculosis drug *S. Waksman*				
1944	Discovry of DNA as the carrier of genes *O.T. Avery* *C.M. MacLeod* *M. McCarty*	1941	Discovery of hormone dependence of prostate cancer *C. Huggins*		
		1948	Development of Pap smear method for cervical cancer screening *G. Papanicolaou*	1946	Use of N-mustard to treat lymphoma *A. Gilman* *L. Goodman*
		1949	Anticancer drug screening using mouse lymphoid leukemia cell line, L1210	1948	Devolopment of antifolates (aminopterin) *S. Farber* Beginning of the anticancer chemotherapy
[1951–1960]					
1953	Discovery of DNA double helix *J. Watson* *F. Crick*			1950	Development of prednisolone *A. Nobile* Development of methotrexate *L.M. Meyer*
				1951	Development of 6-mercaptopurine *G.B. Elion*
1954	"What is true for *E. coli* must also be true for elephants" *J. Monod*	1954	Link between smoking & lung cancer—propose primary prevention of cancer *I. MacLeod*	1955	Establishment of Cancer Chemotherapy National Service Center (CCNSC)

1957	Discovery of interferon inhibiting viral replication *A. Isaacs* *J. Lindemann*			1957	Development of 5-fluorouracil *C. Heidelberger*
1958	"Central Dogma": DNA → RNA → Protein *F. Crick*	1958	Discovery of Epstein-Barr Virus (EBV) causing Burkitt's lymphoma *D.P. Burkitt*	1958	Development of vincristine (vinca alkaloid) *R.L. Noble*
		1958	Treatment of choriocarcinoma with methotrexate: first cure of a solid tumor *R. Hertz* *M.C. Li*		
[1961–1970]					
1961	Discovery of mRNA *S. Brenner* *F. Jacob* *M. Meselson* Deciphering the genetic code *M. Nirenberg* *G. Khorana*				
				1962	First synthesis of tamoxifen

(continued)

Table 2.5 (continued)

Advancement of science		History of cancer		Cancer drug development	
		1964	High-dose combination chemotherapy [VAMP-Vincristine, Amethopterin (methotrexate), Mercaptopurine, Prednisone] *E. Frei* *E. Freireich* *H. Skipper* "Cell kill" hypothesis: A uniform dose of a drug kills a constant fraction of the tumor cells—repeated doses must be administered Combinations of drugs show synergistic effects—lower the chance of resistance *H. Skipper*	1964	FDA approval of Actinomycin D *S. Waksman*
		1965	POMP combination chemotherapy: cure of acute lymphoblastic leukemia (ALL)	1966	Synthesis of etoposide
1970	Discovery of restriction enzyme *H.O. Smithies*	1967	MOPP combination chemotherapy: Cure of Hodgkin's lymphoma	1967	Purification of taxol
1970	Discovery of retrovirus D. Baltimore *H.M. Temin*	1970	Discovery of v-src oncogene *P.H. Duesberg* *G.S. Martin* *P.K. Vogt*		
[1971–1980]					
		1971	The National Cancer Act *R. Nixon* Tumor angiogenesis is proposed *J. Folkman*		
1972	Recombinant DNA *P. Berg*	1971–1984	Cancer treatment with high-dose combination chemotherapy		

		1973	Development of Ames test for screening potential carcinogens *B. Ames*	1973	Development of bleomycin
		1973	Adjuvant chemotherapy to remove residual tumor after surgery		
1975	Development of monoclonal antibody *C. Milstein* *G. Köhler*	1974	Discovery of mechanisms of drug resistance (1): P-glycoprotein/MDR1 efflux pump resistance mechanism	1974	Development of adriamycin
		1975	Anticancer drug screening using tumor xenograft model in immunodeficient mice		
		1975	Adjuvant chemotherapy in early-stage breast cancer: cyclophosphamide, methotrexate and fluorouracil (CMF)		
		1976	Discovery of proto-oncogene *H. Varmus* *M. Bishop*		
1977	Development of DNA sequencing method *W. Gilbert* *F. Sanger*	1976	Cure of testicular cancer with combination of cisplatin, vinblastine, bleomycin		
1978	First production of recombinant synthetic human insulin	1977	Discovery of hepatitis B virus *B. Blumberg*	1977	Development of Tamoxifen AstraZeneca
1980	First production of “transgenic mouse”	1978	Discovery of mechanisms of drug resistance (2): Amplification of dihydrofolate reductase gene	1978	FDA approval of Cisplatin *B. Rosenberg*

(continued)

Table 2.5 (continued)

Advancement of science		History of cancer		Cancer drug development	
[1981–1990]					
1981–1990	Discovery of oncogenes (ras, src, myc, neu, fos, ret, akt, etc.) + anti-oncogenes (p53, Rb, VHL, APC, etc.)	1982	Discovery of *Helicobacter pylori* *B. Marshall* *R. Warren*		
		1982	Discovery of human Ras oncogene *R.A. Weinberg* *M. Barbacid* *M. Wigler*		
		1982	Develpment of Solid Tumor Autologous Marrow Program (STAMP) *E. Frei*		
1983	Development of PCR *K. Mullis*	1983	Discovery of relation between cervical cancer and human papilloma virus (HPV) *H. zur Hausen*	1983	FDA approval of Etoposide
		1984	Introduction of molecular biology (NCI): rapid drug screening, discovery of molecular mechanisms in tumorigenesis		
1986	Development of recombinant hepatitis B vaccine, Production of interferon, the first anticancer drug produced by genetic engineering	1986	Discovery of tumor suppressor gene *R.A. Weinberg*	1986	The first development of the oncogene (APL)-targeted drug, trans-retinoic acid
		1988	Cancer: molecular alterations of genes *B. Vogelstein*		

1990	Human Genome Project began	1990	Development of NCI-60 human tumor cell line panel for anticancer drug screening	1990	Herceptin: development of targeted monoclonal antibody for Her-2 positive breast cancer (Genentech)
		1990	15 % decrease of cancer death rate Lung cancer (primary prevention) Colon & cervical cancer (secondary prevention) Leukemia, lympoma, testicular cancer (chemotherapy) Breast cancer (mammograpy + surgery + adjuvant chemotherapy)		
[1991–2000]					
		1991–2005	Subtle differences between normal and cancer cells Genetic alterations Signal transduction pathways Acquired abilities (angiogenesis, invasion and metastasis)		
		1994	Discovery of BRCA1, 2 muatations increaseing the risk of breast cancer		
1995	Sequencing the genome of *H. influenzae* *C. Venter* *H. Smith*	1995	First human gene therapy clinical trial		

(continued)

Table 2.5 (continued)

Advancement of science		History of cancer		Cancer drug development	
1996	Birth of first cloned sheep, Dolly *I. Wilmut* *K. Campbell*	1997	The caner stem cell theory *J. Dick* *D. Bonnet*	1996	Gleevec: Bcr-Abl kinase inhibitor, treatment of chronic myeloid leukemia ⇒ Introduction of molecule-targeted therapy highly specific to cancer
1998	Completion of the first draft of the human genome containing more than 20,000 genes	2000	The Six Hallmarks of Cancer D. Hananhan R.A. Weinberg Sustaining proliferative signaling Evading growth suppressors Resisting cell death Enabling replicative immortality Inducing angiogenesis Activating invasion and metastasis		
[2001–2010]					
2001	Publication of a draft sequence of human genome *C. Venter* *F. Collins*			2001–2010	Molecular targeted anticancer drugs: dozens of drugs are approved by FDA Avastin: tumor angiogenesis inhibitor Bortezomib (Velcade), etc.
2002	Development of a cervical cancer vaccine				
2003	Completion of the human genome sequence	2004	"Cancer is, in essnece, a genetic disease" *B. Vogelstein*		

2006	Development of induced pluripotent stem cell *S. Yamanaka*	2005	The Cancer Genome Atlas Brain cancer: 40–50 mutations Pancreatic cancer: 50–60 mutations Breast, colon cancer: 50–80 mutations	2005	Dasatinib: new Bcr-Abl kinase inhibitor, target Gleevec-resistant CML (Bristol-Myers Squibb)
		2008	Examination of the dynamics of cigarette smoking *N. Christakis* *J. Fowler*	2009	Olaparib: PARP inhibitor, acts against cancers with BRCA mutations
[2011–present]					
2011		2011	Hallmarks of Cancer: The Next Generation *D. Hanahan* *R.A. Weinberg* Addition of 4 more hallmarks: Avoiding immune destruction Tumor-promoting inflammation Genome instability and mutation Deregulating cellular energetics	2011	Vemurafenib: BRAF kinase inhibitor, treatment of melanoma

reviewed, and the future direction of cancer research and anticancer drug development is proposed.

References

1. Paget S (1889) Distribution of secondary growths in cancer of the breast. Lancet 133:571–573
2. Lister J (1867) On the antiseptic principle in the practice of surgery. Br Med J 2:246–248
3. Halsted W (1894) The results of operations for the cure of cancer of the breast performed at the Johns Hopkins Hospital from June, 1889 to January, 1894. Ann Surg 20:497–555
4. Röntgen W (1896) On a new kind of rays. Science 3:227–231
5. Grubbe EH (1902) X-rays in the treatment of cancer and other malignant diseases. Med Rec 62:692–695
6. Hansemann D (1890) Ueber asymmetrische zelltheilung in epithelkrebsen und deren biologische bedeutung (About asymmetric cell division in epithelial cancer cells and their biological significance). Virchows Arch 119:299–326
7. Boveri T (1914) Zur frage der entstehung maligner tumoren (On the problem of the origin of malignant tumors). Gustav Fisher, Jena
8. Johannsen WL (1909) Elemente der exakten erblichkeitslehre. Molecular and general genetics. Jena: Gustav Fischer
9. Morgan TH et al (1915) The mechanism of Medelian heredity. Henry Holt and Company, New York
10. Müller HJ (1927) Artificial transmutation of the gene. Science 66:84–87
11. Rheinberger H (2007) A short history of molecular biology. Hist Phil Sci Technol 2. EOLSS Publications, Paris
12. Avery OT, MacLeod CM, McCarty M (1944) Studies on the chemical nature of the substance inducing transformation of pneumococcal types. J Exp Med 79:137–158
13. Goodman L et al (1946) Nitrogen mustard therapy. JAMA 132:126–132
14. Farber S et al (1948) Temporary remissions in acute leukemia in children produced by folic acid antagonist, 4-aminopteroyl-glutamic acid(aminopterin). N Engl J Med 238:787–793
15. Noble RL et al (1958) Role of chance observations in chemotherapy: *vinca rosea*. Ann N Y Acad Sci 76:882–894
16. Frei E, Freireich E et al (1961) Studies of sequential and combination antimetabolite therapy in acute leukemia: 6-mercaptopurine and methotrexate. Blood 18:431–454
17. Frei E et al (1965) The effectiveness of combination of antileukemic agents in inducing and maintaining remission in children with acute leukemia. Blood 26:642–656
18. Frei E, Freireich E (1965) Progress and perspectives in the chemotherapy of acute leukemia. Adv Chemother 2:269–298
19. Rodriguez V, Freireich E et al (1973) POMP combination chemotherapy of adult acute leukemia. Cancer 32:69–75
20. Moxley JH, Frei E et al (1967) Intensive combination chemotherapy and X-irradiation in Hodgkin's disease. Cancer Res 27:1258–1263
21. Devita VT, Serpick A, Carbone P (1970) Combination chemotherapy in the treatment of advanced Hodgkin's disease. Ann Intern Med 73:881–895
22. Hertz R, Li MC, Bergenstal DM (1958) Therapy of choriocarcinoma and related trophoblastic tumors with folic acid and purine antagonists. N Engl J Med 259:66–74
23. Crick F (1958) On protein synthesis. Symp Soc Exp Biol 12:138–163
24. Brenner S, Jacob F, Meselson M (1961) An unstable intermediate carrying information from genes to ribosomes for protein synthesis. Nature 190:576–581
25. Martin R, Matthaei JH, Jones OW, Nirenberg MW (1961) Ribonucleotide composition of the genetic code. Biochem Biophys Res Commun 6:410–414

26. Söll D, Cherayil J, Khorana HG et al (1966) sRNA specificity for codon recognition as studied by the ribosomal binding technique. Cold Spring Harb Symp Quant Biol 31:51–61
27. Einhorn LH, Donohue J (1977) Cis-Diamminedichloroplatinum, vinblastine, and bleomycin combination chemotherapy in disseminated testicular cancer. Ann Intern Med 87:293–298
28. MacDonald JS et al (1980) 5-Fluorouracil, coxorubicin, and mitomycin (FAM) combination chemotherapy for advanced gastric cancer. Ann Intern Med 93:533–536
29. Gralla RJ et al (1981) Cisplatin and vindesine combination chemotherapy for advanced carcinoma of the lung: a randomized trial investigating two dosage schedules. Ann Intern Med 95:414–420
30. Frei E (1982) The national cancer chemotherapy program. Science 217:600–606
31. Kelly TJ, Smithies HO (1970) A restriction enzyme from *Hemophilus influenzae* II, base sequence of the recognition site. J Mol Biol 51:393–409
32. Jackson DA, Symons RH, Berg P (1972) Biochemical method for inserting new genetic information into DNA of simian virus 40: circular SV40 DNA molecules containing lambda phage genes and the galactose operon of *Escherichia coli*. Proc Natl Acad Sci U S A 9: 2904–2909
33. Köhler G, Milstein C (1975) Continuous cultures of fused cells secreting antibody of predefined specificity. Nature 7:495–497
34. Maxam HM, Gilbert W (1977) A new method for sequencing DNA. Proc Natl Acad Sci U S A 74:560–564
35. Sanger F, Nicklen S, Coulson AR (1977) DNA sequencing with chain-terminating inhibitors. Proc Natl Acad Sci U S A 74:5463–5467
36. Folkman J (1971) Tumor angiogenesis: therapeutic implications. N Engl J Med 285:1182–1186
37. Povlsen CO, Jacobsen GK (1975) Chemotherapy of a human malignant melanoma transplanted in the nude mouse. Cancer Res 35:2790–2796
38. Schimke RT et al (1978) Amplification of dihydrofolate reductase genes in methotrexate-resistant cultured mouse cells. Cold Spring Harb Symp Quant Biol 42:649–657
39. Nunberc JH et al (1978) Amplified dihydrofolate reductase genes are localized to a homogeneously staining region of a single chromosome in a methotrexate-resistant Chinese hamster ovary cell line. Proc Natl Acad Sol USA 75:5553–5556
40. Ames BN, Durston WE, Yamasaki E, Lee FD (1973) Carcinogens are mutagens: a simple test system combining liver homogenates for activation and bacteria for detection. Proc Natl Acad Sci U S A 70:2281–2285
41. Blumberg BS (1977) Hepatitis-B virus in bedbugs (*Cimex hemipterus*) from Senegal. Lancet 310:217–219
42. Blumberg BS (1977) Non-A, Non-B hepatitis. Ann Intern Med 87:111–113
43. Marshall BJ, Warren JR (1984) Unidentified curved Bacilli in the stomach of patients with gastritis and peptic ulceration. Lancet 323:1311–1315
44. Kelly GL, Papanicolaou GN (1927) The mechanism of the periodical opening and closing of the vaginal orifice in the guinea-pig. Am J Anat 40:387–411
45. Papanicolaou GN (1948) The cell smear method of diagnosing cancer. Am J Public Health 38:202–205
46. Rous P (1911) A Sarcoma of the fowl transmissible by an agent separable from the tumor cells. J Exp Med 13:397–411
47. Burkitt D (1958) A Sarcoma involving the Jaws in African children. Br J Surg 46:218–223
48. zur Hausen H et al (1983) Human Papillomavirus types 6 and 11 DNA sequences in genital and laryngeal papillomas and in some cervical cancers. Proc Natl Acad Sci U S A 80:560–563.
49. Baltimore D (1970) RNA-dependent DNA, polymerase in virions of RNA tumour viruses. Nature 27:1209–1211
50. Temin HM, Mizutani S (1970) RNA-dependent DNA polymerase in virions of Rous sarcoma virus. Nature 27:1211–1213
51. Duesberg PH, Martin GS, Vogt PK (1970) Glycoprotein components of avian and murine RNA tumor viruses. Virology 41:631–646
52. Kleinsmith LJ (2006) Principles of cancer biology. Pearson, San Francisco

53. Stehelin D, Varmus HE, Bishop JM, Vogt PK (1976) DNA related to the transforming gene(s) of avian sarcoma viruses is present in normal avian DNA. Nature 260:170–173
54. Stehelin D, Guntaka RV, Varmus HE (1976) Purification of DNA complementary to nucleotide sequences required for neoplastic transformation of fibroblasts by avian sarcoma viruses. J Mol Biol 5:349–365
55. Bishop JM (1981) Enemies within: the genesis of retrovirus oncogenes. Cell 23:5–6
56. Parada LF, Tabin CJ, Shih C, Weinberg RA (1982) Human EJ bladder carcinoma oncogene is homologue of Harvey sarcoma virus *ras* gene. Nature 297:474–478
57. Reddy EP, Reynolds RK, Santos E, Barbacid M (1982) A point mutation is responsible for the acquisition of transforming properties by the t24 human bladder carcinoma oncogene. Nature 300:149–152
58. Taparowsky E, Suard Y, Fasano O, Shimizu K, Goldfarb M, Wigler M (1982) Activation of the T24 bladder carcinoma transforming gene is linked to a single amino acid change. Nature 300:762–765
59. Weinberg RA, Rapaport JM, Albert DM (1986) A Human DNA segment with properties of the gene that predisposes to retinoblastoma and osteosarcoma. Nature 323:643–646
60. Weinberg RA (1988) Finding the anti-oncogene. Sci Am 259:44–51
61. Gordon JW, Scangos GA, Plotkin DJ, Barbosa JA, Ruddle FH (1980) Genetic transformation of mouse embryos by microinjection of purified DNA. Proc Natl Acad Sci 77:7380–7384
62. Brinster RL, Chen HY, Trumbauer M, Senear AW, Warren R, Palmiter RD (1981) Somatic expression of herpes thymidine kinase in mice following injection of a fusion gene into eggs. Cell 27:223–231
63. Wagner EF, Stewart TA, Mintz B (1981) The Human β-globin gene and a functional viral thymidine kinase gene in developing mice. Proc Natl Acad Sci 78:5016–5020
64. Mukherjee S (2010) Emperor of all Maladies: a biography of cancer. Scribner, New York
65. Vogelstein B et al (1988) Genetic alterations during colorectal-tumor development. N Engl J Med 319:525–532
66. Hanahan D, Weinberg RA (2000) The hallmarks of cancer. Cell 100:57–70
67. Hanahan D, Weinberg RA (2011) Hallmarks of cancer: the next generation. Cell. 144:646–674
68. Hurley LH (2002) DNA and its associated processes as targets for cancer therapy. Nat Rev Cancer 2:188–200
69. Druker BJ (2002) STI571(GleevecTM) as a paradigm for cancer therapy. Trends Mol Med 8:S14–S18
70. Johnson FM (2005) Dasatinib (BMS-354825) tyrosine kinase inhibitor suppresses invasion and induces cell cycle arrest and apoptosis of head and neck squamous cell carcinoma and non-small cell lung cancer cells. Clin Cancer Res 11:6924–6932
71. Chapman PB et al (2011) Improved survival with vemurafenib in melanoma with BRAF V600E mutation. N Engl J Med 364:2507–2516
72. Lander ES et al (2001) Initial sequencing and analysis of the human genome. Nature 409:860–921
73. Venter JC et al (2001) The sequence of the human genome. Science 291:1304–1351
74. Vogelstein B, Kinzler KW (2004) Cancer genes and the pathways they control. Nat Med 10:789–799
75. Vogelstein B et al (2013) Cancer genome landscapes. Science 339:1546–1558
76. Weis SM, Cheresh DA (2011) Tumor angiogenesis: molecular pathways and therapeutic targets. Nat Med 17:1359–1370
77. Chin L, Andersen JN, Futreal PA (2011) Cancer genomics: from discovery science to personalized medicine. Nat Med 17:297–303

Part II
Cancer Drug Discovery: Types and History

Chapter 3
Chronology of Anticancer Drug Development

3.1 A Historical Background of Cancer Chemotherapy

Cancer was not recognized as a major cause of death in western industrialized countries until the nineteenth century, but the cancer-related mortality increased rapidly after the decrease in lethal infectious diseases, such as tuberculosis and typhoid, following national efforts to improve hygiene and public health. The decrease in these diseases also rapidly increased the average life span, and since the twentieth century, cancer has become one of the leading causes of death, demonstrating that it is highly age-dependent. In the United States, life expectancy increased from 47 to 68 years in the first 50 years of the twentieth century, and cancer had been the second most common cause of death since 1933 [1]. Following this, cancer therapy has emerged as a matter of the national concern, and the F.D. Roosevelt administration enacted the world's first National Cancer Act in 1937, which sought the ways to overcome cancer at a national level by establishing the National Cancer Institute (NCI) that specialized in cancer research [2]. Later, European countries started making efforts to stop the spread of cancer, based on their national research institutions.

Until the 1940s, cancer therapies solely relied on surgical resections and radiotherapy, but treatment outcomes remained dismal. These two treatment modalities focused on the local control of cancer and were not able to remove undetectable micrometastases at distant sites; thus, at the beginning of the 1930s, the eradication of cancer was recognized as difficult using these treatments alone. Different opinions about the need for the development of new therapies were expressed, and one physician, W. Meyer, suggested that it is necessary for biological systemic therapies to be added following the local treatments, such as surgical resection and radiotherapy, in order to achieve better patient survival outcomes [3]. The unmet need for such systemic treatments promoted the full-scale development of cancer chemotherapeutic agents.

K.-W. Kim et al., *Cancer Drug Discovery*, DOI 10.1007/978-94-024-0844-7_3

3.2 Development of the Anticancer Drug Screening Systems

Here, we briefly review the history of the drug screening systems, which made the development of the anticancer drugs possible (Fig. 3.1). The establishment of drug screening system is required for the first-line selection process (preclinical testing) of the most clinically effective drugs, among large numbers of drug candidates. The in vivo tumor transplantation method, the transplantation of the tumor tissue or cancer cells into animals, was mainly used to investigate drug efficacy before the cultured cell-based drug screening system, containing 60 human cancer cell lines, was developed in 1990.

Tumor transplantation research began in the late nineteenth century, as the studies regarding the etiology of cancer began, by retrieving tumor tissues from animals with spontaneously occurring tumors and transplanting them to different organisms of the same species. This led to the development of a transplantable tumor model that can induce cancer at a high rate by the early twentieth century. In 1858, Virchow hypothesized [4] that cancer is a disease that occurs following the chronic stimuli (cell stimulus hypothesis), following which, several different hypotheses on the causes of cancer emerged. In 1876 German microbiologist, R. Koch formulated the pathogen-derived disease hypothesis, after discovering *Bacillus anthracis*, the cause of anthrax [5]. This hypothesis greatly affected cancer research, leading to the studies investigating the possibility that pathogens may cause cancer; hence, experimental biology and the animal experimentation methods, which include the transplantable animal tumor model, developed [6].

3.2.1 Transplantable Tumor Models in Animals

The first tumor transplantation was reported by M.A. Novinsky from St. Petersburg College, Russia, in 1877 [7]. In order to study the pathogen-derived disease hypothesis, Novinsky transplanted naturally occurring canine nasal tumor and venereal

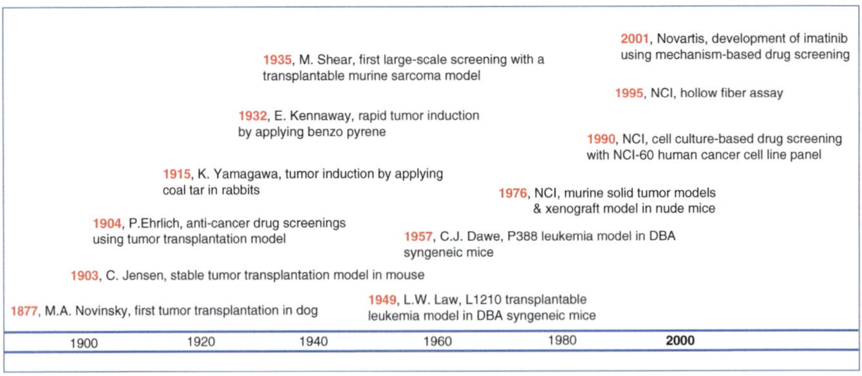

Fig. 3.1 Key advances in tumor models and anticancer drug screening systems

sarcoma into the skin of a puppy and succeeded in maintaining them at over two consecutive generations. Subsequently, several other laboratories in Europe succeeded in transplanting tumors in other animals, such as mice, rabbits, and rats. In 1903, C. Jensen at the Copenhagen Institute of Agricultural and Aquatic Medicine, Denmark, was the first to establish a stable tumor-transplantation mouse model over multiple generations [8]. Following this, P. Ehrlich in Germany improved Jensen's tumor transplantation model, increasing the cancer incidence rate, from 1904 to 1908, and utilized this model for anticancer drug screenings [9]. He examined anticancer efficacy of various compounds, including dyes and arsenic compounds. Despite these efforts, Ehrlich was not successful in discovering an active anticancer compound, but he did establish the theoretical background and systematic methodology for anticancer drug screenings, and provided an insight about the need for developing anticancer drugs, which would have low toxicity toward normal cells while having highly selective toxicity toward continuously proliferating cancer cells.

In the USA, H.R. Gaylord and G. Clowes at the Roswell Park Memorial Institute, New York, established a tumor transplantation model in 1910, using C. Jensen's model, and founded the basis for the full-scale anticancer drug development [10].

3.2.2 *Chemical Tumor Induction and Anticancer Drug Screening Using Inbred Mice*

In 1910, P. Rous at Rockefeller University, USA, discovered the Rous sarcoma virus, which causes chicken sarcoma [11], but this discovery did not receive a lot of attention at that time, because scientists considered this virus non-oncogenic. Later, in 1915, K. Yamagawa, Virchow's disciple, at Tokyo University, Japan, succeeded in causing squamous cell carcinoma for the first time using chemical methods, based on the cell stimulation theory, by applying coal tar to the ears of a rabbit [12]. Owing to the development of this cancer induction system, it became possible to overcome the inaccuracy of evaluation of anticancer drugs caused by the rejection of transplanted tumors when using spontaneous tumor models.

Transplantable tumor models were established in several laboratories, but because between the 1910s and the early 1930s separation and purification techniques of natural substances and synthesis techniques of organic chemicals were still at early stages of development, there were limited numbers of compounds available for these studies. Anticancer effects of only a small number of compounds, such as natural dyes or cellular respiratory toxins like ferricyanide, were investigated.

Full-scale anticancer drug screening was initiated by M. Shear at the Cancer Research Institute, the United States Public Health Service affiliate, which was the origin of the NCI [13]. The anticancer effects of a wide variety of bacterial polysaccharides were tested after the establishment of a large-scale screening system using a transplantable murine sarcoma model in 1935, and afterward, by 1953, more than 3,000 kinds of plant extracts and synthetic compounds were examined for anticancer effects. These studies failed to lead to the development of any clinically approved drugs.

However, it was determined that N-mustard (by L.S. Goodman and A. Gilman in 1946), aminopterin (by S. Farber in 1948), and 6-mercaptopurine (by G. Elion in 1951) have anticancer activities. This led to an active promotion of chemotherapeutic cancer treatment studies, and a large-scale national program for the development of anticancer drugs was conducted by the US National Cancer Chemotherapy Service Center (NCCSC) in 1955. During the following 10 years (1955–1964), hundreds of thousands of synthetic chemical species, fermentation products, plant extracts, and their derivatives have been tested as potential candidates. This program was led by M. Shear at the NCI, and it was conducted in collaboration with the Memorial Sloan Kettering Cancer Center in New York, Southern Research Institute in Alabama, Dana-Farber Cancer Institute in Boston, and Chester Beatty Research Institute in London.

The rejection of tissue transplants frequently occurred, because transplanted tumors used in the initial drug screenings were often not derived from inbred mice, and various authors argued that precise drug tests were not possible using this model. This led to studies aiming to establish an inbred mouse transplantation model, in order to prevent tissue rejection. In the early twentieth century, several inbred mouse strains, such as DBA, BALB/c, and C57BL, were established. In 1932, J.W. Cook and E. Kennaway discovered that carcinogenic benzopyrene from coal tar components can cause cancer in mice in less time compared with the coal tar [14]. Using these inbred mice and polycyclic aromatic cancer inducers, the transplantable leukemia models, L1210 and P388, were established by L.W. Law at NCI in 1949 [15] and C.J. Dawe and M. Potter in 1957 [16] from the DBA inbred mice, respectively. This made screening of cytotoxic anticancer agents quick and reproducible, and these animal models have been actively used in NCCSC program between the 1950s and 1960s.

3.2.3 Solid Tumor Animal Models and Xenograft Screening Methods

By using L1210 and P388 leukemia models, various types of anticancer agents, such as busulfan and cyclophosphamide, have been developed during the 1950s and 1960s. It was shown that these anticancer agents were effective in clinical treatments of leukemia and lymphoma, but not in solid cancer treatments, which have a much higher incidence, and there was a growing need for the development of solid tumor animal model system. In 1976, the NCI adopted solid cancer mouse transplant models, such as B16 (melanoma), C38 (colon cancer), Lewis (lung carcinoma), and three types of new human solid cancer xenograft screening systems, LX-1 for human lung cancer, CX-1 for human colon cancer, and MX-1 for human breast cancer [17]. Xenograft studies began in 1966 by establishing immunodeficient nude mice with T-cell deficiency caused by thymic hypoplasia, by S.P. Flanagan at the Animal Genetics Institute, UK [18]. In 1969, J. Rygaard and C.O. Povlsen, at the Institute of Pathological Anatomy, Denmark, established the first xenograft model by succeeding in harvesting colon-cancer patient tissues and transplanting them to nude mice [19]. Solid tumor screening systems allowed the identification of the drugs that were missed in previous leukemia model screenings, such as paclitaxel. About 30 % of substances previously eliminated in the inbred mice transplanting system studies have been reported to have activity in a xenograft model upon retesting [20].

3.2.4 Anticancer Drug Screening Methods Based on Human Cancer Cell Lines

In 1983, several researchers, including M.J. Staquet, reported that solid tumor models were still not highly relevant for the clinical efficacy of the investigated anticancer agents [21]. Although solid tumor animal models reflected well clinical efficacy of the cytotoxic compounds, they did not present the appropriate screening models for new drug classes, such as cytostatic agents or angiogenesis inhibitors. Additionally, these models required a great amount of time and resources, in order to screen large numbers of different synthetic drugs, and the influence of social movements from animal advocates gradually restricted the use of large numbers of animals for drug screening. Therefore, in 1989, NCI developed NCI-60, a panel of 60 diverse human cancer cell lines mainly composed of solid tumor cell lines [22], and established a high-speed, large-scale, and tumor type-oriented drug development system, which has been used as a main drug screening system since 1990.

Additionally, in 1995, the hollow fiber assay, which complements the weaknesses of drug efficacy tests in the cell culture system, was adopted by various researchers, including M.G. Hollingshead at the NCI [23]. In this method, hollow fiber filled with human cancer cells are transplanted into nude mice, and recovered several days following the treatment with the investigated compound. The drug efficacy is assessed by cell number analysis. This method has the advantage of the rapid assessment of the drug efficacy in vivo, so that lower numbers of the nude mice are sacrificed, and therefore, it is more cost-effective and does not violate animal ethical standards.

3.2.5 Mechanism-Based Anticancer Agent Screening Method

Since the 1980s, the studies of cancer pathogenesis at the gene level began to accumulate rapidly, which led to the development of targeted anticancer agents that specifically inhibit oncogenic protein activities. Targeted anticancer agent discovery depended on the mechanism-based screening methods, established at private research institutions, such as pharmaceutical companies and universities. Imatinib appeared in 2001: it was discovered through a screening method developed by Novartis [24]. Mechanism-based screening method is a technology for identifying candidate compounds by examining the compound efficacy against the target protein at the cellular level. This is generally achieved through the chemical design of a compound via structural protein analyses, and using high-throughput screening techniques. When a candidate drug is discovered by these methods, preclinical drug candidates are further evaluated in order to examine in vivo anticancer effects by using xenograft models or more advanced animal models, such as the orthotopic transplantation model, which involves transplantation of human cancer cells from human organs to the same organ of nude mice [25], or genetically engineered cancer mouse model [26].

3.3 Chronology of the Anticancer Drug Development

An overview of the history of anticancer drugs developed by the end of 2013, based on the described screening systems, is shown in Fig. 3.2. The emergence of chemotherapy began in 1946 from nitrogen mustard, an alkylating agent, and it was accelerated when aminopterin, a folic acid antagonist, was introduced for the treatment of pediatric leukemia patients in 1948, by S. Farber. Anticancer agents that were later developed can be divided into six categories, depending on their activities against cancer cells, as follows: (1) alkylating agents, (2) antimetabolites, (3) plant alkaloids and natural compounds that contain antibiotics, (4) immunotherapeutic anticancer agents and other anticancer agents, (5) hormonal anticancer agents, and (6) molecular targeted anticancer agents. Anticancer agents that belong to each of these groups exhibit a distinct development pattern, as shown in Fig. 3.2.

Alkylating agents cause DNA damage and suppress continuous cell proliferation, which is a typical hallmark of cancer, and they had been intensively developed from the 1940s until the early 1970s. Antimetabolites were being developed from the late 1940s until recently. These drugs, due to the similarity in structure to precursors required for DNA synthesis, inhibit cell growth, by acting as bait molecules for several enzymes, and preventing DNA replication.

The development of plant alkaloids, starting with vincristine and anticancer antibiotics such as dactinomycin, had begun in the 1960s, because of large-scale anticancer drug screening conducted by the NCCSC in 1954, and the trend has continued into the 1990s. Synthetic derivatives of these natural compounds were being investigated at the same time, and a variety of synthetic anticancer drugs was developed from the mid-1960s through the mid-2000s. Most of these anticancer agents were focused on DNA synthesis and replication, which are essential for cell proliferation, and substances that inhibit DNA precursor synthesis, and stimulate the inhibition of DNA damage repair process, were called conventional chemotherapeutic agents (Fig. 3.3). However, these anticancer agents were developed without the understanding of basic cancer biology, such as the molecular etiology, complexity, and

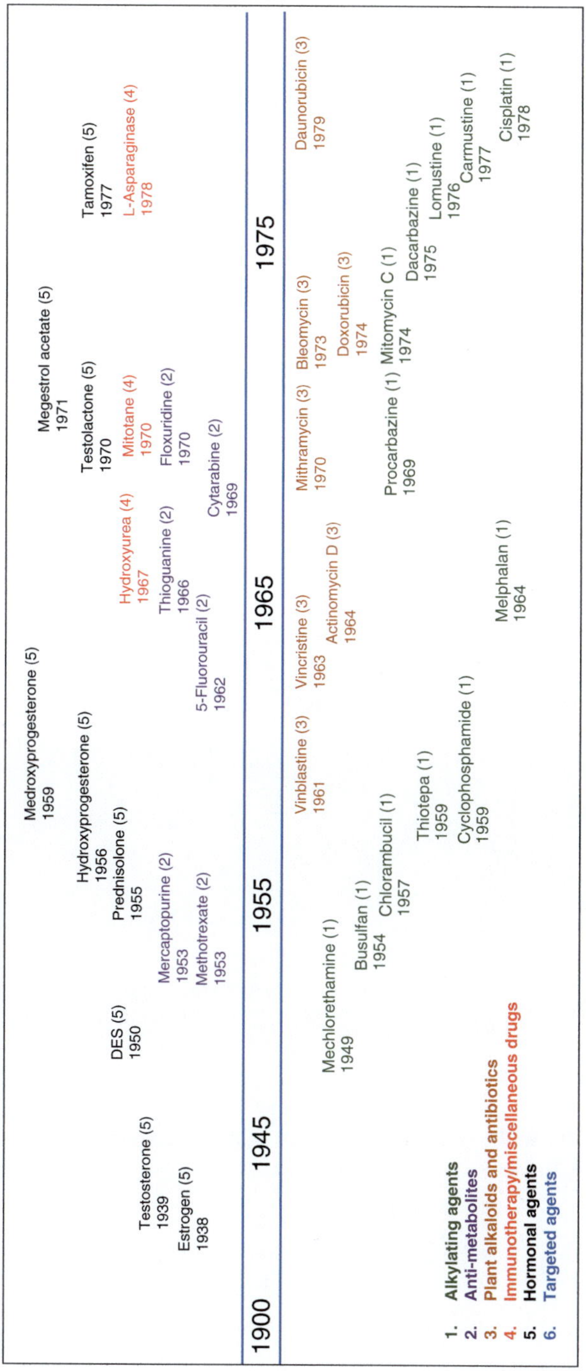

Fig. 3.2 Types of anticancer drugs and a timeline of their development

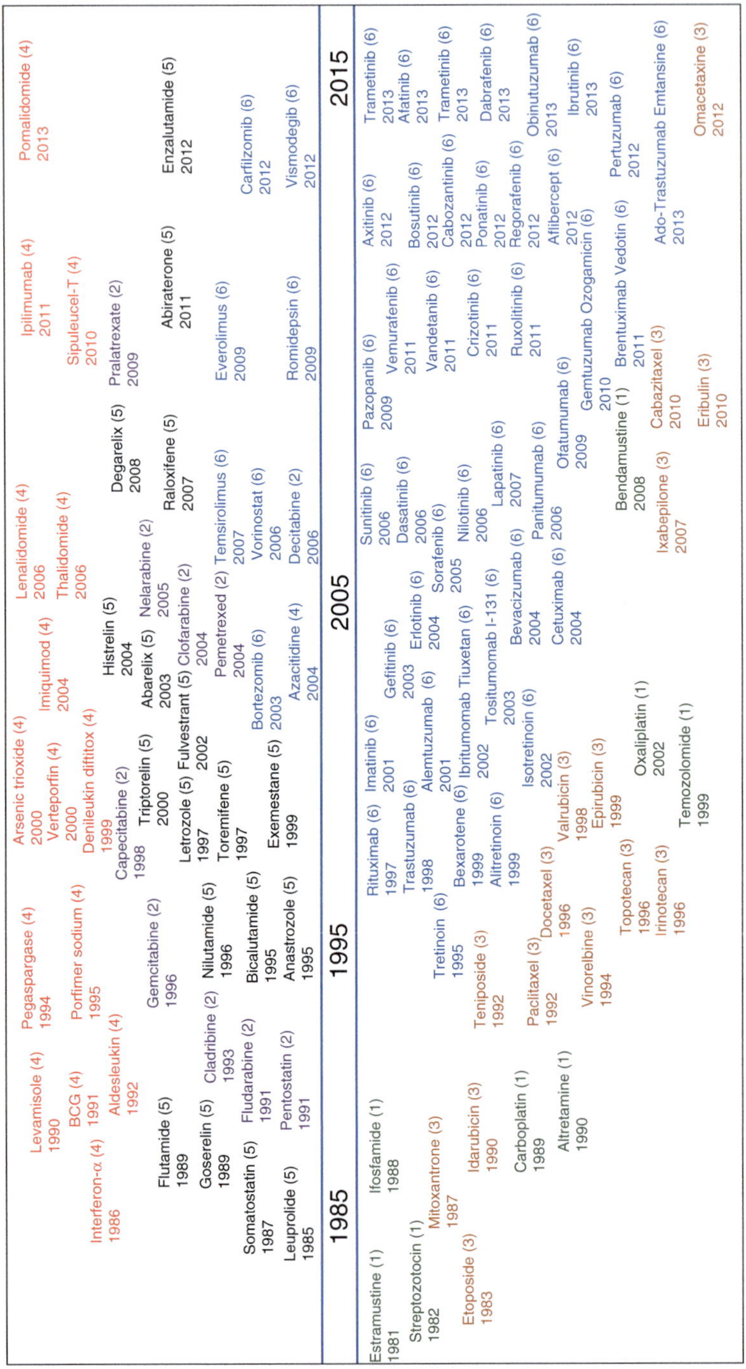

Fig. 3.2 Continued

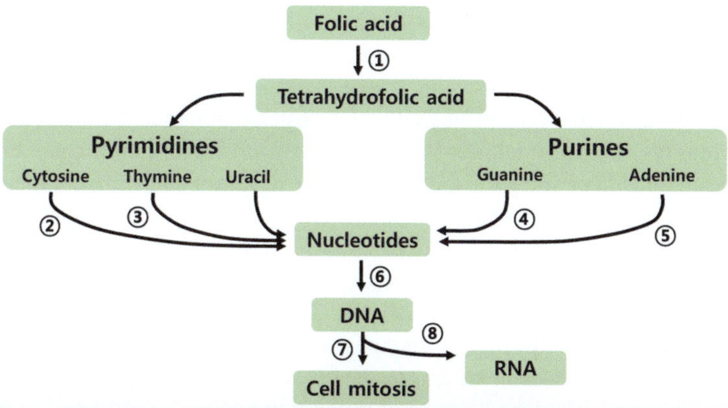

Site of drug action	Anticancer drug
①	Methotrexate
②	Hydroxyurea
③	5-fluorouracil
④	Thioguanine
⑤	Mercaptopurine
⑥	Hydroxyurea, Alkylating agents
⑦	Mitotic disrupters
⑧	Antibiotics

Fig. 3.3 Target sites of conventional chemotherapeutic agents

diversity of cancer, which resulted in less than expected treatment efficacy and serious side effects for normal cells in the treatment of large number of cancers, with the exception of certain types of chemosensitive cancers such as leukemia and lymphoma.

The fourth anticancer agent category covers immunotherapeutic and miscellaneous anticancer drugs. Immunotherapeutic anticancer drugs have been steadily developed through the 1980s and 1990s up to the present, with aim of eliminating cancer cells by stimulating immune system components including cytokines such as interferon-α, humanized antibody therapeutics, and dendritic cells. Miscellaneous anticancer drugs such as asparaginases had been developed since the mid-1960s up to the 2000s.

Before the emergence of molecular targeted anticancer agents, which have been developed based on the biological understanding of normal and cancer cells, hormonal anticancer agents have been developed based on the knowledge about the cancer biology, for the treatment of particular types of cancer. Testosterone and estrogen were found to be frequently involved in the development of prostate and breast cancer, respectively, and this led to the development of hormonal anticancer drugs, such as diethylstilbestrol (DES) or tamoxifen. The development of these drugs began in the 1940s, and they are still regularly used in clinical practice.

Since the 1990s, a new concept of molecular targeted anticancer drugs began to develop rapidly. The accumulation of the results from the in-depth basic biological research on cancer since the 1980s made the development of this anticancer drug category possible. As the details of molecular mechanisms of tumorigenesis became elucidated, because of studies that used molecular biology tools, and as many factors that play important roles in various cancer types have been discovered, targeted drug development had accelerated. These anticancer drugs have constituted an important drug category since the twenty-first century. Characteristics of these six drug categories, including the development process and structure, pharmacological actions, and toxicity are described in detail in the following chapter.

3.4 Clinical Application of Anticancer Drugs

The anticancer agents are applied in three major ways during the cancer treatment. Palliative chemotherapy is applied for the treatment of the advanced cancer cases, where it is impossible to apply only local treatment, such as surgery, due to the cancer metastases, and this chemotherapy is used to delay the progression of cancer, prolonging survival and alleviating cancer-related symptoms [27]. However, in some cases of the certain types of solid tumors, full recovery is possible even in the advanced cancer stages, such as in adult Hodgkin's lymphoma, acute myeloid leukemia, reproductive system cancers, chorionic cancer, acute infant lymphoma, Burkitt's lymphoma, and Wilm's tumor.

Neoadjuvant chemotherapy is used for maximizing the therapeutic efficacy of surgery, reducing tumor size, and eliminating micrometastases by preoperative chemotherapy in locally advanced cancers, which are not amenable to complete surgical resection [28].

Adjuvant chemotherapy is used after the surgical removal of the local cancer. Performing postoperative chemotherapy on patients with no visible lesions, in order to remove undetectable micrometastases, leads to the decrease in tumor recurrence and ultimately improves disease-free survival. After the first successful postoperative application of CMF therapy, which consists of cyclophosphamide, methotrexate (MTX), and 5-fluorouracil (5-FU) for breast cancer treatment, in 1975 [29], the role of adjuvant chemotherapy in improving the overall survival in colon, stomach, non-small cell lung cancer, and osteosarcoma has been established. The cure rate using various antitumor agents is shown in Table 3.1.

Table 3.1 The curability of cancers with chemotherapy

Curable with conventional chemotherapy
1. Acute lymphocytic leukemia, 2. Hodgkin lymphoma 3. Germ cell tumor: embryonal carcinoma, teratoma, seminoma or dysgerminoma, choriocarcinoma 4. Gestational Trophoblastic neoplasia 5. Pediatric cancer: Wilm's tumor, Ewing sarcoma, neuroblastoma, embryonal rhabdomyosarcoma 6. Small cell lung cancer 7. Ovarian carcinoma
Curable with concurrent chemoradiotherapy
1. Head and neck squamous cell carcinoma 2. Anal squamouse cell carcinoma 3. Esophageal squamous cell carcinoma 4. Uterine cervix cancer 5. Non-small cell lung cancer (stage III) 6. Small cell lung cancer
Curable with surgical resection and adjuvant chemotherapy
1. Breast cancer 2. Colorectal cancer 3. Osteosarcoma 4. Soft tissue sarcoma
Curable with high dose chemotherapy and hematopoietic stem cell transplantation
1. Relapsed leukemia and lymphoma 2. Chronic myelogenous leukemia 3. Multiple myeloma

References

1. National Center for Health Statistics. Leading causes of death, 1900–1998. http://www.cdc.gov/nchs/data/dvs/lead1900_98.pdf
2. Shimkin MB (1977) As memory serves – an Informal History of the National Cancer Institute, 1937–57. J Natl Cancer Inst 59(Suppl 2):559–600
3. Meyer W (1932) Inoperable and malignant tumors. Ann Surg 96:891–892
4. Virchow R (1858) Reizung und Reizbarkeit. Arch Pathol Anat Physiol Klin Med 14:1–63
5. Koch R (1876) Die Ätiologie der Milzbrandkrankheit, begründet auf die Entwicklungsgeschichte des Bacillus Anthracis. Beiträge zur Biologie der Pflanzen 2:277–310
6. Triolo VA (1964) Nineteenth century foundations of cancer research origins of experimental research. Cancer Res 24:4–27
7. Novinsky M (1877) On the question of the inoculation of malignant neoplasms (experimental investigations). Thesis, St. Petersburg
8. Jensen CO (1903) Experimental researches on cancer in the mouse. Hospitalstidende 11:549
9. Ehrlich P (1906) Über ein transplantables Chondrom der Mause. Arb Kgl Inst Exp Ther 1:63

10. Triolo VA, Riegel IL (1961) The American Association for Cancer Research, 1907–1940 – historical review. Cancer Res 21:137–167
11. Rous P (1911) A Sarcoma of the fowl transmissible by an agent separable from the tumor cells. J Exp Med 13:397–411
12. Yamagawa K, Ichikawa K (1915) Über die kunstliche Erzeugung von Papillom. Verh Jap Path Ges 5:142–148
13. Shear MJ, Hartwell JL, Peters VB et al (1947) Some aspects of a joint institutional research program on chemotherapy of cancer: current laboratory and clinical experiments with bacterial polysaccharide and with synthetic organic compounds. In: Moulton FR (ed) Approaches to tumor chemotherapy. American Association for the Advancement Science, Washington, DC, pp 236–284
14. Cook JW, Hieger I, Kennaway EL, Mayneord WV (1932) The production of cancer by pure hydrocarbons – Part I. Proc Royal Soc Lond B Biol Sci 111:455–484
15. Law LW, Dunn DB, Boyle PJ, Miller JH (1949) Observations on the effect of a folic-acid antagonist on transplantable lymphoid leukemias in mice. J Natl Cancer Inst 10:179–192
16. Dawe CJ, Potter M (1957) Morphologic and biologic progression of a lymphoid neoplasm of the mouse *in vivo* and *in vitro*. Am J Pathol 33:603
17. Venditti JM, Wesley RA, Plowman J (1984) Current NCI preclinical antitumor screening *in vivo*: results of tumor panel screening, 1976–1982, and future directions. In: Garrattini S, Goldin A, Hawking F (eds) Advances in pharmacology and chemotherapy, vol 20. Academic, Orlando, p 20
18. Flanagan SP (1966) "Nude", a new hairless gene with pleiotropic effects in the mouse. Genet Res Camb 8:295–309
19. Rygaard J, Povlsen CO (1969) Heterotransplantation of a human malignant tumor to "nude" mice. Acta Pathol Microbiol Scand 77:758–760
20. Suggitt M, Bibby MC (2005) 50 years of preclinical anticancer drug screening: empirical to target-driven approaches. Clin Cancer Res 11:971–981
21. Staquet MJ, Byar DP, Green SB, Rozencweig M (1983) Clinical predictivity of transplantable tumor systems in the selection of new drugs for solid tumors: rationale for a three-stage strategy. Cancer Treat Rep 67:753–765
22. Double JA, Bibby MC (1989) Therapeutic index: a vital component in selection of anticancer agents for clinical trial. J Natl Cancer Inst 81:988–994
23. Hollingshead MG, Alley MC, Camalier RF, Abbott BJ, Mayo JG, Malspeis L, Grever MR (1995) *In vivo* cultivation of tumor cells in hollow fibers. Life Sci 57:131–141
24. Druker BJ, Tamura S, Buchdunger E, Ohno S, Segal GM, Fanning S et al (1996) Effects of a selective inhibitor of the Abl tyrosine kinase on the growth of Bcr-Abl positive cells. Nat Med 2:561–566
25. Naito S, Von Eschenbach AC, Giavazzi R, Fidler IJ (1986) Growth and metastasis of tumor cells isolated from a surgical specimen of a human renal cell carcinoma subsequent to implantation into different organs of nude mice. Cancer Res 46:4109–4115
26. Stewart TA, Pattengale PK, Leder P (1984) Spontaneous mammary adenocarcinomas in transgenic mice that carry and express MTV/myc fusion genes. Cell 38:627–637
27. Karnofsky DA, Abelson WH, Craver LF, Burchenal JH (1948) The use of nitrogen mustards in the palliative treatment of carcinoma. Cancer 1:634–656
28. Goldie JH (1987) Scientific basis for adjuvant and primary (neoadjuvant) chemotherapy. Semin Oncol 14:1–7
29. Bonadonna G, Brusamolino E, Valagussa P, Rossi A, Brugnatelli L, Brambilla C et al (1976) Combination chemotherapy as an adjuvant treatment in operable breast cancer. N Engl J Med 294:405–410

Chapter 4
Alkylating Anticancer Drugs

Alkylating agents are the first chemotherapeutic anticancer agents developed, and account for the largest drug group among conventional cytotoxic chemotherapeutics. This class is largely divided into three subgroups: classical alkylating agents, nonclassical alkylating agents, and alkylating-like agents. Classical alkylating agents include nitrogen mustards, nitroso ureas, aziridines, and alkyl sulfonates. Nonclassical alkylating agents include hydrazine, triazene, and altretamines. In addition, the alkylating-like agent group, which functions by crosslinking with DNA similarly to alkylating agents, includes platinum compounds (Fig. 4.1).

Alkylating anticancr agents form electrophilic substances when dissolved in aqueous solution and trigger alkylation of nucleophilic functional groups on macromolecules such as sulfhydryl groups, amino groups, hydroxyl groups, carboxyl groups, and phosphate groups, thereby transforming biomacromolecules. Cytotoxicity of this class occurs mainly by alkylation reaction with DNA molecule more than the various other biomacromolecules. Alkylation of DNA impairs its function as a template and blocks replication of new DNA or inhibits transcription to mRNA for protein synthesis, which are essential for cell survival and function. This alkylation of DNA occurs mostly on N^7 and weakly on O^6 of the guanine base. Depending on the drug, such alkylation can occur only on one base, or on two bases within the same strand inducing crosslinking, or can occur on two bases from the complementary strands inducing interstrand crosslink (Fig. 4.2). Crosslinking between complementary strands prevents the separation of two DNA strands during replication and thereby halts cell division. Most classical alkylating agents and platinum compounds display cytotoxicity by inducing DNA crosslinking. In comparison, streptozotocin and nonclassical alkylating agents such as dacarbazine, procarbazine, and temozolomide induce methylation of O^6 or N^7 on the guanine base and do not trigger DNA crosslinking. Hence, methylation occurring on a single strand leads to mismatched base pairing of the transformed guanine with thymine instead of

K.-W. Kim et al., *Cancer Drug Discovery*, DOI 10.1007/978-94-024-0844-7_4

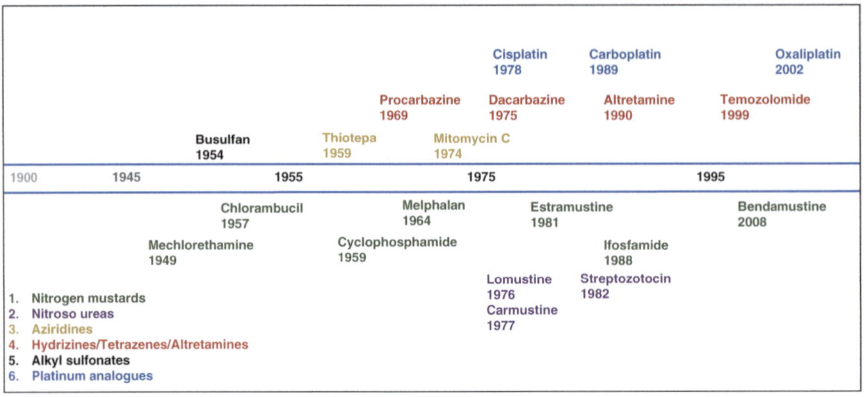

Fig. 4.1 Types of alkylating drugs and a chronology of their development

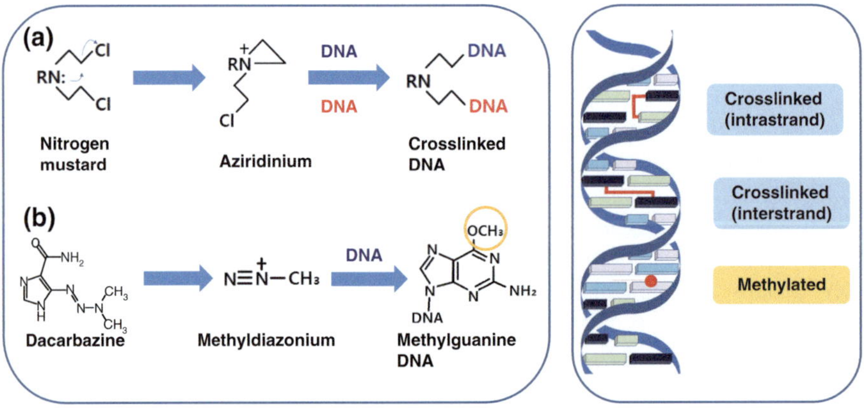

Fig. 4.2 General mechanisms of action for alkylating anticancer agents. (**a**) Conventional nitrogen mustard alkylating anticancer agents undergo an intramolecular cyclization reaction to form the electrophilic substance aziridinium, before causing an alkylating reaction at the nucleophilic N^7 of guanine. This reaction can induce cross-linking when it occurs at two bases on complementary or identical strands. (**b**) The unconventional alkylating anticancer agent dacarbazine forms a methyldiazonium ion that induces methylation by reacting with O^6 in guanine. This reaction causes errors during base pairing in the course of DNA replication

cytosine during replication. This results in DNA truncation by DNA repair enzymes, leading to suppression of cell cyle progression or induction of apoptosis.

Although reactions of such alkylating agents are not specific to one phase of the cell cycle, their toxicity is particularly strong in late G1 phase and S phase when DNA replication occurs. It is also known that alkylating agents function as carcinogens, and can cause secondary hematologic malignancies.

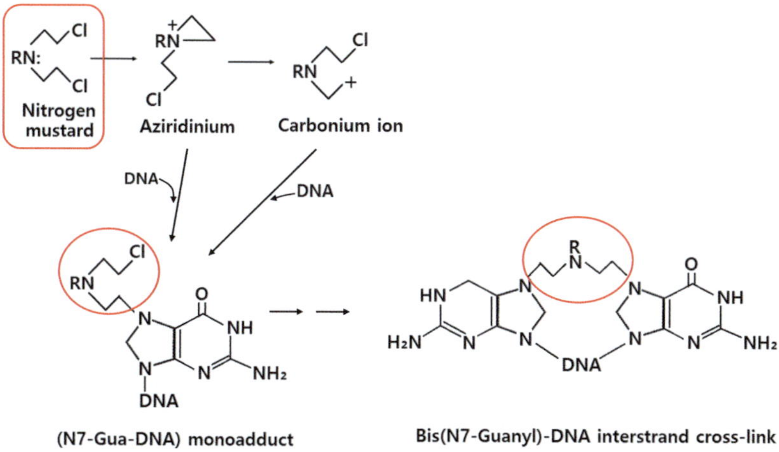

Fig. 4.3 Nitrogen mustard mechanism of action. Once nitrogen mustards are absorbed into the body and hydrated, they form an aziridinium ion through an intramolecular cyclization reaction before causing an alkylating reaction at guanine's nucleophilic N, either directly or after conversion to a carbonium ion. This reaction can induce cross-linking when it occurs at two bases on complementary or identical strands

4.1 Classical Alkylating Drugs

When classical alkylating drugs are absorbed into the body and hydrated, it forms an aziridinium ion, which is an electrophilic cyclic ion that induces DNA alkylation either directly or through conversion to a carbonium ion. DNA structural change caused by alkylation is recognized as an abnormal signal by the DNA repair system, which halts cell growth, depending on the type and degree of the structural change, and either repairs the abnormal region or induces apoptosis. DNA change caused by classical alkylating agents involves the formation of widespread interstrand cross-links, and they therefore exert their anticancer effect through apoptosis rather than DNA repair (Fig. 4.3).

4.1.1 Bis Amine/Nitrogen Mustards

Nitrogen mustard was the first agent clinically approved. Representative drugs of this kind include mechlorethamine, cyclophosphamide, ifosfamide, melphalan, and chlorambucil, which are still clinically used (Fig. 4.4). They all have a bischloroethyl group, which induces alkylation by attacking the highly nucleophilic N^7 in the guanine base and the remaining chlorine triggers secondary alkylation, generating interstrand cross-links (ICLs). DNA regions with interstrand crosslink formation disrupt DNA separation during DNA replication, thereby inhibiting mitosis and causing cytotoxcitiy (Fig. 4.3).

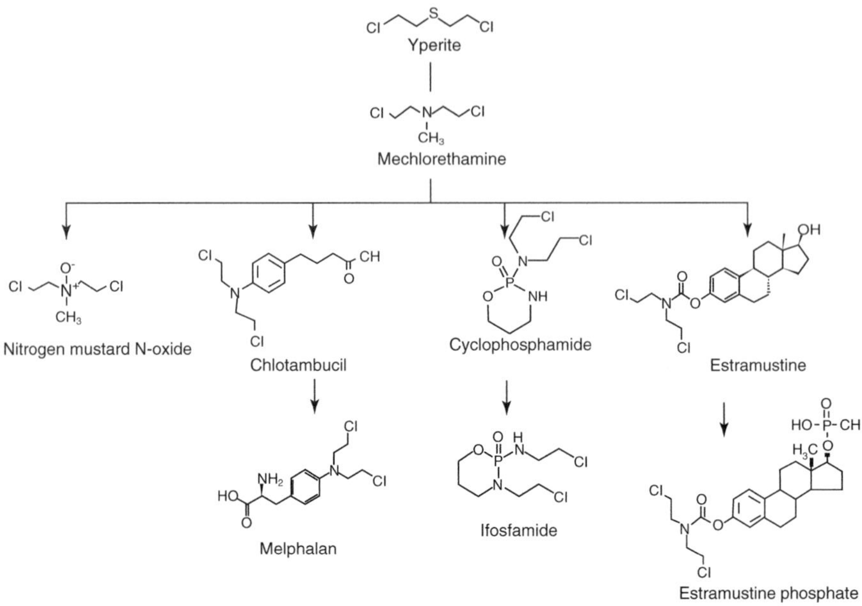

Fig. 4.4 The structure of bis amine/nitrogen mustard drugs and the process of their development

4.1.1.1 Mechlorethamine (Mustine)

Development of nitrogen mustard began from the influence of World War I, which is one of the wars with the most victims in human history. Yperite (sulfur mustard gas), a toxic gas, was first introduced by the Germans in the form of bombs dropped on the camps of the Allied Forces in the Ypres front line in Belgium from July 1917, which caused large numbers of casualties. In 1919 when World War I was over, the husband and wife team of E.B. Krumbhaar and H.D. Krumbhaar, who were pathologists in the U.S., investigated the long-term effect of this toxic gas on survivors who had been exposed to yperite used by the Germans, and discovered severe suppression of bone marrow and lymphoid organs as well as a markedly reduced number of blood cells [1]. Later, in 1929, I. Berenblum at the University of Leeds in England, who was studying mechanisms of carcinogenesis, predicted that because sulfur mustard gas has a blood congestion effect by intensely stimulating the skin like tar, it would have a boosting effect on skin cancer caused by tar. He applied sulfur mustard gas to mouse ears along with tar and analyzed the effect, which led him to discover that sulfur mustard inhibited the development of skin cancer, unlike his prediction that it would accelerate cancer growth [2]. This was the first report of the anticancer effect exerted by mustard gas experimently. Later, Berenblum observed that it also inhibits carcinogenesis by another carcinogen, dibenzanthracene. Based on these results, F.E. Adair and H.J. Bagg at the Memorial Hospital in New York confirmed the anticancer effect of sulfur mustard gas in animals with chemically induced cancer and conducted clinical tests of applying sulfur mustard gas on the affected skin of cancer patients with melanoma and squamous cell carcinoma, reporting a therapeutic effect in 1931 [3].

It was L. Goodmman and A. Gilman at Yale University who developed this mustard gas from its proposed potential as an anticancer agent into the actual anticancer drug. Between World War I and World War II, Germany developed nitrogen mustrand gas in addition to sulfur mustard gas. In order to reduce the damage caused by these chemical weapons, the Allied Forces decided to investigate the mechanism and detoxification of these chemicals. Goodman and Gilman participated in this study in 1942. They studied the toxic effect of nitrogen mustard in animals and became interested in its selective cytotoxicity against hematopoietic cells. Gilman predicted that sulfur mustard gas would be hard to be developed as a systemic therapeutic agent as it displays strong toxicity in the gastrointestinal tract, kidney, and bone marrow, but it would be feasible to develop nitrogen mustard as a drug since its toxicities were more tolerable. This difference in toxicity between these two compounds was speculated to be due to the higher electrophilicity of the sulfur atom in sulfur mustard gas compard to the nitrogen atom in nitrogen mustard, which increases the reactivity. Moreover, nitrogen mustard forms crystals as a hydrochloride, and dissolving it in aqueous solution enables whole body treatment through injection.

Thus, along with their university collegue T. Dougherty, they studied the therapeutic effect of nitrogen mustard in a mouse leukemia model using intravenous injection. They found that the tumor regressed in the first mouse injected with the drug just after two treatments, and that the median survival duration after cancer transplantation was prolonged from 3 weeks to 12 weeks, an increase of 9 weeks. However, additional experiment showed that this anti-cancer effect was transient and the recurrence was observed in all the mice injected with nitrogen mustard [4]. Nevertheless, even this degree of therapeutic efficacy was an extremely dramatic result at the time, and therefore a clinical study on the anticancer effects of nitrogen mustard in humans was led by G. Lindskog, a thyroid surgeon at New Haven Hospital, on patients with various late stage hematologic malignancies, including Hodgkin's lymphoma, starting in late 1942. The first patient had late stage lymphosarcoma, and his neck mass almost completely disappeared 10 days after the treatment. However, similarly to mice, the tumor relapsed and the patient died after the third cycle treatment. An early therapeutic response was observed in other patients, but the effect was also transient.

The nitrogen mustard used in the early stage of drug development was tris (β-chloroethyl)-amine, but mechlorethamine [methyl-bis (β-chloroethyl)-amine] began to be used as a investigational drug from 1943 when the clinical trials were further expanded. Clinical trials proceeded with collaboration of researchers from various hospitals, including M. M. Wintrobe from the Salt Lake County General Hospital. They observed that, among numerous cancer patients treated with mechlorethamine, the anticancer effect was maintained for at least several weeks in a patient with Hodgkin's lymphoma, although it was not a complete remission [5]. This study on the anticancer effect of nitrogen mustard was the first demonstration of the therapeutic potential of chemotherapy, showing that cancer could be potentially treated with drugs. Later, further clinical studies observed similar therapeutic effects, and mechlorethamine was approved by the FDA as the first chemotherapeutic anticancer durg in 1949. Although it is rarely used today, due to the continuous development of other anticancer agents, it still holds significance as the very first chemotherapeutic anticancer agent.

The mechanisms of mechlorethamine action were studied later, and in 1946, C. Golumbic et al. at Oxford Univeristy discovered that the chloroethyl group becomes cyclized and forms an aziridinium ion with high reactivity, triggering chemical reactions with intracellular components [6]. In addition, W.C.J. Ross's group at the Chester Beatty Research Institute (the former incarnation of the Institute of Cancer Research (ICR), London, England, observed that alkylating drugs induced chromosomal abnormalities and proposed crosslinking of chromatin threads as a cytotoxic mechanism of alkylating drugs [7].

The therapuetic effect of mechlorethamine spurred studies of new anticancer agents in various laboratories worldwide. In 1951, J.H. Burchenal et al. at the Memorial Center for Cancer and Allied Diseases in New York synthesized approximately 30 new kinds of nitrogen mustard derivatives and investigated their anticancer effects. They discovered 1,4-Bis (2-chloroethyl)-1,4-piperazine and N,N′-Bis (2-chloroethyl)-N,N′-diethylethylenediamine exerting effects comparable to mechlorethamine [8].

4.1.1.2 Chlorambucil

The development of alkylating drugs with more selective cytotoxicity against cancer cells and lower toxicities on normal tissues was intensively undertaken by A. Haddow, a director of the Chester Beatty Research Institute [former Institute of Cancer Research (ICR)], and his researcher W.C.J. Ross. They first replaced the methyl group of mechlorethamine with various aromatic compounds and synthesized bromoethyl aryl amine derivatives whose chlorine group was substituted with bromine group, and β-chloroalkyl aryl amine derivatives whose ethyl group was substituted with other alkyl groups, and analyzed the therapeutic effects of these compounds using Walker carcinosarcoma 256 animal cancer models in 1948 [9]. They observed from this study that aromatic nitrogen mustard, which generates a carbonium ion but not an aziridinium ion, displayed effective anticancer effects.

Later, W.C.J. Ross et al. continued with this study and developed chlorambucil in 1953 [10], which had milder toxicities and was approved by the FDA as the first aromatic nitrogen mustard drug in 1957. Because of the reduced electrophilicity of the nitrogen, the aromatic ring in chlorambucil does not form a cyclic aziridinium ion, which is generated as an intermediate in aliphatic nitrogen mustards, and therefore the drug exhibits lower toxicity than aliphatic nitrogen mustards. This low reactivity increased the chemical stability of chlorambucil and allowed it to function for a long time after the drug administration, which increased its potential to reach the DNA of the target cancer cells, and enabled oral administration of the drug.

The efficacy of chlorambucil has been examined in various cancers and therapeutic effects have been observed in Hodgkin's lymphoma and ovarian sarcoma, which led to its approval as an anticancer agent. Although therapeutic effects have additionally been reported in chronic myeloid leukemia, Polycythemia Vera (PV), trophoblastic neoplasms, and ovarian sarcoma, it is currently rarely used.

4.1.1.3 Melphalan

In 1954, F. Bergel and J.A. Stock at the ICR developed melphalan, which is another aromatic nitrogen mustard, in addition to chlorambucil [11]. Melphalan was synthesized using a chemical design in order to develop a drug with reduced bone marrow toxicity and higher cancer cell specificity. Under the assumption that cancer cells would have high demands for amino acids due to active proliferation, melphalan was developed by conjugating phenylalanine in place of the methyl group in mechlorethamine so that the drug could be delivered specifically to cancer cells through the L-phenylalanine active transport system. Melphalan's therapeutic effect through oral administration was observed in multiple myeloma (MM) and ovarian cancer, and the drug was approved by the U.S. FDA as the second aromatic nitrogen mustard in 1964. It is currently widely used for the treatment of multiple myeloma.

4.1.1.4 Cyclophosphamide

An alkylating anticancer agent with another strategy to lower the toxicities on normal cells and increase the specificity for cancer cells was attempted by O.M. Friedman and A.M. Seligman at Harvard University in 1949. Based on the previous finding that cancer cells have higher phosphamidase activity, they predicted that if the activity of this enzyme were used to develop a drug that existed as an innocuous prodrug that becomes activated by phosphoamidases inside the cancer cells, this could specifically eliminate cancer cells [12]. To verify this hypothesis, they synthesized bis-β-chloroethyl-phosphamide-dichloride, which is a prodrug in the form of nitrogen mustard, and evaluated its anticancer effect in animal models in 1954, but unlike their prediction, this drug did not show satisfactory therapeutic effects [13].

Later, a study of an anticancer agent with the strategy proposed by Friedman and Seligman was fully executed by N. Brock's research team at ASTA Inc. (now Baxter Oncology) in Germany. Because bis-β-chloroethyl-phosphamide-dichloride was a chemically stable prodrug that was difficult to be activated, H. Arnold and F. Bourseaux at ASTA Inc. tried to attach a cyclic compound to the N′ position for easier activation. Hence in 1958, they synthesized cyclophosphamide, a prodrug with a cyclic structure, by reacting alkanolamine to bis-β-chloroethyl-phosphamide-dichloride, which was observed to have excellent anticancer effect through conversion to its active form with higher rate [14, 15]. However, it was later determined that this active form is generated by a different drug metabolic pathway, contrary to the initial assumption that phosphamidases would be involved. In other words, cyclophosphamide is mostly activated to 4-hydroxycyclophosphamide by cytochrome P450 enzymes in the liver microsomes, secreted to the bloodstream, and absorbed by cancer cells. It undergoes

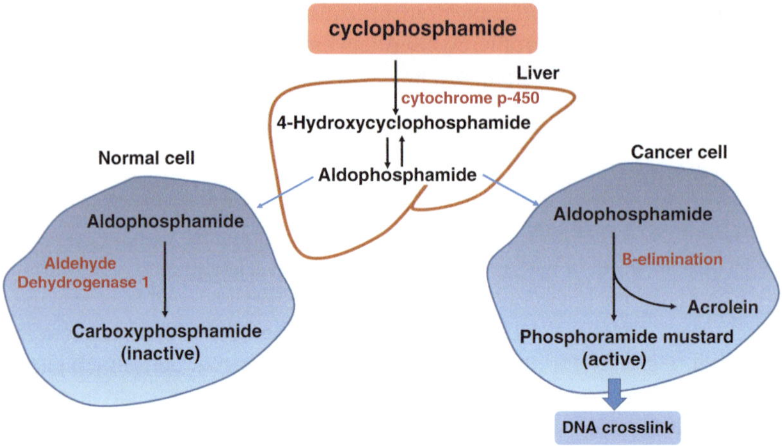

Fig. 4.5 Cyclophosphamide metabolism and mechanism of action. Cyclophosphamide is activated as 4-hydroxycyclophosphamide by cytochrome p-450 in the liver, after which it readily changes into its isomer aldophosphamide. These two intermediary metabolites readily spread into cells. In normal hematopoietic stem cells, where there is ample aldehyde dehydrogenase, 4-hydroxycyclophosphamide and aldophosphamide are oxidized by this enzyme to produce carboxyphosphamide, which is not cytotoxic. However, in cancer cells, aldophosphamide is broken down into the cytotoxic phosphoramide mustard and the by-product acrolein. Phosphoramide mustard causes cytotoxicity by inducing DNA cross-linking between guanine molecules

spontaneous hydrolysis in cancer cells and subsequent converstion to phosphoramide mustard, an efficacious substance, inducing DNA alkylation and triggering a cytotoxic effect (Fig. 4.5) [16, 17]. Cyclophosphamide was observed to have less toxicity in normal tissues such as liver, bone marrow, and intestinal epidermal cells compared to previous alkylating drugs. This is because these tissues have an abundant amout of aldehyde dehydrogenase (ALDH), which converts 4-hydroxycyclophosphamide into non-toxic compounds.

With the therapeutic effect of cyclophosphamide verified in clinical tests on patients with malignant lymphoma, it was registered as an FDA-approved lymphoma anticancer agent in 1959. Later, cyclophosphamide has been widely used in anticancer treatment for not only lymphocytic leukemia such as Hodgkin's lymphoma, Burkitt lymphoma, childhood acute lymphoblastic leukemia, chronic granulocytic leukemia, acute myeloid leukemia, and multiple myeloma, but also solid cancers such as breast cancer, ovarian cancer, and sarcoma.

4.1.1.5 Ifosfamide

H. Arnold at ASTA Inc. developed a new drug ifosfamide in 1967 by modifying cyclophosphamide [18]. This drug, which is a structural isomer of cyclophosphamide, was not only effective for leukemia treatment but also showed a superior efficacy compared to cyclophosphamide in solid tumor such as testicular cancer and

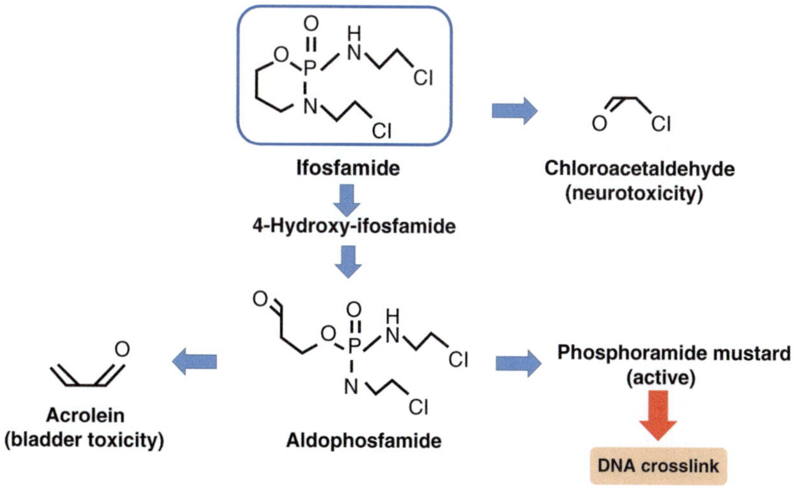

Fig. 4.6 Ifosfamide metabolism and mechanism of action. Ifosfamide induces DNA alkylation by conversion to neurotoxic chloroacetaldehyde or by forming aldophosfamide, which has an anticancer effect, via 4-hydroxy-ifosfamide. Ifosfamide undergoes the same processes of metabolization and activation as cyclophosphamide, but oxidation of the outer chain occurs more readily, meaning that it produces more acrolein; thus, higher toxicity has been observed in the kidneys and bladder

sarcoma. Therefore, it obtained FDA approval as a therapeutic agent for testicular cancer and sarcoma in 1988. Although ifosfamide undergoes drug metabolism and activation processes similar to those of cyclophosphamaide and forms isofosforamide mustard in cancer cells, it was found to have the disadvantage of increased toxicity in the bladder and nervous system since oxidation of its side chain occurs more easily, leading to enhanced formation of acrolein, a toxic byproduct (Fig. 4.6) [19]. In 1981, while searching for approaches to lower the toxicity of ifosfamide, N. Brock et al. discovered that sodium-2-mercaptoethane sulfonate (mesna), which contains a thiol group, can convert acrolein into a non-toxic compound and thereby effectively prevent bladder toxicity (hemorrhagic cystitis). Since then, mesna has been used until today to clinically prevent the side effects of ifosfamide [20].

4.1.1.6 Estramustine

Estramustine was developed by I. Niculescu-Duvaz et al., researchers at the Oncological Institute in Bucharest, Romania, to treat estrogen-dependent breast cancer by conjugating estrogen to nitrogen mustard in 1967 [21]. Because the drug binds to estrogen receptors (ER), it was initially predicted to have a therapeutic effect in breast cancer with high expression of estrogen receptors. However, the effect was observed to be weak, and a similar effect was observed in breast cancer that does not express estrogen receptors [22]. Later, P.O. Gunnarsson et al. at Uppsala University Hospital observed that estramustine showed selective drug accumulation in the prostate in 1981 [23], which immediately led to clinical tests and validation of its therapeutic effect in prostate cancer. In 1981, estramustine was approved as a prostate cancer therapeutic agent. In 1985, H.J. Nelde et al. found that estramustine binds more strongly to estramustine binding protein (EMBP), which is highly expressed in the prostate tissues, than to estrogen receptors [24]. Furthermore, it is known that the inhibitory effect of microtubule formation is more important than alkylation for the cytotoxic effect of estramustine [25].

4.1.1.7 Bendamustine

Bendamustine is a drug developed by W. Ozegowski and D. Krebs, researchers at the Institute for Microbiology and Experimental Therapy in Jena, former East Germany, by conjugating a benzimidazole ring to nitrogen mustard in 1963 [26]. Because of the benzimidazole ring, which has the properties of a purine antimetabolite drug, this drug was found to have the advantage of exerting cytotoxic effects in cancer cells that are resistant to alkylating anticancer agents [27]. Clinical trials in East Germany demonstrated an efficacy in various cancers such as chronic lymphobastic leukemia, Hodgkin's lymphoma, non-Hodgkin's lymphoma, multiple myeloma, and lung cancer. Also in the U.S., an excellent therapeutic effect was observed in patients with chronic lymphoblastic leukemia, extending progression-free survival by 1 year compared to chlorambucil, and so bendamustine was approved by FDA as a therapeutic agent for chronic lymphoblastic leukemia and B-lymphocyte non-Hodgkin's lymphoma in 2008, and is still used clinically.

4.1.2 Alkyl Sulfonate: Busulfan

In 1948, as R.J. Goldacre et al. reported that more than two alkylation reactive groups of various nitrogen mustard anticancer agents induce crosslinking to biomacromolecules including DNA, widespread studies were conducted on chemical compounds with similar mechanisms. In 1951, A. Haddow and G.M. Timmis at the Chester Beatty Research Institute focused on the alkyl sulfonate drugs that induce alkylation at both ends. They synthesized a series of dimethanesulfonate compounds that have hydrocarbon chains with various lengths and examined their effects in cancer transplantation animal models. As a result, they identified busulfan, a new alkylating drug with a superior efficacy and reduced bone marrow suppression than nitrogen mustard anticancer agents. As busulfan has methanesulfonic acid at both ends of the buthane chain and can thereby effectively act on both strands of DNA, it triggers crosslinking between DNA strands, causing cytotoxicity (Fig. 4.7) [28].

In 1953, an outstanding therapeutic effect of busulfan specific to chronic myeloid leukemia (CML) was reported [29], and the FDA approved it as a therapeutic agent for CML in 1954. Busulfan had been widely used as a CML therapeutic agent until imatinib emerged recently, in 2001.

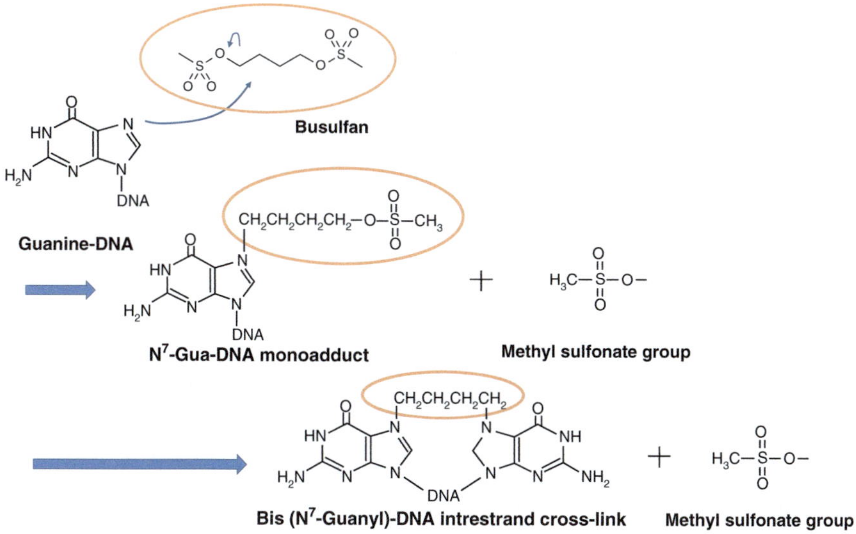

Fig. 4.7 Mechanism of action of busulfan. Busulfan has a linear symmetrical chemical structure and readily forms cross-links. Unlike other mustards and aziridines that can only react with DNA after producing active substances, busulfan binds directly with guanine's N, releasing a methyl sulfonate group and forming DNA monoadducts and biadducts

4.1.3 Aziridines (Ethylenimines)

Aziridine (ethylenimine) alkylating drugs, which are similar to nitrogen mustards, induce alkylation but unlike aziridinium intermediates in the nitrogen mustard group, they are not charged and display much weaker reactivity. These aziridine compounds are known to assault cancer cells by triggering DNA interstrand cross-linking, similarly to nitrogen mustards, and the major drugs in this group include thioTEPA and mitomycin C.

4.1.3.1 ThioTEPA

In 1950, a study was published on triethylenemelamine (TEM), which induces crosslinking with more than two alkylating groups. A.L. Walpole's research group at the Imperial Chemical Industries Inc. in England and J.H. Burchenal's group at the Sloan-Kettering Cancer Center reported the anticancer effect of aziridine compounds independently in 1950. They predicted that ethylenimine (aziridine ring) compounds, which have a similar structure to the ethylenimonium (aziridinium) intermediates generated by nitrogen mustard alkylating drugs, would act similarly to aziridinium ions and exert an anticancer effect. They examined the anticancer activity of various kinds of ethylenimine compounds and found that triethylenemelamine (TEM) which has 3 aziridine rings showed an anticancer effect similar to nitrogen mustard in various animal cancer models [30, 31].

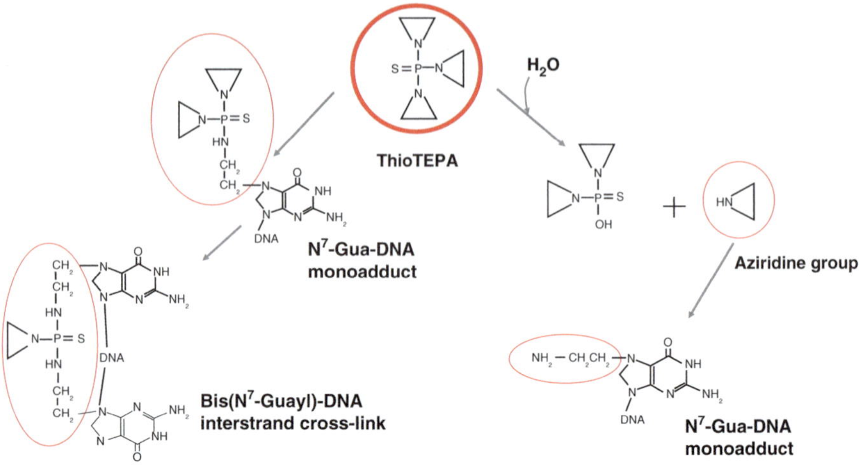

Fig. 4.8 Mechanism of action of ThioTEPA. ThioTEPA acts through two mechanisms. The first mechanism of ThioTEPA is forming cross-links through serial reactions. The second mechanism of ThioTEPA involves hydrolysis to produce an aziridine group, which then forms DNA monoadducts, separating the DNA strands and inducing apoptosis

However, as no prominent therapeutic effects of TEM were observed in further clinical tests, Burchenal's group synthesized various additional TEM derivatives and examined their anticancer effects through collaboration with the American Cyanamid Company. As a result, triethylene phosphoramide (TEPA) was developed, an organic phosphate compound showing excellent effect in various kinds of cancer [32]. TEPA was modified to a more chemically stable derivative, triethylene thiophosphoramide (thioTEPA), and clinical tests were performed for various cancers (Fig. 4.8) [33]. The results showed therapeutic effects for thioTEPA against various solid cancers such as breast cancer, ovarian cancer, and bladder cancer, and it was registered as an FDA-approved drug in 1959. It is currently a widely used drug for conditioning chemotherapy in patients with bone-marrow transplantation.

4.1.3.2 Mitomycin C

In 1956, T. Hata et al. at the Kitasato Institute in Japan isolated mitomycin C from *Streptomyces caespitosus* and observed that this antibiotic had an anticancer effect in animal cancer models [34]. Later, in 1964, W. Szybalski and V.N. Iyer at the University of Wisconsin in the U.S. discovered the mechanism of its cytotoxicity against cancer cells, which was DNA crosslinking induced by the aziridine ring of mitomycin C [35]. As mitomycin C undergoes reduction inside cells, carbon-1 of the aziridine ring alkylates the highly nucelophilic nitrogen-2 in the guanylic acid of DNA, which then causes migration of the activated carbamate group of carbon-10 in mitomycin C. This reacts with amino nitrogen of the guanylic acid in the opposite DNA strand, leading to interstrand crosslinking.

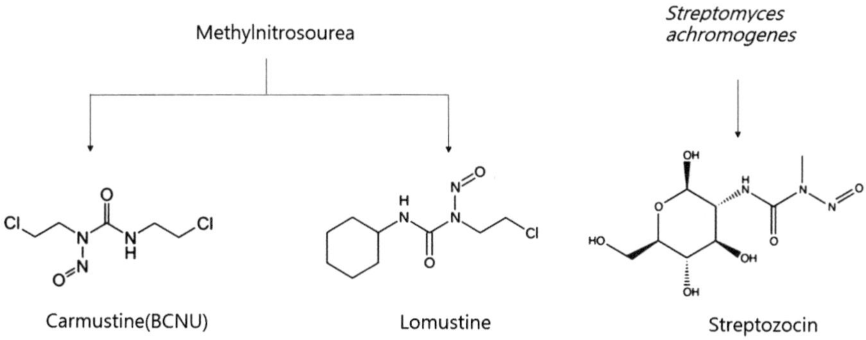

Fig. 4.9 The structure of nitrosourea drugs and the process of their development

The therapeutic efficacies of mitomycin C were observed in various solid tumors from clinical tests performed in the 1960s, and it was finally approved by FDA as a therapeutic agent for lung cancer and pancreatic cancer in 1974. The therapeutic effects of mitomycin C were further observed in the treatment of bladder cancer and non-small cell lung cancer. However, due to toxicities such as hemolysis, and the introduction of other superior anticancer agents, its clinical use has largely declined.

4.1.4 Nitrosoureas

Nitrosourea alkylating anticancer agents have a nitroso (R-NO) group and urea bound together, and undergo spontaneous hydrolysis inside the body producing substances that have alkylating and carbamoylating activities. Alkylating substances induce DNA alkylation and carbamoylating substances transform proteins. Representative drugs include carmustine (BCNU) and lomustine (CCNU), which are mainly used in the treatment of brain tumors such as glioblastoma multiforme, as their high lipophilicity allows them to easily penetrate blood-brain barrier (BBB) (Fig. 4.9).

Development of nitrosourea drugs was led by the National Cancer Chemotherapy Service Center (NCCSC) in the U.S. In 1959, A. Goldin et al. at NCCSC discovered the anticancer activity of 1-methyl-2-nitro-1-nitrosoguanidine (MNNG), which provided the crucial basis for the development of nitrosourea anticancer agents [36]. The NCI was interested in MNNG as a new class of alkylating drugs and made a contract with the Southern Research Institute (SRI) for developing nitrosourea anticancer agents. Later, in 1961, H.E. Skipper at SRI led a collaborative study with the Sloan-Kettering Cancer Center and developed N-methyl-N-nitrosourea (MNU), which demonstrates superiority compared to MNNG in the L1210 mouse leukemia model. He also found that MNU functioned effectively in L1210 cancers transplanted into the brain, and suggested the potential of nitrosourea anticancer agents for the treatment of brain carcinoma [37].

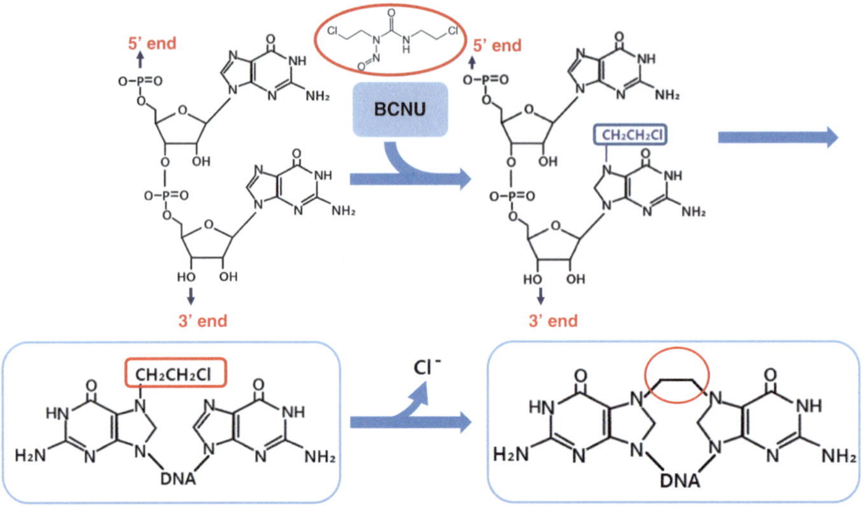

Fig. 4.10 Mechanism of action of BCNU (carmustine). BCNU forms unstable 2-chloroethyl diazene hydroxide, which undergoes spontaneous breakdown to produce a chloroethyl carbonium ion, which causes alkylation of N or O in guanine, inducing DNA cross-links and thereby inhibiting replication and transcription of DNA. Because BCNU is highly hydrophobic, it can readily cross the blood-brain barrier and is used as a treatment for patients with brain cancers

4.1.4.1 BCNU (Carmustine)

T.P. Johnston and J.A. Montgomery at SRI reported in 1963 that 1,3-Bis (2-chloroethyl)-1-nitrosourea (BCNU, Carmustine), in which the methyl group of MNU was replaced with a 2-chloroethyl group, had a superior anticancer efficacy, which led carmustine to become the first clinical nitrosourea drug (Fig. 4.10) [38]. Clinical studies were conducted on various cancers at NCI in 1965, and improvement of symptoms by carmustine was confirmed in various cancers. In particular, due to the outstanding therapeutic effect in patients with brain tumor, carmustine was approved by the FDA in 1977 as a therapeutic agent for brain tumor, and is still clinically used.

4.1.4.2 CCNU (Lomustine)

In 1966, J.A. Montgomery's research team developed N-(2-chloroethyl)-N′-cyclohexyl-N-nitrosourea (CCNU, Lomustine), a new nitrosourea anticancer agent in which a cyclohexyl group was conjugated to the N′ position of BCNU [39]. It was observed in 1972 that lomustine had a superior effect to carmustine on L1210 cancer transplanted into mouse brain. Although lomustine was predicted to be effective for brain tumor as it has higher lipid solubility, which is associated with penetration of blood-brain barrier, clinical test results comparing the two drugs showed similar therapeutic effects. However, because lomustine had the advantage of oral administration compared to carmustine, it was approved by the FDA as a brain tumor therapeutic agent in 1976. In addition to brain tumor, therapeutic effects of lomustine were observed in blood cancers such as Hodgkin's lymphoma, non-Hodgkin's lymphoma, and multiple myeloma and various solid cancers such as malignant melanoma and gastrointestinal tumor. However, it is rarely used today, except for in the treatment of brain tumor.

4.1.4.3 Streptozotocin (STZ)

Streptozotocin is an antibiotic containing nitrosourea identified from *Streptomyces achromogenes* by J.J. Vavra, a researcher at Upjohn Inc (merged with Pfizer) in the U.S., in 1959 [40]. Unlike carmustine or lomustine which are chloroethyl nitrosoureas (CENU), STZ is a methylnitrosourea similar to MNU. Hence, whereas CENU causes chloroethylation and crosslinking between guanine and cytocine bases in DNA, STZ forms diazomethane hydroxide and only induces methylation of guanine.

Moreover, because STZ is a glucosamine-nitrosourea compound with a sugar structure, it selectively binds to GLUT2, a glucose transporter, and enters into cells. Due to this characteristic, STZ was shown to exert a selective toxicity against pancreatic beta islet cells. The anticancer effects of STZ were first observed by S.P. Owen in 1965. In 1968, I.M. Murray-Lyon et al. at King's College Hospital in England focused on the pancreatic tissue-specific toxicity and reported that STZ showed an excellent therapeutic effect in insulinoma, a type of pancreatic cancer [41]. Later, R.M. Bukowski et al. proved its therapeutic effect in the treatment of metastatic pancreatic cancer using combination therapy with 5-fluorouracil, adriamycin, and mitomycin C. Streptozotocin was approved by FDA as a pancreatic cancer therapeutic agent in 1982, but it is rarely used today.

4.2 Nonclassical Alkylating Drugs

Nonclassical alkylating agents, which include hydrazines and triazenes, are synthetic inorganic nitrogen compounds that bind to biomacromolecue by forming alkyl diazonium intermediates with high alkylation activity either spontaneously or through the action of enzymes. Among the compounds in this class, most of those approved as anticancer agents induce methylation of guanine bases, and therefore do not have the DNA crosslinking activity shown in classical alkylating agents. The anticancer agents in this class are as follows.

4.2.1 Hydrazine: Procarbazine

The first alkylating anticancer agent approved by the FDA among hydrazines was procarbazine, developed at Hoffmann-La Roche. In the late 1950s, while studying derivatives of methylhydrazine, an inhibitor of monoamine oxidase being developed as a sympathetic nervous system stimulant, the company discovered that 1-methyl-2-benzylhydrazine had an anticancer effect in a cancer transplanation mouse model. In 1963, P. Zeller and W. Bollag, researchers at Hoffmann-La Roche, reported that, among numerous derivatives synthesized to develop drugs with high efficacy, procarbazine exhibited the strongest anticancer effect in various cancer transplantation mouse models [42, 43]. It was later discovered that the drug exerts its anticancer effect by generating a methyldiazonium ion through spontaneous hydrolysis and inducing DNA methylation, which leads to truncation of chromatin threads and apoptosis. Procarbazine showed a therapeutic efficacy for the treatment of Hodgkin's lymphoma in combination therapy with MOPP (mechlorethamine, vincristine, procarbazine, prednisone), and became an FDA-approved drug in 1969. Procarbazine is still used clinically today.

4.2.2 Triazenes

4.2.2.1 Dacarbazine

The anticancer effect of triazene drugs was first reported by D.A. Clarke et al. at the Sloan-Kettering Institute in 1955. His research team observed an inhibitory effect of 1-aryl-3, 3-dialkyltriazene on cancer cell growth in a cancer transplantation mouse model [44]. Later, in 1961, while studying synthetic derivaties of 5-aminoimidazole-4-carboxamide, which was developed as a metabolic antagonist anticancer agent, J.A. Montgomery and Y.F. Shealy at the Southern Research Institute discovered that 5-diazoimidazole-4-carboxamide (dacarbazine), a triazene derivative, exhibited a strong anticancer effect [45].

Thereafter, the metabolism and mechanisms of dacarbazine were investigated. Dacarbazine acts as a prodrug, and when absorbed into the body, it becomes demethylated by cytochrome P450 (CYP3A4) detoxification enzyme and converted into an activated monomethyl compound. As this compound undergoes spontaneous hydrolysis, it generates 5-aminoimidazole-4-carboxamide and diazomethane, and ultimately, a methyl diazonium ion derived from diazomethane methylates guanine in DNA, causing cytotoxicity (Fig. 4.11). These findings indicated that, unlike the prediction, dacarbazine displays its anticancer effect by a DNA alkylation reaction, rather than acting as a metabolic antagonist.

Clinical trials of dacarbazine have been conducted in various cancers, and since therapeutic efficacies were observed in melanoma and Hodgkin's lymphoma, it was approved by the FDA as therapeutic agents for these diseases in 1975. Currently, it is used as a first-line drug in melanoma rather than Hodgkin's lymphoma.

4.2.2.2 Temozolomide

Dacarbazine has the disadvantages that it needs to be directly injected into the blood vessels, since it is extremely unstable in aqueous solution, and that it shows strong toxicity against normal tissues. Therefore, studies on more stable and less toxic

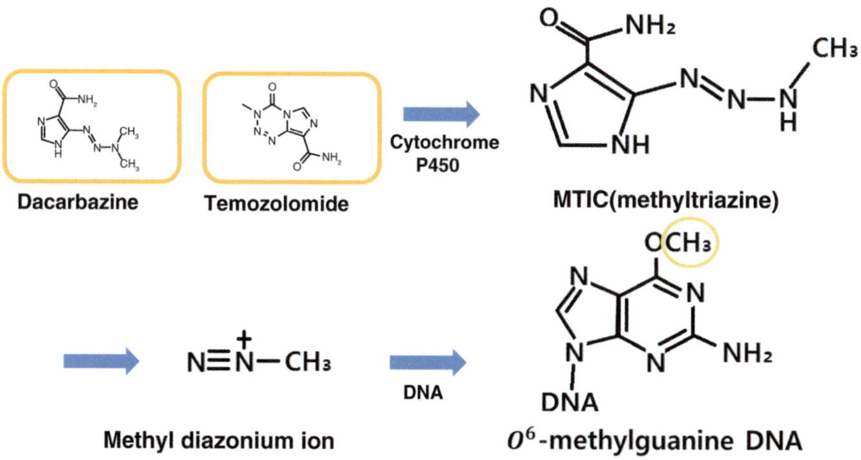

Fig. 4.11 Mechanism of action of dacarbazine and temozolomide. Dacarbazine and temozolomide are similar imidazotetrazine drugs. Both drugs are converted to MTIC by cytochrome p450 in the liver, which forms methyl diazonium ions that cause a methylation reaction at the O of guanine. During DNA replication, O-methylguanine causes the addition of a thymidine instead of a cytosine in new DNA strands

derivatives have been performed by various groups. Among them, the most successful drug, temozolomide, was developed by M.F.G. Stevens at Aston University in England.

In 1984, while conducting a collaborative research project with May & Baker Inc., Stevens developed imidazotetrazinone derivatives by reacting dacarbazine and aryl isocyanate [46]. Among them, mitozolomide, which was conjugated with a chloroethyl group, showed a superior anticancer activity in murine tumor implantation models, and subsequent clinical trials were performed. However, severe myelosupression was observed in human, which had not been seen in mice, and so the compound could not be approved as an anticancer agent. This side effect was speculated to be caused by the chloroethyl carbonium ion, which is produced by spontaneous hydrolysis of the mitozolomide prodrug in the human body and induces DNA crosslinking, unlike the methyl carbonium ion derived from diazomethane, triggering severe toxicity in normal bone marrow [47, 48].

Later, in 1987, together with the Cancer Research Campaign (CRC, UK), Stevens synthesized imidazotetrazine compounds in which the chloroethyl group was substituted with an alkyl group in order to lower the side effects of mitozolomide [49]. Analysis of its anticancer effect in animal models showed that temozolomide, in which a methyl group was substituted, had the best efficacy. Temozolomide produces a methyl carbonium ion when hydrolyzed inside the body, similar to dacarbazine, but it was observed to be far more stable than dacarbazine (Fig. 4.11). Thus, oral administration is possible for temozolomide, and bone marrow toxicity shown in dacarbazine or mitozolomide were significantly improved.

Interestingly, because temozolomide also has the characteristic of penetrating blood-brain barriers, its therapeutic effects were observed in phase I clinical trial on patients with brain tumors such as astrocytoma or glioblastoma multiforme [50]. Large scale clinical trials began later and it was approved by the U.S. FDA as an astrocytoma therapeutic agent in 1999 and glioblastoma multiforme therapeutic agent in 2005. It is still widely used against brain tumors.

The anticancer effect of temozolomide depends on the level of DNA methylation on tumor. It is reported that certain brain tumor cells exhibit resistance against temozolomide due to DNA alkyltransferase (AKT) expressed by the MGMT gene. Conversely, epigenetic silencing of MGMT gene in brain tumor cells is known to be a predictive factor for response to temozolomide treatment. Based on these results, studies are currently ongoing to apply temozolomide after selecting patient groups who are predicted to have a favorable therapeutic response by examining MGMT expression level.

4.2.3 *Altretamines*

Altretamine (Hexamethylmelamine) is an s-triazine derivative, which was studied as a material for synthetic resins in its early development. However, during the process of searching for anticancer agents among ethylenimine analogue-related compounds, A.L. Walpole's group at ICI in England and C.P. Rhoads's group at the Memorial Center for Cancer and Allied Disease first reported that altretamine exhibited anticancer effects in the mouse cancer model in 1951 and 1952, respectively [51, 52]. Nevertheless, because altretamine did not have an outstanding anticancer effect compared to triethylenemelamine (TEM) from the same search, it did not receive much attention.

In the early 1960s, the NCI decided to reinvestigate the anticancer effect of altretamine in a search for new anticancer agent candidates, and conducted a clinical trial in 1965 [53]. In a clinical trial conducted by W.L. Wilson et al. at the University of Wisconsin, altretamine showed an excellent anticancer effect with lower toxicities compared to the previously developed alkylating anticancer agents such as chlorambucil, cyclophosphamide, and melphalan, and its clinical trials were actively conducted for various cancers. Among them, it was found to have a superior therapeutic efficacy in ovarian cancer, and the FDA approved altretamine as an ovarian cancer therapeutic agent in 1990.

Although its mechanism has not been clearly determined, it is speculated that altretamine is first oxidized by hepatic cytochrome P450 monooxygenase, undergoes an intermediate state as an iminium ion, before spontaneous demethylation to form formaldehyde, with weak methylation activity, reacting with DNA.

4.3 Alkylating-Like Agents: Platinum Compounds

Platinum compounds are known to have similar mechanisms to alkylating drugs. These compounds are coordination complexes of platinum with a planar structure that can form covalent bonds with electrophilic atoms similarly to alkylating drugs. It is known that they bind to N^7 of the guanine base in DNA and induce intrastrand or interstrand crosslinks, which inhibit replication or transcription of DNA, resulting in an anticancer activity. As well as the first-generation cisplatin, the second-generation carboplatin and the third-generation oxaliplatin platinum compounds are widely used in clinics.

4.3.1 Cisplatin

Cisplatin is one of the most widely used anticancer agents today, and because its discovery was made coincidentally, it is called the "penicillin of cancer treatment." In 1965, B. Rosenberg, a biophysicist at Michigan State University, was studying the effect of electric fields on bacterial proliferation. He discovered by chance that bacterial proliferation was inhibited in the culture medium with an electric current. In an additional experiment conducted later, he found that the inhibitory effect on proliferation depends on the type of metallic electrodes used to generate the electric field, rather than the electric field itself. It was discovered that, among the metallic electrodes, platinum electrodes released platinum ions that react with ammonium ions and chlorine ions, chemical components in the culture medium, to create the platinum complex cisplatin, and this has an inhibitory effect on bacterial proliferation [54].

Focusing on this potent inhibitory effect of cisplatin on bacterial proliferation, Rosenberg conductd an experiment to test its anticancer effects using a mouse sarcoma model in 1969, which confirmed its inhibtory effect on cancer proliferation [55]. Later, from 1971, clinical trials on cisplatin were conducted in various hospitals. The potential of cisplatin as an anticancer therapeutic agent was confirmed by L. Einhorn at the Indiana University Medical Center who was concentrating on the treatment of malignant testicular cancer. He observed a dramatic therapeutic effect in approximately 20 testicular cancer patients between 1974 and 1975 using a combination therapy with cisplatin, vinblastine, and bleomycin. It was later found that some of the patients were completely cured. This was the second example of cure in solid cancer [56]. In addition to metastatic testicular cancer, effects of cisplatin were observed in clinical trials for metastatic ovarian cancer, invasive bladder cancer, and non-small cell lung cancer. It was approved by the FDA in 1978 as a therapeutic agent for these cancers.

Cisplatin has a very simple molecular structure, having a platinum atom in the center, with two amine groups and two chlorine groups all located on the same side (*cis* position). Cisplatin is hydrolyzed in cancer cells, and the two chlorine groups become detached, after which the platinum ion, now with increased reactivity, forms crosslinks with two guanine bases in DNA. As a result, it inhibits DNA replication, exerting an anticancer activity (Fig. 4.12). Cisplatin is effective only when the two chlorine molecules are located in the same side, allowing DNA crosslinking. The *trans* form of cisplatin is known to have no effect as an anticancer agent.

Cisplatin is currently widely used in various cancers as a combination therapy with other cytotoxic chemotherapeutics, including gastric cancer, lung cancer, head and neck cancer, ovarian cancer, sarcoma, endometrial cancer, and cervical cancer. Although cisplatin is an excellent anticancer agent, effective in many different

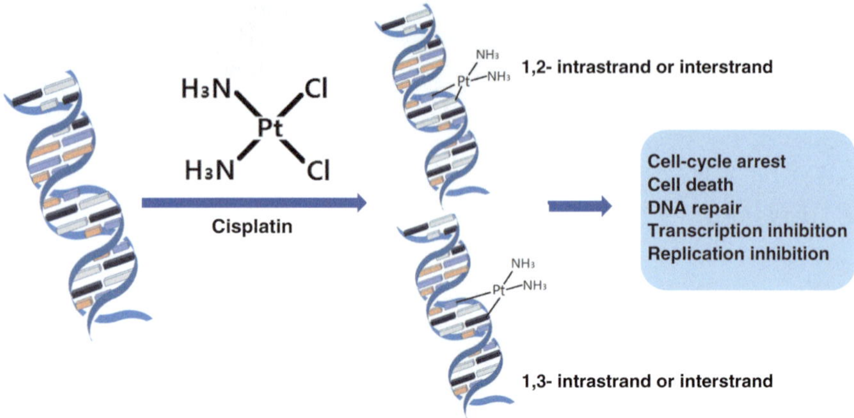

Fig. 4.12 Mechanism of action of cisplatin. When cisplatin is absorbed into cells, it undergoes a hydration reaction to form $[Pt\ (NH_3)_2Cl\ (OH_2)]^+$ and $[Pt\ (NH_3)_2\ (OH_2)_2]^{2+}$. Subsequently, cisplatin's Pt forms a ionic bond with the N of guanine, producing 1,2- intrachain, 1,3-intrachain, 1,2-interchain, and 1,3-interchain cross-links

cancers, it has many side effects such as nausea, vomiting, and nephrotoxicity, and so pretreatment is required before cisplatin administration to reduce the tocixity and most toxicities are manageable and tolerable today.

4.3.2 *Carboplatin*

Although cisplatin has a superior anticancer activity, because it has strong toxicity in the kidney and nervous system, induces severe nausea and vomiting, and because drug resistance in tumor cells has also been reported, there have been attempts to develop new platinum compound. Although thousands of derivatives were synthesized and their effects were examined, two new platinum compounds - carboplatin and oxaliplatin—are used clinically. Carboplatin (cis-diammine-1,1′-cyclobutane dicarboxylate platinum) was first developed by B. Rosenberg as a second-generation drug in the early 1970s, and the Bristol-Myers Squibb Company developed it fully as an anticancer agent in the 1980s [57].

As the cyclobutane ring of carboplatin has higher stability, and therefore lower reactivity, compared to the chlorine in cisplastin, it was shown to have lower toxicities in animal models, including nephro- and neurotoxicity, myelosuppression, and vomiting. Drug resistance was also improved compared to cisplatin [58]. Clinical trials of carboplatin were conducted in the Royal Marsden Hospital in England and the NCI in the U.S., and it was approved by the FDA for treatment of ovarian cancer in 1989. Later, through numerous clinical trials, its effect on non-small cell lung cancer has been also verified and the drug is widely used.

4.3.3 *Oxaliplatin*

Emergence of the limitations of carboplatin in clinical application due to its low solubility in aqueous solution led to the development of oxaliplatin, which is a third-generation platinum compound anticancer agent. This drug was first synthesized by Y. Kidani at Nagoya University in Japan in 1976, and was fully developed as a third-generation platinum compound by Sanofi-Aventis Inc [59].

In addition to enhanced solubility, oxaliplatin was shown to have an effect on cancer cells showing resistance to cisplastin and carboplatin while having low side effects [60]. Furthermore, clinical trials on oxaliplatin have been conducted in various cancers, and prominent effects have been reported from a clinical phase II trial in metastatic cololectal cancer in 1997, in which numerous cancer centers participated [61]. Subsquently, a clinical phase III trial was conducted with various conditions, and oxaliplatin became approved as a therapeutic agent for metastatic cololectal cancer as a combination therapy with 5-fluorouracil (5-FU)/leucovorin (LV) in 2002. It is also widely used in adjuvant chemotherapy after colorectal cancer surgery. Moreover, it is used in adjuvant chemotherapy after lung cancer surgery and as a therapeutic agent for metastatic lung cancer, as well as in anticancer therapy for pancreatic cancer and biliary tract cancer.

References

1. Krumbhaar EB, Krumbhaar HD (1919) Blood and bone marrow in yellow cross gas (mustard gas) poisoning. J Med Res 40:497–506
2. Berenblum I, Riley-Smith (1929) The modifying influence of dichloroethyl sulphide on the induction of tumours in mice by tar. J Pathol Bacteriol 32:424–434
3. Adair FE, Bagg HJ (1931) Experimental and clinical studies on the treatment of cancer by dichlorethylsulphide (mustard gas). Am J Surg 93:190–199
4. Gilman A, Philips FS (1946) The biological actions and therapeutic applications of the B-chloroethyl amines and sulfides. Science 103:409–415
5. Goodman LS, Wintrobe MM, Dameshek W et al (1946) Nitrogen mustard therapy: use of methyl-bis (b-chloroethyl) amine hydrochloride and tris (b-chloroethyl) amine hydrochloride for Hodgkin's disease, lymphosarcoma, leukemia, and certain allied and miscellaneous disorders. J Am Med Assoc 132:126–132
6. Golumbic C, Fruton JS, Bergmann M (1946) Chemical reactions of the nitrogen mustard gases. I. The transformations of methyl-bis (b-chloroethyl) amine in water. J Org Chem 11:518–535
7. Goldacre RJ, Loveless A, Ross WCJ (1949) Mode of production of chromosome abnormalities by the nitrogen mustards. Nature 163:667–669
8. Burchenal JH, Burchenal JR, Johnston SF (1951) Chemotherapy of leukemia. III. Further studies on the effects of nitrogen mustards and related compounds on transmitted mouse leukemia. Cancer 4:353–356
9. Haddow A, Kon AR, Ross WCJ (1948) Effects upon tumors of various haloalkylaryl amines. Nature 162:824–825
10. Everett J, Robertson JJ, Ross WCJ (1953) Aryl-2-halogenalkylamines. Part XII. Some carboxylic derivatives of N,N-di-2-chloroethylamines. J Chem Soc 2386–2390

11. Bergel F, Stock JA (1954) Cyto-active amino-acid and peptide derivatives. Part I. Substituted phenylalanines. J Chem Soc 2409–2417
12. Seligman AM, Nachlas MM, Manheimer LH, Friedman OM, Wolf G (1949) Development of new methods for the histochemical demonstration of hydrolytic intracellular enzymes in a program of cancer research. Ann Surg 130:333–341
13. Friedman OM, Seligman AM (1954) Preparation of N-phosphorylated derivatives of bis b-chloroethylamine. J Am Chem Soc 76:655–661
14. Arnold H, Bourseaux F (1958) Synthese und abbau zytostatisch wirksamer zyklischer N-phosphamidester des bis-(chloroethyl)-amins. Angew Chem 70:539–544
15. Arnold H, Bourseaux F, Brock N (1958) Chemotherapeutic action of a cyclic nitrogen mustard phosphoramide ester (B 518-ASTA) in experimental tumours of the rat. Nature 181:931
16. Brock N, Hohorst HJ (1967) Metabolism of cyclophosphamide. Cancer 20:900–904
17. Horch RF, Valente RR (1991) Synthesis, activation and cytotoxicity of aldophosphamide analogues. J Med Chem 34:3052–3058
18. Arnold H (1967) Uber die chemie neuer zytostatisch wirksamer N-chlor-aethyl-phosphorsauresterdiamide. Vortrag auf dem V. Internat. Kongreb flir Chemotherapie, Wien. Verlag der Wiener Medizinische Akademie Abstr A IV-1a/5
19. van Dyk JJ, Falkson HC, van der Merwe AM, Falken G (1972) Unexpected toxicity in patients treated with ifosfamide. Cancer Res 32:921–924
20. Brock N, Pohl J, Stekar J (1981) Studies on the urotoxicity of oxazaphosphorine cytostatics and its prevention. 2. Comparative study on the uroprotective efficacy of thiols and other sulfur compounds. Eur J Cancer Clin Oncol 17:1155–1163
21. Niculescu-Duvaz I, Cambani A, Tarnauceanu E (1967) Potential anticancer agents. II Urethane-type nitrogen mustards of some natural sex hormones. J Med Chem 10:172–174
22. Tew KD (1983) The mechanism of action of estramustine. Semin Oncol 10:21–26
23. Gunnarsson PO, Forshell GP, Fritjoesson A, Norlen BJ (1981) Plasma Concentrations of estramustine phosphate and its major metabolites in patients with prostatic carcinoma treated with different doses of estramustine phosphate. Scand J Urol Nephrol 153:201–206
24. Nelde HJ, Fluchter SH, Harzmann R, Bichler KH (1985) Immunohistologischer Nachweis des Estramustin-bindenden Proteins (EMBP) in der Prostata. In: Experimentelle Urologic. Springer, Berlin, Heidelberg, pp 332–340
25. Hartrey-ASP B (1984) Estramustine-induced mitotic arrest in two human prostatic carcinoma cell lines, DU 145 and PC-3. Prostate 5:93–100
26. Ozegowski W, Krebs D (1963) W-[bis-(chlorethyl)-amino-benzimidazolyl-(2)]-propionic or butyric acids as potential cytostatic agents. J Prakt Chem 20:178–186
27. Ozegowski W, Krebs D (1971) IMET 3393, gamma-(1-methyl-5-bis-(ß-chlorathyl)-amino-benzimidazolyl(2)-buttersäure-hydrochlorid, ein neues Zytostatikum aus der Reihe der Benzimidazol-Loste. Zbl Pharm 110:1013–1019
28. Haddow A, Timmis GM (1951) Bifunctional sulfonic acid esters with radiomimetic activity. Acta Unio Int Contra Cancrum 7:469
29. Galton DA (1953) Myleran in chronic myeloid leukaemia; results of treatment. Lancet 264:208–213
30. Rose FL, Hendry JA, Walpole AL (1950) New cytotoxic agents with tumour-inhibitory activity. Nature 165:993–996
31. Burchenal JH, Crossley ML, Stock CC, Rhoads CP (1950) The action of certain ethyleneimine (aziridine) derivatives on mouse leukaemia. Arch Biochem 26:321
32. Burchenal JH, Johnstone SC, Parker RP, Crossley ML, Kuh E, Seeger DR (1952) Effects of N-ethylene substituted phosphoramides on transplantable mouse leukaemia. Cancer Res 12:251–252
33. Sykes MP, Karnofsky DA, Philips FS, Burchenal JH (1953) Clinical studies on triethylenephosphoramide and diethylenephosphoramide, compounds with nitrogen-mustard-like activity. Cancer 61:142–148

34. Hata T, Sano Y, Sugawara R, Matsumae A, Kanamori K, Shima T, Hoshi TJ (1956) Mitomycin, a new antibiotic from Streptomyces. J Antibiot 9:141–146
35. Szybalski W, Iyer VN (1964) Cross-linking of DNA by enzymatically or chemically activated mitomycins and porfiromycins, bifunctionally "alkylating" antibiotics. Fed Proc 23:946–957
36. Goldin A, Venditti JM, Kline I (1959) Evaluation of antileukemic agents employing advanced leukemia L1210 in mice. Cancer Res 19:429–466
37. Skipper HE, Schabel FM Jr, Trader MW, Thomson JR (1961) Experimental evaluation of potential anticancer agents vi. Anatomical distribution of leukemic cells and failure of chemotherapy. Cancer Res 21:1154–1164
38. Johnston TP, McCaleb GS, Montgomery JA (1963) The synthesis of antineoplastic agents. XXXII. N-Nitrosoureas. J Med Chem 6:669–681
39. Johnston TP, McCaleb GS, Montgomery JA (1966) The synthesis of potential anticancer agents. XXXVI. N-Nitrosoureas. II. Haloalkyl derivatives. J Med Chem 9:892–911
40. Vavra JJ, Deboer C, Dietz A, Hanka LJ, Sokolski WT (1959) Streptozotocin, a new antibacterial antibiotic. Antibiot Annu 7:230–235
41. Murray-Lyon IM, Eddleston AL, Williams R, Brown M, Hogbin BM, Bennett A, Edwards JC, Taylor KW (1968) Treatment of multiple-hormone-producing malignant islet-cell tumour with streptozotocin. Lancet 292:895–898
42. Bollag W, Grunberg E (1963) Tumour inhibitory effects of a new class of cytotoxic agents: methylhydrazine derivatives. Experientia 19:130–131
43. Zeller P, Gutmann H, Hegedus B et al (1963) Methylhydrazine derivatives, a new class of cytotoxic agents. Experientia 19:129
44. Clarke DA, Barclay RK, Stock CC, Rondestvedt CS Jr (1955) Triazenes as inhibitors of mouse sarcoma 180. Proc Soc Exp Biol Med 90:484–489
45. Shealy YF, Struck RF, Holum LB, Montgomery JA (1961) Synthesis of Potential Anticancer Agents. XXIX. 5-Diazoimidazole-4-carbox amide and 5-Diazo-c-triazole-4-carboxamide. J Org Chem 26:2396–2401
46. Stevens MFG, Hickman JA, Stone R et al (1984) Antitumour imidazotetrazines. 1. Synthesis and chemistry of 8-carbamoyl-3-(2-chloroethyl)imidazo[5,1-d]-1,2,3,5-tetrazin-4(3H)-one, a novel broad-spectrum antitumour agent. J Med Chem 27:196–201
47. Hickman JA, Stevens MFG, Gibson NW et al (1985) Experimental antitumour activity against murine tumor model systems of 8-carbamoyl-3-(2-chloroethyl)imidazo[5,1-d]-1,2,3,5-tetrazin-4(3H)-one (mitozolomide), a novel broad-spectrum agent. Cancer Res 45:3008–3013
48. Newlands ES, Blackledge G, Slack JA et al (1985) Phase I clinical trial of mitozolomide. Cancer Treat Rep 69:801–805
49. Stevens MFG, Hickman JA, Langdon SP et al (1987) Antitumour activity and pharmacokinetics in mice of 8-carbamoyl-3-methylimidazo[5,1-d]-1,2,3,5-tetrazin-4(3H)-one (CCRG81045; M&B 39831), a novel drug with potential as an alternative to dacarbazine. Cancer Res 47:5846–5852
50. Newlands ES, Blackledge GRP, Slack JA et al (1992) Phase I trial of temozolomide (CCRG 81045: M&B 39831: NSC 362856). Br J Cancer 65:287–291
51. Hendry JA, Homer RF, Rose FL, Walpole AL (1951) Cytotoxic agents. III. Derivatives of ethyleneimine. Brit J Pharmacol 6:357–410
52. Buckley SM, Stock CC, Crossley ML, Rhoads CP (1952) Inhibition of the crocker mouse sarcoma 180 by certain ethylenimine derivativesand related compounds. Cancer 5:144–152
53. Wilson WL, de la Garza JG (1965) Phase I study of hexamethylmelamine (NSC-13875). Cancer Chemotherapy Rept 48:49–52
54. Rosenberg B, Van Camp L, Krigas T (1965) Inhibition of cell division in *Escherichia coli* by electrolysis products from a platinum electrode. Nature 205:698–699
55. Rosenberg B, Van Camp L, Trosko JE, Mansour VH (1969) Platinum compounds: a new class of potential anti-tumor agents. Nature 222:385–386

56. Einhorn LH, Donohue J (1977) Cis-diamminedichloroplatinum, vinblastine and bleomycin combination chemotherapy in disseminated testicular cancer. Ann Intern Med 87:293–298
57. Harrap KR (1985) Preclinical studies identifying carboplatin as a viable cisplatin alternative. Cancer Treat Rev 12(Suppl A):21–33
58. Rose WC, Schurig JE (1985) Preclinical antitumor and toxicologic profile of carboplatin. Cancer Treat Rev 12(Suppl A):1–19
59. Mathe G, Kidani Y, Noji M, Maral R, Bourut C, Chenu E (1985) Antitumor activity of 1-OHP in mice. Cancer Lett 27:135–143
60. Kelland LR et al (1999) Mini-review: discovery and development of platinum complexes designed to circumvent cisplatin resistance. J Inorg Biochem 77:111–115
61. Becouarn Y, Ychou M, Ducreux M et al (1997) Oxaliplatin (l-OHP) as 1st-line chemotherapy in metastatic colorectal cancer patients: preliminary activity/toxicity report. Proc Am Soc Clin Oncol 16:229a

Chapter 5
Antimetabolic Anticancer Drugs

Antimetabolic drugs bind to a specific enzyme and prevent normal metabolites from interacting with the enzymes, leading to inhibition of a specific metabolic pathway. Especially, the antimetabolic anticancer drugs interfere with DNA synthesis at multiple levels by inhibiting enzymes that utilize folic acid or synthesize the precursors of pyrimidine and purine, which are necessary for cell growth. In addition, some antimetabolites are directly incorporated into DNA, which inhibits DNA synthesis (Fig. 5.1). Therefore, these drugs are largely classified into folic acid derivatives that inhibit enzymes of folate pathway such as dihydrofolate reductase (DHFR), pyrimidine or purine derivatives that inhibit pyrimidine or purine synthesis, and direct inhibitors of DNA synthesis (Fig. 5.2).

5.1 Folic Acid Derivatives

Folic acid derivatives are cytotoxic drugs used not only as anticancer drugs but also as anti-inflammatory drugs or as immunosuppressants, inhibiting the function of folic acid. Folic acid provides the methyl group in the reactions of various methyltransferases such as the synthesis of thymidine and methionine. When folic acid analogs inhibit these enzymes, cell division is suppressed because the precursors of biopolymers such as DNA and protein are not synthesized. Methotrexate (MTX), pemetrexed, and pralatrexate are folic acid derivatives used as anticancer drugs. They act mainly as inhibitors of DHFR, but some of them can inhibit thymidylate synthase (TS) or other enzymes (Fig. 5.3).

K.-W. Kim et al., *Cancer Drug Discovery*, DOI 10.1007/978-94-024-0844-7_5

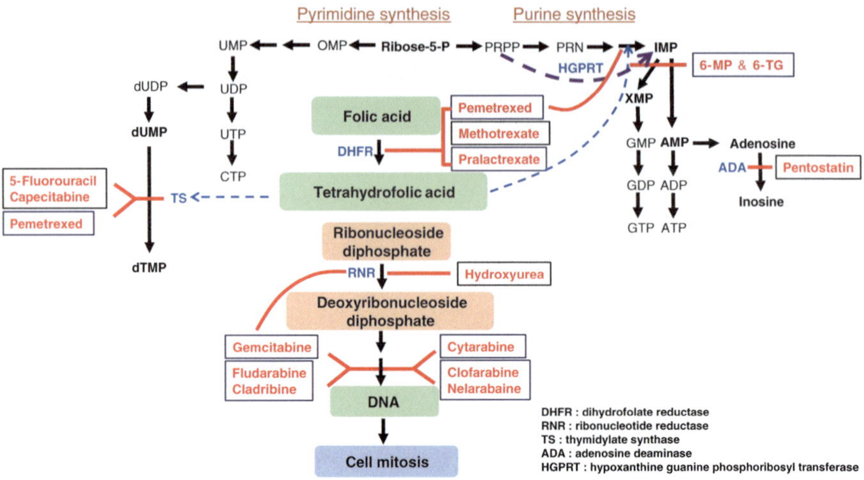

Fig. 5.1 Intracellular sites of action for various anticancer antimetabolites

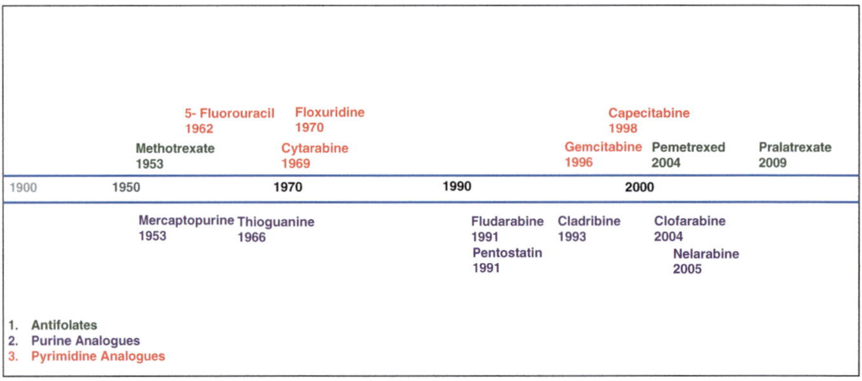

Fig. 5.2 Types of anticancer antimetabolite and a chronology of their development

5.1.1 *Methotrexate*

Aminopterin is the second drug developed as a chemotherapy agent. It is an antagonist of folic acid, a substrate of DHFR that is important in DNA synthesis. Folic acid was discovered in 1928 by the British physician L. Wills, who was working in Bombay, India [1]. Wills used yeast extracts to treat pernicious anemia due to chronic malnutrition in pregnant women working in textile factories in Bombay, and discovered that folic acid was the effective component.

After hearing of folic acid being effective against anemia, S. Farber of Harvard Medical School assumed that it could restore malignant blood cells into normal ones and administered folic acid to a pediatric lymphocytic leukemia patient in 1947. However, folic acid increased the proliferation of malignant blood cells and

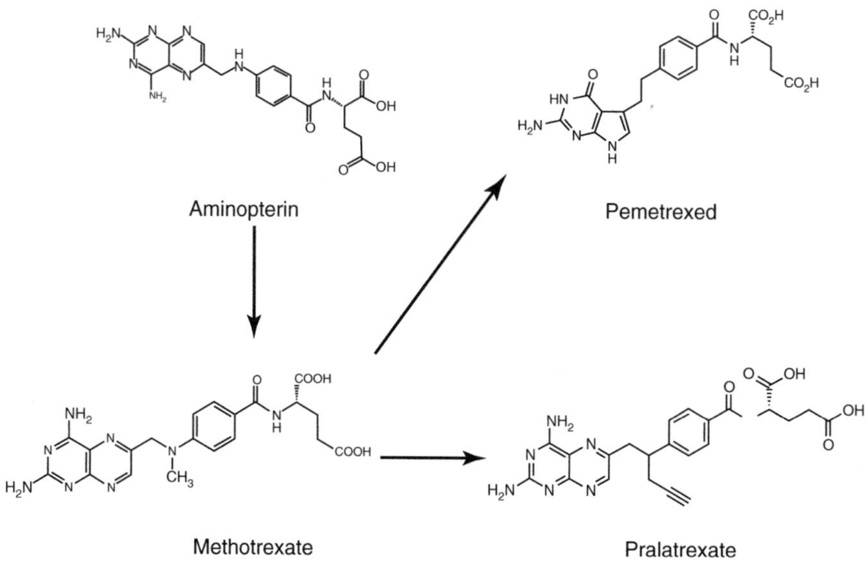

Fig. 5.3 Types of folate-derivative anticancer agents and the process of their development

worsened the patient's condition [2]. Based on this observation, Farber modified his hypothesis that a folic acid antagonist could treat leukemia. In 1948, he conducted a clinical trial with aminopterin, a folic acid antagonist synthesized by the synthetic chemist D. Seeger of the American Cyanamid Company. Aminopterin improved the symptoms and controlled leukemia in 10 out of 16 children and extended the lives of one-third of the 16 patients by 4 months [3, 4]. Thereafter, D. Seeger and Y. Subbarow, synthetic chemists of the American Cyanamid Company, reported the synthesis of MTX in 1949, which showed greater efficacy against cancer cells than that shown by aminopterin [5]. The FDA approved MTX for the treatment of acute lymphocytic leukemia in 1953.

Later, MTX was also found to be useful in treating other carcinomas. In 1951, J.C. Wright of the New York City Harlem Hospital Cancer Research Center observed that MTX relieved symptoms of breast cancer, and proposed the possibility of chemotherapy for solid tumors for the first time [6], Curative effects of MTX were also observed in ovarian, bladder, head, and neck cancers. In 1956, M.C. Li of the National Cancer Institute (NCI) used MTX to treat choriocarcinoma, a rare cancer that develops in the placenta [7] and achieved the first cure for solid cancer in 1958. Li administered MTX four times to confirm visible necrosis of choriocarcinoma, and administered it further until the chorionic gonadotropin secreted by the choriocarcinoma cells completely disappeared, which led to full recovery from choriocarcinoma. Furthermore, in 1974, E. Frei of the NCI effectively treated osteosarcoma with high-dose MTX combination therapy. MTX is still used widely for various carcinomas, despite its long history.

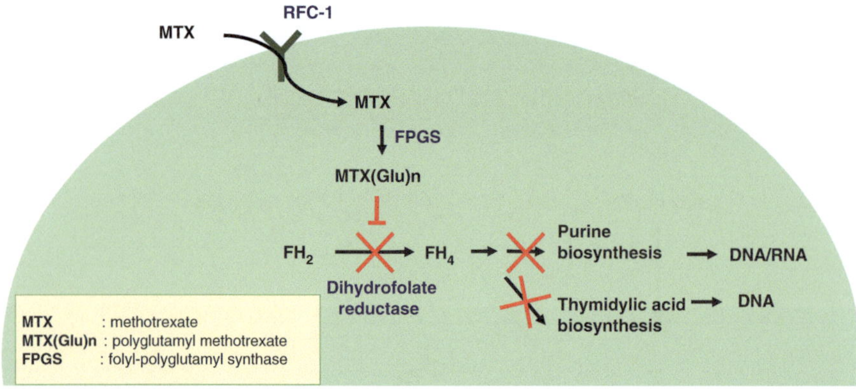

Fig. 5.4 Mechanism of action of methotrexate. Methotrexate is transported into the cell by reduced folate carrier type-1 (*RFC-1*), a membrane protein involved in the transport of folic acid. Some methotrexate is converted into polyglutamyl methotrexate [*MTX (Glu)n*] by folly-polyglutamyl synthase (*FPGS*), after which polyglutamyl methotrexate inhibits dihydrofolate reductase, thereby suppressing synthesis of tetrahydrofolic acid (*FH4*) from folic acid (*FH2*) and ultimately inhibiting DNA synthesis because of a deficiency of thymidylic acid and purine nucleotide within the cell

In 1958, M. Osborn and F. Heunnekens of the University of Washington defined the mechanisms underlying MTX actions. MTX binds DHFR and inhibits the reduction of folic acid (FH2) to tetrahydrofolic acid (FH4), eventually inhibiting DNA synthesis due to the lack of thymidylic acid in cells (Fig. 5.4) [8]. Metabolic studies of MTX revealed that the drug enters the cell through the reduced folate carrier type-1 (RFC-1), and is partly converted to polyglutamyl methotrexate via folyl-polyglutamyl synthase (FPGS) in the cell. Polyglutamyl methotrexate inhibits not only DHFR but also efflux pumps that cause drug resistance, enabling efficient MTX activity within the cell and inhibition of TS and glycinamide ribonucleotide formyltransferase (GARFT).

5.1.2 *Pemetrexed*

After the anticancer efficacy of MTX was established, many inhibitors that target enzymes responsible for the action of MTX have been synthesized. Among those, pemetrexed was discovered during the search for GARFT inhibitors in a joint study conducted by E.C. Taylor of Princeton University and Eli Lilly and Company. In 1992, it was found to have an anticancer effect by strongly inhibiting TS [9]. Pemetrexed inhibits DHFR about 1/1,000 times more weakly than MTX, and inhibits TS more strongly when converted to polyglutamyl pemetrexed by FPGS (Fig. 5.5). In clinical trials, pemetrexed showed clinical efficacy in various cancers such as breast, bladder, colon, and non-small-cell lung cancers, and was especially effective against malignant mesothelioma [10]. In 2004, FDA approved the combination therapy of pemetrexed and cisplatin for the treatment of malignant mesothelioma. Later, in 2008, the FDA further approved the use of this combination therapy

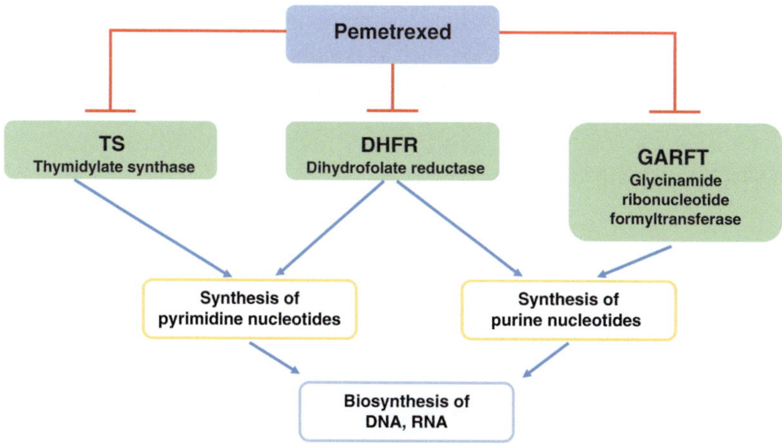

Fig. 5.5 Mechanism of action of pemetrexed. Pemetrexed is an antifolate agent that inhibits the action of enzymes involved in the pyrimidine and purine cycle. Pemetrexed interferes with dihydrofolate reductase (*DHFR*) and thymidylate synthase (*TS*), thereby inhibiting pyrimidine synthesis. Pemetrexed also inhibits purine synthesis by interfering with the action of DHFR and glycinamide ribonucleotide formyl transferase (*GARFT*). Therefore, pemetrexed inhibits DNA and RNA synthesis by reducing the abundance of pyrimidines and purines

for patients with locally advanced or metastatic non-small-cell lung cancer (excluding squamous cell carcinoma). Pemetrexed was also approved for use in maintenance therapy after first-line therapy for lung cancer. Currently, it is a potent anticancer drug widely used in lung adenocarcinoma patients.

5.1.3 *Pralatrexate*

Pralatrexate, an MTX analog, was synthesized in the 1950s at the Stanford Research Institute (SRI) International, and showed anticancer activity in animal models. In the 1970s, F.M. Sirotnak of the Memorial Sloan Kettering Cancer Center observed that several types of cancer cells showed high absorption of folic acid in the cell and that the membranous protein RFC-1, involved in such a phenomenon, was overexpressed in cancer cells [11]. Sirotnak started to develop antimetabolic drugs that strongly bind to RFC-1 and are transferred into the cell more easily than folic acid or MTX, consequently inhibiting the DHFR in the cancer cells. In the joint study of SRI International and the Southern Research Institute to discover a substance that could bind to RFC-1 more strongly than MTX, they discovered a 10-deaza derivative in 1984, which is an N^{10} substituent of aminopterin [12]. The efficacy of this drug was further improved by synthesizing a 10-deaza-ethyl derivative in 1987 and 10-deaza propargyl derivative named pralatrexate in 1998 [13, 14].

Pralatrexate has high affinity for RFC-1 than MTX (14 times more). Compared to MTX, pralatrexate shows 10-fold conversion to the polyglutamylated form, thus having the advantage of much greater accumulation in cells. The accumulated polyglutamylated pralatrexate effectively inhibits DHFR, suppressing DNA synthesis and leading to cell death. Later clinical studies reported that pralatrexate is exceptionally effective in hematologic cancers such as lymphoma and leukemia. In 2009, it was approved as a treatment for peripheral T-cell lymphoma.

5.2 Purine Analogs

Purine antimetabolites such as 6-mercaptopurine (6-MP), 6-thioguanine (6-TG), fludarabine, pentostatin, cladribine, clofarabine, and nelarabine have been developed and used clinically (Fig. 5.6).

5.2.1 6-Mercaptopurine and 6-Thioguanine

The purine antimetabolite 6-MP was the second antimetabolite drug developed. Biochemist G. Hitchings of the New York Burroughs Wellcome & Company (now GlaxoSmithKline) assumed that nucleic acids such as DNA and RNA might have important roles in cell division as biopolymers, and developed some nucleic acid

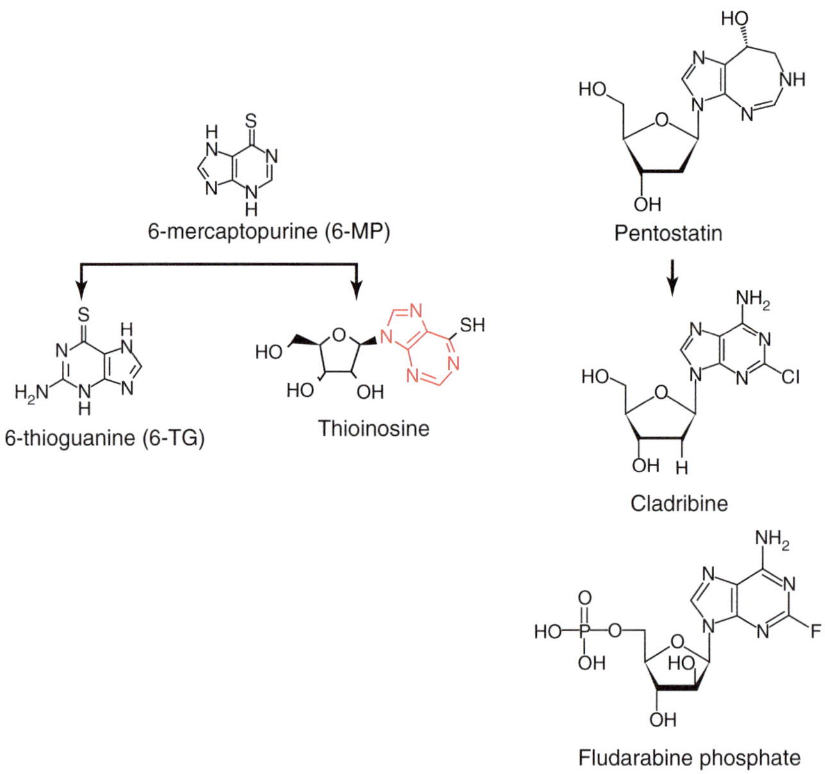

Fig. 5.6 Types of purine analogs and the process of their development

synthesis inhibitors, expecting that these antimetabolite drugs could treat bacterial infectious diseases or cell proliferative diseases such as cancer. G. Elion of this research team focused on purine, one of the DNA precursors, and synthesized a purine analog to study its inhibitory effect on the proliferation of *Lactobacillus casei* [15]. In 1951, Elion discovered that 6-MP strongly suppressed bacterial proliferation. The Sloan-Kettering Institute confirmed its anticancer activity in an animal cancer model [16]. 6-MP is a purine derivative with the 6-OH of hypoxanthine substituted with a thiol (-SH) group. 6-TG was developed later on by substituting guanine similarly [17].

In 1953, J.H. Burchenal conducted a clinical trial of 6-MP on patients with acute lymphoblastic leukemia and observed a durable anticancer effect for 1 year median survival that was superior to that of MTX [18]. Based on this result, the FDA approved 6-MP in 1953 as a drug for acute lymphoma. The clinical efficacy of 6-MP was also observed in patients whose lymphoma progressed even after aminopterin treatment, which suggested the different mechanisms of action for these two drugs. This marked the start of the combination therapy that has since been widely used for cancer treatment. Based on these findings, E. Frei et al. of NCI treated pediatric acute lymphocytic leukemia with POMP combination therapy of 6-MP, MTX, prednisone, and vincristine in 1965, thereby ushering the age of combination chemotherapy. 6-MP is still widely used. G. Elion and G.H. Hitchings developed another purine analog named 6-thioguanine, which was approved by FDA in 1966 as a therapeutic agent for leukemia.

6-MP acts as a prodrug and is converted to thioinosine monophosphate (TIMP) by hypoxanthine-guanine phosphoribosyltransferase within the body. It has been revealed that TIMP suppresses the enzyme that acts in the early stages of purine biosynthesis and induces cell death since its structure that is similar to that of nucleoside monophosphates such as adenine or guanine [19, 20].

5.2.2 Fludarabine

J.A. Montgomery and K. Hewson of the Southern Research Institute developed 2-fluoroadenosine in 1957 by adding fluorine to adenosine, taking a cue from 5-fluorouracil, which C. Heidelberger developed earlier as an anticancer drug [21]. However, this drug could not be used as an anticancer drug because of its strong toxicity, which was observed in an animal tumor transplant model.

In 1960, B.R. Baker et al. of the Stanford Research Institute developed the adenine arabinoside derivative, vidarabine (ara-A) for anticancer drugs [22]. However, it was ineffective as an anticancer drug because it is rapidly deaminated by adenosine deaminase. It was then developed as an antiviral drug because it inhibited viral proliferation.

The Montgomery group developed fludarabine (F-ara-A) in 1969, a derivative of vidarabine with fluorine attached at C-2, to avoid deamination. It was based on the fact that 2-fluoroadenosine was not deaminated by adenosine deaminase [23]. Later on, studies on the mechanism of action of F-ara-A revealed that it inhibits DNA polymerase and ribonucleotide reductase as well, leading to blockage of ribonucleotide conversion to deoxyribonucleotide [24]. This action of F-ara-A eventually inhibits normal DNA synthesis, suppressing cancer cell growth (Fig. 5.7).

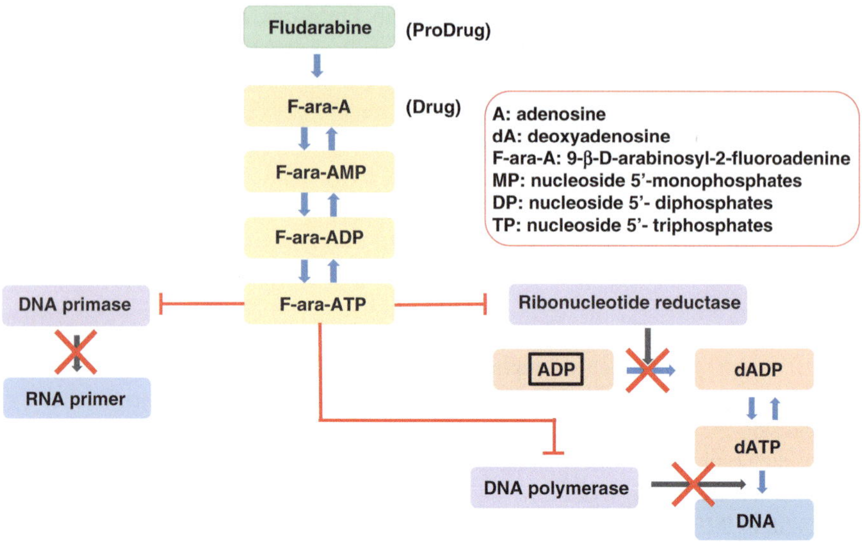

Fig. 5.7 Mechanism of action of fludarabine. The action of fludarabine requires conversion of the drug to F-ara-ATP. The main effect of F-ara-ATP is suppression of DNA synthesis via inhibition of various DNA synthesis-related enzymes. In particular, F-ara-ATP acts as a competitive inhibitor of dATP and inhibits DNA polymerase. F-ara-ATP also interferes with the action of DNA primase, which synthesizes RNA primers required for DNA polymerase to recognize the point at which synthesis of the DNA strand begins. Moreover, F-ara-ATP inhibits the action of ribonucleotide reductase, decreasing the pool of the deoxyribonucleotide maintained within the cell by this enzyme, leading to an increase in the effect of fludarabine on DNA synthesis. The effects of F-ara-ATP described above bring about the blockage of DNA synthesis and cause apoptosis

Fludarabine showed an excellent efficacy in treating B cell chronic lymphoma in clinical trials, for which it was approved by FDA in 1991. It is also widely used in combination chemotherapy for non-Hodgkin's lymphoma and acute myelogenous leukemia.

5.2.3 Pentostatin (2'-deoxycoformycin)

P.W.K. Woo et al. of Parke Davis & Co., a pharmaceutical company in the U.S., discovered a strong inhibitor of adenosine deaminase (ADA) named pentostatin (deoxycoformycin and covidarabine) in the culture medium of *Streptomyces antibioticus* in 1974 [25]. Pentostatin suppresses adenosine deaminase because its structure is similar to the transition state of the deamination reaction of adenosine by adenosine deaminase.

Adenosine deaminase is an enzyme involved in the catabolism of adenosine and deoxyadenosine. In 1972, geneticist E.R. Giblett et al. of Seattle's King County Central Blood Bank Inc. and H.J. Meuwissen et al. of New York Albany Medical College discovered that the genetic disease, severe combined immunodeficiency (SCID), was induced by mutation of adenosine deaminase [26]. In 1978, M.S. Coleman et al. of the Kentucky Medical Center studied the pathogenesis of SCID and discovered adenosine deaminase deficiency in the patient's erythrocytes and lymphocytes, accompanied by accumulation of dATP in the cells. They predicted that the high dATP concentration would disturb lymphocyte development and proliferation [27].

Based on these discoveries, K.R. Harrap of the United Kingdom's Institute of Cancer Research assumed that treatment of lymphocytic leukemia would be possible through suppression of adenosine deaminase, and first reported, in 1979, that the adenosine deaminase inhibitor pentostatin might have an anticancer effect [28]. Later, in 1981, M.R. Grever et al. of Ohio State University observed the curative effect of pentostatin in T lymphocytic leukemia patients [29]. Large-scale clinical trials showed the excellent efficacy of pentostatin in hairy-cell leukemia, a type of B lymphocytic leukemia, which resulted in its FDA approval in 1991. Pentostatin also showed remission in other hematologic cancers such as chronic and acute lymphocytic leukemia, acute promyelocytic leukemia, and acute myelocytic leukemia. This drug is still frequently used for the treatment of these cancers.

Pentostatin inhibits adenosine deaminase, which leads to the accumulation of dATP in the cells and then the accumulated dATP perturbs the activity of ribonucleotide reductase, resulting in the death of cancer cells.

5.2.4 *Cladribine*

Toxicities such as hepatotoxicity, nephrotoxicity, and neurotoxicity were reported for pentostatin. This led to research on purine analogs with fewer side effects. As a result, cladribine (2-chlorodeoxyadenosine), with fewer side effects, was discovered (Fig. 5.8). Cladribine contains chlorine bound to the C-2 of deoxyadenosine.

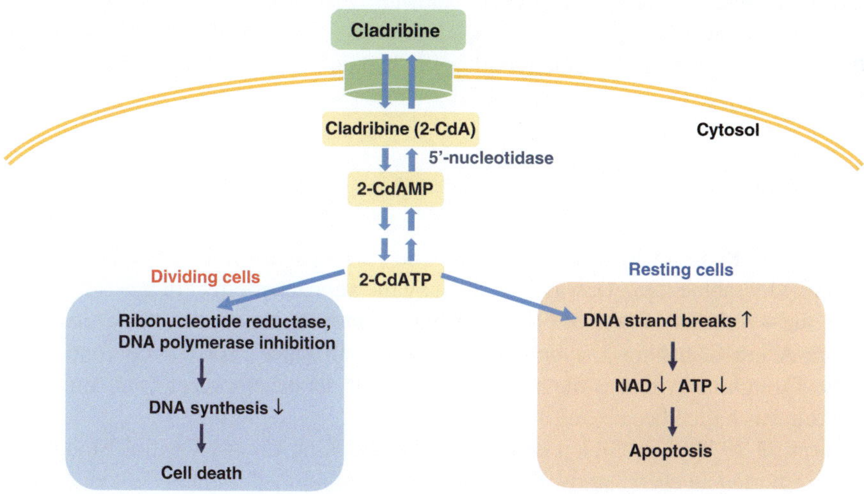

Fig. 5.8 Mechanism of action of cladribine. Cladribine (2-CdA) enters lymphocytes via a membrane transporter. Subsquently, cladribine is phosphorylated by deoxycytidine kinase, forming 2-CdATP, which is toxic to lymphocytes. In proliferating cells, accumulation of 2-CdATP interferes with ribonucleotide reductase and DNA polymerase, inhibiting DNA synthesis and causing apoptosis. In resting cells, cladribine induces apoptosis by depleting NAD and ATP

L.F. Christensen et al. of the University of Utah developed it in 1972, and its anticancer effect was studied in an L-1210 murine leukemia model [30].

In the 1980s, hematologist D. Carson of Scripps Research Institute searched for a metabolic toxic drug that could treat lymphocytic leukemia using the deoxycytidine kinase expressed in lymophocytes, and found that cladribine had such efficacy [31]. It was revealed in 1988 that this drug acts as a stable substrate analog of adenosine deaminase and inhibits its activity. It was further shown to suppress the activity of ribonucleotide reductase when converted to 2-CdATP through phosphorylation by deoxycytidine kinase [32]. D. Carson and E. Beutler conducted clinical trials that showed the clear effect of cladribine in hairy-cell leukemia, due to which it received FDA approval in 1993 as a drug against hairy-cell leukemia [33].

5.2.5 Clofarabine

Fludarabine and cladribine are not degraded by adenosine deamination, but the loss of their efficacy due to the phosphorolysis caused by purine nucleoside phosphorylase (PNP) was not resolved. In addition, the serious neurotoxicity of fludarabine led to the development of a drug that could overcome these drawbacks.

J.A. Montgomery group of the Southern Research Institute synthesized various 2′-fluoro-2-halo derivatives from 9-β-D-arabinofuranosyladenine and examined their anticancer efficacy. They discovered clofarabine with less susceptibility for phosphorolysis and low neurotoxicity [34].

Clofarabine showed an anticancer activity by inhibiting ribonucleotide reductase and DNA polymerase after phosphorylation [35]. Clinical trials that targeted refractory acute lymphocytic leukemia patients showed reduction in side effects and improved treatment efficacy. Accordingly, clofarabine received FDA approval in 2004 as a therapeutic drug for acute lymphocytic leukemia. It is still widely used.

5.2.6 Nelarabine

L. Goodman of Stanford Research Institute, who participated in the development research on vidarabine (ara-A), was motivated by the anticancer effect of ara-A and reported the synthesis of ara-G (9-β-D-arabinofuranosylguanine) in 1964 [36]. Unlike ara-A, ara-C, and ara-T, which exist as natural substances, ara-G is not found naturally. Though its synthesis method was developed, its development as an anticancer drug was halted because of its low solubility.

However, in 1975, E.R. Giblett et al. of the Seattle King County Central Blood Bank Inc. reported a genetic study, which proved that combined immunodeficiency disease (CID) was not caused by deficiency of adenosine deaminase (ADA) but that of purine nucleoside phosphorylase (PNP) [37]. PNP was revealed as an enzyme involved in the metabolism of purine nucleosides into the base and the ribose-1-phosphate. dGTP was accumulated in T lymphocytes specifically in this genetic disease, inducing T-cell lymphopenia.

Based on these findings, researchers studied the possibility of treating T-cell acute lymphocytic leukemia (T-ALL) through dGTP accumulation by the inhibition of PNP. Among them, L. J. Gudas et al. of University of California, San Francisco (UCSF) reported in 1978 that, deoxyguanosine inhibited DNA synthesis in T-ALL cells leading to leukemic cell death [38].

However, deoxyguanosine could not be used as an anticancer drug because PNP rapidly degrades deoxyguanosine *in vivo*. Therefore, there were attempts to develop a PNP-resistant deoxyguanosine analog ara-G into drugs. However, ara-G has low solubility, so researches continued to solve this problem.

In 1995, C.U. Lambe and T.A. Krenitsky et al. of Burroughs Wellcome Co. developed a prodrug of ara-G called nelarabine, the solubility of which was eight times higher than that of ara-G, and confirmed its efficacy in animal tumor models [39]. Nelarabine was converted to ara-G, forming ara-GTP, which interfered with the DNA synthesis, but the precise anticancer mechanism is unknown. Nelarabine showed a curative effect in a clinical trial that targeted T-ALL and T-cell lymphoblastic lymphoma (T-LBL) patients, and received FDA approval as the therapeutic agent for T-ALL and T-LBL in 2005. It is currently used clinically.

5.3 Pyrimidine Analogs

Starting with the development of 5-fluorouracil (5-FU), pyrimidine analog anticancer drugs such as capecitabine, cytarabine, and gemcitabine have been developed and are now being used clinically (Fig. 5.9).

5.3.1 Fluoropyrimidines

5.3.1.1 5-Fluorouracil (5-FU) and 5-Fluorodeoxyuridine Monophosphate (FdUMP)

5-FU is one of the early anticancer drugs to be developed, but it is an effective drug still widely used for solid tumors. In the mid-1950s, C. Heidelberger of the University of Wisconsin focused on the study of fluoro-substituted bioorganic molecules as fluorine is reported to have various physiologic effects. Various fluoro substituted bioorganic compounds were screened for anticancer properties.

Heidelberger heard that A. Cantarow and K. Paschkis of Jefferson Medical College reported the selective absorption of radioisotope-traced uracil by liver can-

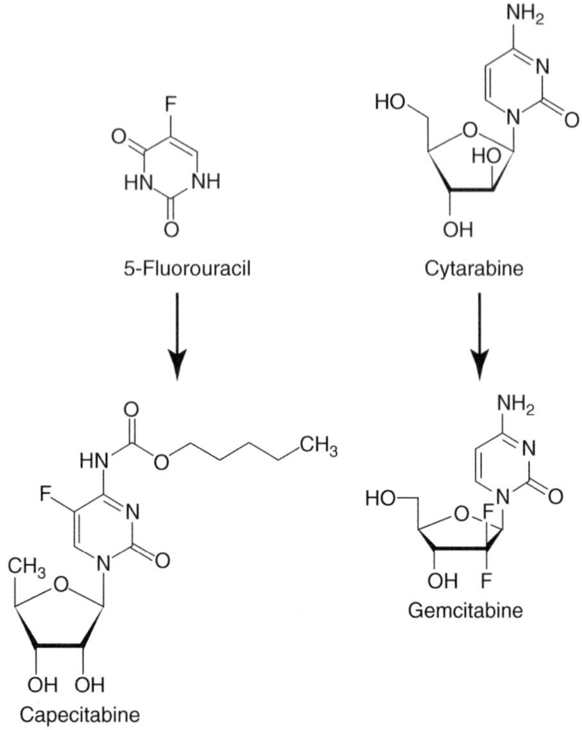

Fig. 5.9 Types of pyrimidine analogs and the process of their development

cer cells than normal liver cells in a mouse in 1954 [40]. Hence, Heidelberger decided to investigate the anticancer effect of the fluorine substituent uracil derivatives. Various fluoropyrimidine derivatives were synthesized and examined for their efficacy in transplant tumor animal models in a joint study conducted by R. Duschinsky and R. Schnitzer of Hoffmann-LaRoche. They reported potent anticancer activities of 5-FU and 5-fluoroorotic acid in 1957 [41].

Later, in 1959, Heidelberger studied the mechanism of 5-FU's anticancer effect. It was revealed that 5-FU is converted into FdUMP *in vivo* and inhibits DNA synthesis by targeting thymidylate synthase (TS) (Fig. 5.10) [42, 43]. Moreover, in 1974, D.V. Santi et al. of UCSF revealed the molecular mechanism by which TS covalently binds with FdUMP, then reacts with the methylene group provided by 5,10-methylene tetrahydrofolate, forming a TS-FdUMP-CH_2H_4folate complex and suppressing the activity of TS [44].

Clinical trials of 5-FU were conducted against various types of cancer. It showed clinical efficacy in epithelial cancers of the colon, rectum, breast, stomach, and pancreas. Thus, FDA approved 5-FU in 1962. Heidelberger also synthesized 5-fluorodeoxyuridine monophosphate (FdUMP), the intermediate product of 5-FU and found its anticancer effect [45]. The clinical trial data showed the curative effect of FdUMP in gastrointestinal adenocarcinoma patients, and hence approved by FDA in 1970 for gastrointestinal adenocarcinomas.

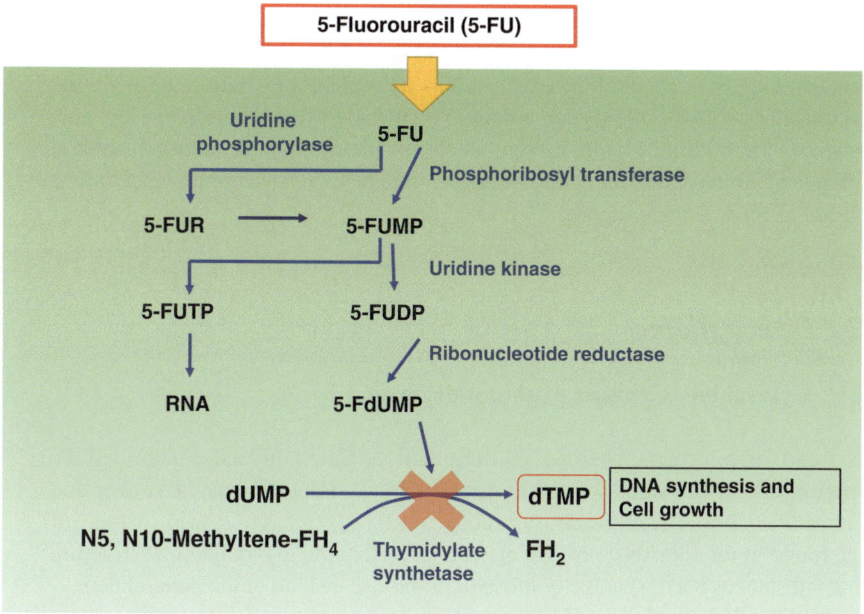

Fig. 5.10 Mechanism of action of 5-fluorouracil. 5-Fluorouracil (5-FU) is converted to 5-FdUMP via several biochemical reactions, after which it prevents the formation of thymidylate, an important DNA precursor, by inhibiting thymidylate synthetase. 5-FU also interferes with transcription by inserting itself in place of uracil during the process of RNA synthesis

Interestingly, the mechanism and toxicities of 5-FU are also known to be affected by the 5-FU infusion method. 5-FU shows an anticancer effect by suppressing RNA synthesis when given in bolus, with more hematologic toxicity due to bone marrow suppression. On the other hand, 5-FU mainly suppresses TS and causes oral mucositis or hand-foot syndrome when continuously infused. The 5-FU plus oxaliplatin (FOLFOX) therapy, which uses both types of infusion, is currently mainly used to treat colon and gastric cancer.

5.3.1.2 Capecitabine

5-FU was found to have very low bioavailability due to its short half-life since it is metabolized by dihydrouracil dehydrogenase, in liver. In 1998, Nippon Roche Company developed an orally administered prodrug of 5-FU named fluoropyrimidine carbamate (capecitabine), which had 70–80 % higher bioavailability than that of 5-FU [46]. This drug caused cytotoxicity by forming 5-FU through a three-step reaction. Especially, the thymidine or uridine phosphorylases acting in the last step are more active in cancer cells than normal cells. Hence, the prodrug is selective towards cancer cells.

Capecitabine was approved in 1998 as a therapeutic agent for colon cancer. It is also effectively used against breast, gastric, and pancreatic cancer.

The advantage of capecitabine over 5-FU is its oral administration with comparable anticancer effect. Patients can continue their daily life without long-term hospitalization. In addition, side effects such as chemotherapy-induced nausea, vomiting, and alopecia, are reduced. This has led to the extensive use of capecitabine than 5-FU as an anticancer agent.

5.3.2 *Deoxycytidine*

5.3.2.1 Cytarabine (Cytosine Arabinoside, ara-C)

In 1951 and 1955, organic chemist W. Bergmann of Yale University identified the new pyrimidine nucleosides spongothymidine (3-β-D-arabofuranosylthymine) and spongouridine (3-β-D-arabofuranosyluracil) from *Cryptotethia crypta*, a type of sponge found in the Florida coast. He also revealed that the glycochemical structure of these substances had a specific pentose of arabinose instead of the general deoxyribose used in DNA synthesis [47].

In 1956, biochemist S. Cohen of University of Pennsylvania observed the *E. coli* growth inhibition effect of spongothymidine and proposed the possibility to develop this unusual nucleoside as an anticancer drug [48]. After that, several groups chemically synthesized arabinose nucleoside. Among them, C. Dekker's group at the University of California, Berkeley synthesized an arabinosyl cytosine, cytarabine, in 1959 [49]. Later, C.J. Kensler et al. of the Boston University School of Medicine reported cytarabine's curative effect in several animal cancer models in 1965 [50].

In the late 1960s, cytarabine showed an excellent effect in various hematologic malignancies, including pediatric acute lymphocytic leukemia (ALL), chronic myelogenous leukemia (CML), and acute myelogenous leukemia (AML). FDA approved cytarabine against hematologic malignancies in 1969, and it is still widely used.

Cohen et al. studied the mechanism of cytarabine, and revealed in 1968 that cytarabine is converted to ara-CTP through phosphorylation in cancer cells, suppressing the DNA polymerase and inducing cell death (Fig. 5.11) [51].

5.3.2.2 Gemcitabine (2′, 2′-difluoro-2′-deoxycytidine, dFdC)

Cytarabine had the shortcoming of rapid inactivation by cytidine deaminase into ara-U, which has no anticancer effect, when it is absorbed by the body. Thus, studies were pursued to overcome this problem. L. Hertel of Eli Lilly and Company, who was developing antiviral drugs, reported in 1968 various novel compounds with two fluorines instead of hydrogens attached to C-2′ of deoxyribopyrimidine and deoxyarabinopyrimidine [52]. Later, in 1990, his team found that the 2′, 2′-difluoro-2′-deoxycytidine (gemcitabine) showed an anticancer effect superior to that of cytarabine in various animal tumor models [53].

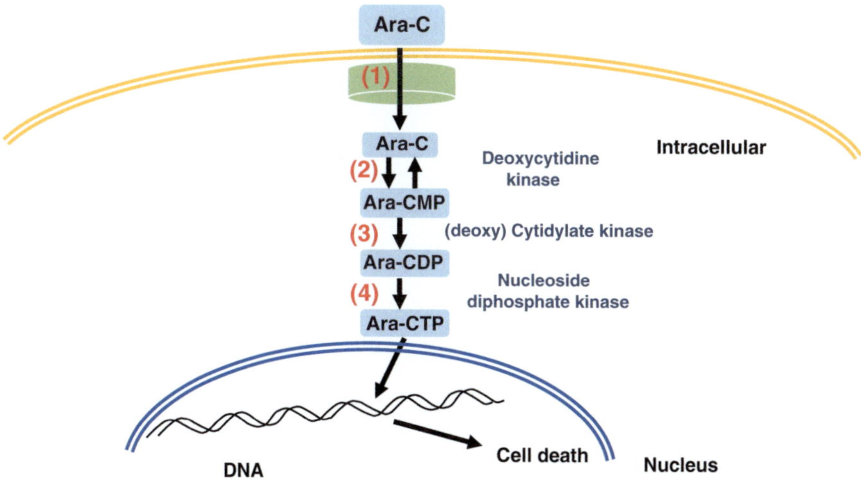

Fig. 5.11 Mechanism of action of cytarabine. Nucleoside transporter (*hENT1*) promotes the entry of cytarabine (*ara-C*) into the cell (*1*). Once inside the cell, cytarabine (ara-C) is phosphorylated by deoxycytosine kinase (dCK) to form ara-CMP (*2*). Subsequently, ara-CTP is produced by (deoxy) cytidylate kinase (UMP-CMPK) (*3*) and nucleoside diphosphate kinase (NDK) (*4*). The resulting ara-CTP causes apoptosis by inserting itself into DNA during DNA synthesis

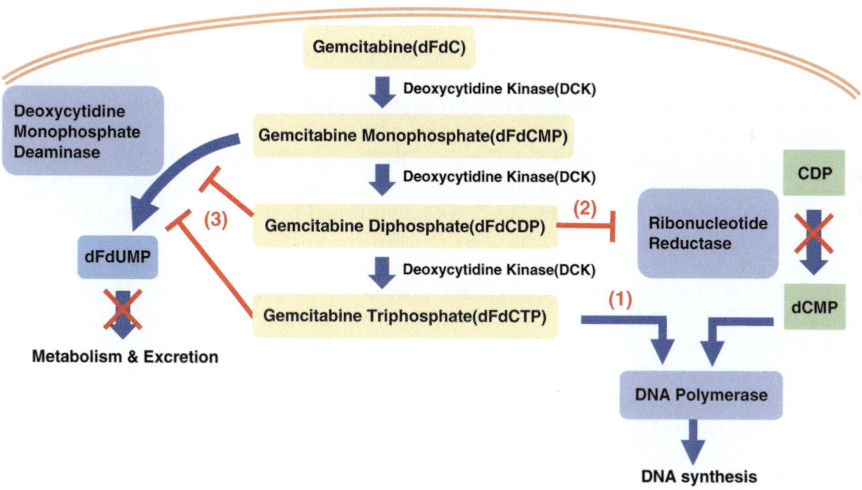

Fig. 5.12 Mechanism of action of gemcitabine. Gemcitabine (*dFdC*) undergoes phosphorylation by deoxycytidine kinase to form gemcitabine diphosphate (*dFdCDP*), followed by conversion to gemcitabine triphosphate (*dFdCTP*), which inserts itself into DNA and interferes with DNA synthesis (*1*). dFdCDP also inhibits ribonucleotide reductase and blocks formation of deoxycytidine monophosphate (*dCMP*) (*2*), which acts as a substrate in the process of DNA replication. Additionally, because dFdCDP inhibits deoxycytidine monophosphate deaminase, gemcitabine is not dgraded and acts continuously (*3*). *dFdC* 2′-deoxy-2′,2′-difluorocytidine, *dFdUMP* 2′-deoxy-2′,2′-difluorouridine monophosphate, *CDP* cytidine diphosphate, *dCMP* deoxycytidine monophosphate

Gemcitabine has a longer half-life than cytarabine, and is converted to dFdCDP and dFdCTP, as is cytarabine, suppressing ribonucleotide reductase that is involved in the dCTP synthesis required in DNA replication. It also inhibits cell growth by suppressing the DNA polymerases α/ε (Fig. 5.12) [54, 55]. Gemcitabine showed an outstanding anticancer properties in clinical trials of various solid carcinomas, unlike cytarabine, which shows little effect in solid tumors, and was approved for malignant pancreatic cancer treatment in 1996. Since then, it has been approved for the treatment of non-small-cell lung cancer, breast cancer, biliary tract cancer, ovarian cancer, etc. It is still widely used.

References

1. Wills L (1978) A biographical sketch. J Nutr 108:1379–1383
2. Farber S, Cutler EC, Hawkins JW, Harrison JH, Peirce EC 2nd, Lenz GG (1947) The action of pteroylglutamic conjugates on man. Science 106:619–621
3. Seeger D, Smith J, Hultquist M (1947) Antagonist for pteroylglutamic acid. J Am Chem Soc 69:2567
4. Farber S, Diamond LK, Mercer RD et al (1948) Temporary remission in acute leukaemia in children produced by folic acid antagonists. N Engl J Med 238:787–793
5. Seeger D, Cosulich DB, Smith JM Jr, Hultquist M (1949) Analogs of pteroylglutamic acid. III. 4-Amino derivatives. J Am Chem Soc 71:1753–1758
6. Wright JC, Prigot A, Wright BP, Weintraub S, Wright LT (1951) An evaluation of folic acid antagonists in adults with neoplastic diseases. A study of 93 patients with incurable neoplasms. J Natl Med Assoc 43:211–240
7. Li MC, Li R, Spencer DB (1956) Effect of methotrexate upon choriocarcinoma. Proc Soc Exp Biol Med 93:361–366
8. Osborn MJ, Freeman M, Huennekens FM (1958) Inhibition of dihydrofolic reductase by aminopterin and amethopterin. Proc Soc Exptl Biol Med 97:429–431
9. Taylor EC, Kuhnt D, Shih C, Rinzel SM, Grindey GB, Barredo J, Jannatipour M, Moran RG (1992) A dideazatetrahydrofolate analogue lacking a chiral center at C-6, N-[4-[2-(2-amino-3,4 dihydro-4-oxo-7H-pyrrolo[2,3-d]pyrimidin-5-yl)ethyl] benzoyl]-L-glutamic acid, is an inhibitor of thymidylate synthase. J Med Chem 35:4450–4454
10. Vogelzang NJ et al (2003) Phase III study of pemetrexed in combination with cisplatin versus cisplatin alone in patients with malignant pleural mesothelioma. J Clin Oncol 21:2636–2644
11. Sirotnak FM, Donsbach RC (1976) Kinetic correlates of methotrexate transport and therapeutic responsiveness in murine tumors. Cancer Res 36:1151–1158
12. Sirotnak FM, DeGraw JI, Moccio DM, Samuels LL, Goutas LJ (1984) New folate analogs of the 10-deaza-aminopterin series. Basis for structural design and biochemical and pharmacologic properties. Cancer Chemother Pharmacol 12:18–25
13. Sirotnak FM, Schmid FA, Samuels LL et al (1987) 10-Ethyl-10-deaza-aminopterin: structural design and biochemical, pharmacologic, and antitumor properties. NCI Monogr 15:127–131
14. Sirotnak FM, DeGraw JI, Colwell WT et al (1998) A new analogue of 10-deazaaminopterin with markedly enhanced curative effects against human tumor xenografts in mice. Cancer Chemother Pharmacol 42:313–318
15. Elion GB, Hitchings GB, Vanderwerff H (1951) Antagonists of nucleic acid derivatives. VI. Purines. J Biol Chem 192:505–518
16. Clarke DA, Philips FS, Sternberg SS, Stock CC, Elion GB, Hitchings GH (1953) 6-Mercaptopurine: effects in mouse sarcoma 180 and in normal animals. Cancer Res 13:593–604
17. Elion GB, Hitchings GH (1955) The synthesis of 6-thioguanine. J Am Chem Soc 77:1676

18. Burchenal JH, Murphy ML, Ellison RR et al (1953) Clinical evaluation of a new antimetabolite, 6 mercaptopurine in the treatment of leukemia and allied diseases. Blood 8:965–999
19. Skipper HE (1954) On the mechanism of action of 6-mercaptopurine. Ann NY Acad Sci 60:315–321
20. Elion GB (1967) Biochemistry and pharmacology of purine analogs. Fed Proc 26:898–904
21. Montgomery JA, Hewson K (1957) Synthesis of potential anticancer agents. X. 2-Fluoroadenosine. J Am Chem Soc 79:4559–4560
22. Lee WW, Benitez A, Goodman L, Baker BR (1960) Potential anticancer agents. XL. Synthesis of the b-anomer of 9-(d-arabinofuranosyl)-adenine. J Am Chem Soc 82:2648–2649
23. Montgomery JA, Hewson K (1969) Nucleosides of 2-fluoroadenine. J Med Chem 12:498–504
24. Tseng WC, Derse D, Cheng Y-C et al (1982) *In vitro* activity of 9-b-D-arabinofuranosyl-2--fluoroadenine and the biochemical actions of its triphosphate on DNA polymerases and ribonucleotide reductase from HeLa cells. Mol Pharmacol 21:474–477
25. Woo PWK, Dion HW, Lange SM, Dahi LF, Durham LJ (1974) A novel adenosine ara-A deaminase inhihitor, (R)-3-(2-deoxy-b-D-erythro-pentofuranosyl)-3.6.7.8-trtrahydro-imidazo[4.5-d][1,3]diazepin-8-ol. J Heterocycl Chem 11:641–643
26. Giblett ER, Anderson JE, Cohen F, Pollara B, Meuwissen HJ (1972) Adenosine-deaminase deficiency in two patients with severely impaired cellular immunity. Lancet 320:1067–1069
27. Coleman MS, Donofrio J, Hutton JJ, Hahn L, Daoud A, Lampkin B, Dyminski J (1978) Identification and quantitation of adenine deoxynucleotides in erythrocytes of a patient with adenosine deaminase deficiency and severe combined immunodeficiency. J Biol Chem 253:1619–1626
28. Paine RM, Smyth JF, Harrap KR (1979) Biochemical consequences of treatment with the adenosine deaminase inhibitor 2'-deoxycoformycin. Adv Exp Med Biol 122:365–371
29. Grever MR, Siaw MF, Jacob WF et al (1981) The biochemical and clinical consequences of 2′-deoxycoformycin in refractory lymphoproliferative malignancy. Blood 57:406–417
30. Christensen LF, Broom AD, Robins MJ, Bloch A (1972) Synthesis and biological activity of selected 2,6-disubstituted-(2-deoxy-a-and-b-D-erythro-pentofuranosyl) purines. J Med Chem 5:735–739
31. Carson DA, Wasson DB, Beutler E (1984) Antileukemic and immunosuppressive activity of 2-chloro-2'-deoxyadenosine. Proc Natl Acad Sci 81:2232–2236
32. Parker WB, Bapat AR, Shen JX et al (1988) Interaction of 2-halogenated dATP analogs (F, Cl and Br) with human DNA polymerases, DNA primase, and ribonucleotide reductase. Mol Pharmacol 34:485–491
33. Piro LD, Carrera CJ, Carson DA, Beutler E (1990) Lasting remissions in hairy-cell leukemia induced by a single infusion of 2-chlorodeoxyadenosine. N Engl J Med 322:1117–1121
34. Montgomery JA, Shortnacy-Fowler AT, Clayton SD, Riordan JM, Secrist JA 3rd (1992) Synthesis and biologic activity of 2′-fluoro-2-halo derivatives of 9-b-D-arabinofuranosyladenine. J Med Chem 35:397–401
35. Parker WB, Shaddix SC, Rose LM et al (1999) Comparison of the mechanism of cytotoxicity of 2-chloro-9-(2-deoxy-2-fluoro-β-D-arabinofuranosyl) adenine, 2-chloro-9-(2-deoxy-2-fluoro-β-D-ribofuranosyl) adenine, 2-chloro-9-(2-deoxy-2,2-difluoro-β-D-ribofuranosyl) adenine in CEM cells. Mol Pharmacol 55:515–520
36. Reist EJ, Goodman L (1964) Synthesis of 9-β-D-arabinofuranosylguanine. Biochemistry 3:15–18
37. Giblett ER, Ammann AJ, Wara DW, Sandman R, Diamond LK (1975) Nucleoside-phosphorylase deficiency in a child with severely defective T-cell immunity and normal B-cell immunity. Lancet 325:1010–1013
38. Gudas LJ, Ullman B, Cohen A, Martin DW Jr (1978) Deoxyguanosine toxicity in a mouse T lymphoma: relationship to purine nucleoside phosphorylase-associated immune dysfunction. Cell 14:531–538
39. Lambe CU, Averett DR, Paff MT et al (1995) 2-Amino-6-methoxypurine arabinoside: an agent for T-cell malignancies. Cancer Res 55:3352–3356

40. Rutman RJ, Cantarow A, Paschkis K (1954) Studies in 2-acetylaminofluorene carcinogenesis. III. The utilization of uracil-2-C14 by preneoplastic rat liver and rat hepatoma. Cancer Res 14:119–123
41. Heidelberger C, Chaudhuri NK, Danneberg P et al (1957) Fluorinated pyrimidines, a new class of tumor-inhibitory compounds. Nature 179:663–666
42. Harbers E, Chaudhuri NK, Heidelberger C (1959) Studies on fluorinated pyrimidines: VIII. Further biochemical and metabolic investigations. J Biol Chem 234:1255–1262
43. Heidelberger C, Kaldor G, Muererjee KL, Danneberg PB (1960) Studies on fluorinated pyrimi dines. XI. In vitro studies on tumor resistance. Cancer Res 20:903–909
44. Santi DV, McHenry CS, Sommer H (1974) Mechanism of interaction of thymidylate synthetase with 5-fluorodeoxyuridylate. Biochemistry 13:471–482
45. Heidelberger C, Griesbach L, Cruz O et al (1958) Fluorinated pyrimidines. VI. Effects of 5-fluorouridine and 5-fluoro-2'-deoxyuridine on transplanted tumors. Proc Soc Exp Biol Med 97:470–475
46. Miwa M, Ura M, Nishida M, Sawada N, Ishikawa T, Mori K, Shimma N, Umeda I, Ishitsuka H (1998) Design of a novel oral fluoropyrimidine carbamate, capecitabine, which generates 5-fluorouracil selectively in tumours by enzymes concentrated in human liver and cancer tissue. Eur J Cancer 34:1274–1281
47. Bergmann W, Burke DC (1955) Contributions to the study of marine products. XXXIX. The nucleosides of sponges. III. Spongothymidine and spongouridine. J Org Chem 20:1501–1507
48. Cohen SS, Barner HD (1956) Studies on the induction of thymine deficiency and on the effects of thymine and thymidine analogues in *Escherichia coli*. J Bacteriol 71:588–597
49. Walwick R, Roberts W, Dekker C (1959) Cyclization during the phosphorylation of uridine and cytidine. Proc Chem Soc 3:84
50. Wodinsky I, Kensler CJ (1965) Activity of cytosine arabinoside (NSC 63878) in a spectrum of rodent tumors. Cancer Chemother Rept 47:65–68
51. Furth JJ, Cohen SS (1968) Inhibition of mammalian DNA polymerase by the 5'-triphosphate-1-b-d-arabinofuranosylcytosine and the 5'-triphosphate of 9-b-d-arabinofuranosyladenine. Cancer Res 28:2061–2067
52. Delong DC, Hertel LW, Tang J et al (1986) Antiviral Activity of 2',2'-difluorodeoxycytidine. American Society of Microbiology, Washington, DC, March, Meeting abstract
53. Hertel LW, Boder GB, Kroin JS et al (1990) Evaluation of the antitumor activity of gemcitabine (2',2'-difluoro-2'-deoxycytidine). Cancer Res 50:4417–4422
54. Heinemann V, Xu YZ, Chubb S et al (1990) Inhibition of ribonucleotide reductase in CCRF-CEM cells by 2',2'-difluorodeoxycytidine. Mol Pharmacol 38:567–572
55. Huang P, Chubb S, Hertel LW et al (1991) Action of 2',2'-difluoroxdeoxycytidine on DNA synthesis. Cancer Res 51:6110–6117

Chapter 6
Natural Product Anticancer Drugs

Natural product anticancer drugs that are used clinically include compounds isolated from plants such as the vinca alkaloids, taxane/taxane analogues, podophyllotoxin derivatives, and camptothecin derivatives, as well as anticancer antibiotics isolated from various *Streptomyces* species such as anthracycline/anthracenedione, bleomycin, and actinomycin (Fig. 6.1). Vinca alkaloids and taxane/taxane analogues exhibit anticancer effects by inhibiting the microtubule function of spindle fibers, which is related to chromosome segregation, while podophyllotoxin derivatives, camptothecin derivatives, and other antibiotics cleave DNA bases, causing DNA damage through the suppression of topoisomerase I or II and the production of free radicals.

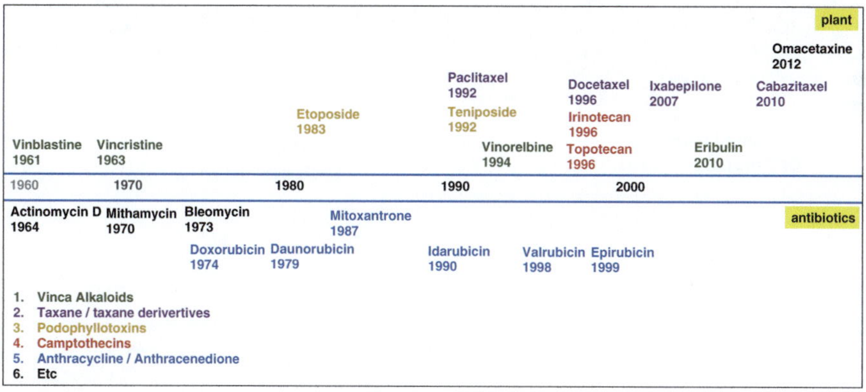

Fig. 6.1 Types of natural product-derived anticancer agents and a chronology of their development

K.-W. Kim et al., *Cancer Drug Discovery*, DOI 10.1007/978-94-024-0844-7_6

6.1 Plant-Derived Anticancer Drugs

6.1.1 Vinca Alkaloids

A number of plant extracts were used in initial anticancer drug development; vinblastine and vincristine are vinca alkaloids, the first approved anticancer drugs derived from plant extracts. Thereafter, vinorelbine, a semisynthetic derivative, was developed with less side effects (Fig. 6.2). Vinca alkaloids exhibit anticancer effects by inhibiting microtubule formation. Halichondrin B, a macrolide with a similar anticancer mechanism, was extracted from sea sponges. Eribulin, an analogous synthetic compound of halichondrin, are clinically used.

6.1.1.1 Vinblastine and Vincristine

The history of anticancer treatment derived from plant extracts in Western literature was first recorded in the book "De Materia Medica (Regarding Medical Materials)" written by P. Dioscorides, an ancient Greek doctor, around first century AD. It described about 400 medicinal plants, and identified *Colchicum autumnale*, a plant

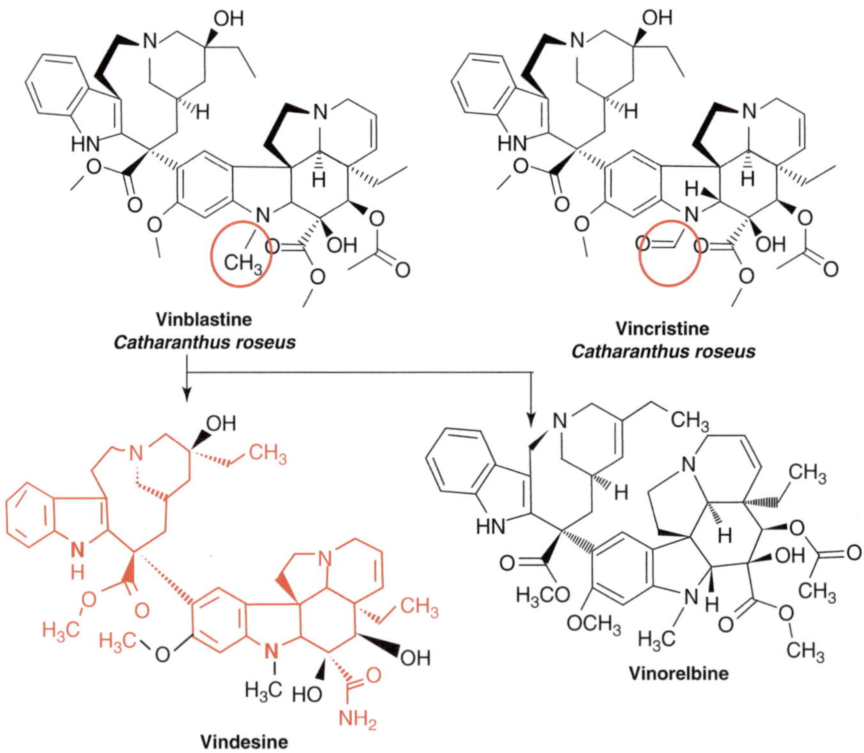

Fig. 6.2 Types of vinca alkaloid and the process of their development

belonging to the liliaceae family, as a treatment for cancer and gout. P.S. Peletier and J. Caventon, French chemists, isolated colchicine, a plant alkaloid and the effective component of *C. autumnale* in 1820.

Thereafter, in 1934, F.J. Lits at Yale University studied the effects of colchicine on cells. He carefully investigated the effect of colchicine treatment on cells of various murine tissues, and observed mitotic arrest in hematopoietic cells and basal cells of epithelium [1].

In 1934, A.P. Dustin et al. of Chicago University reported that colchicine demonstrated anticancer activity in an animal tumor transplantation model by arresting the growth of cancer cells at mitosis [2]. However, marked toxicity was observed in clinical trial, and thus, colchicine's development as a clinical drug was halted. Nonetheless, colchicine provided an opportunity to uncover the functional principles of anticancer drug action at the cellular level, thus playing a fundamental role in the development of vinblastine and vincristine and in identifying the mechanisms of other anticancer effects. Colchicine was approved by the FDA as a gout medicine in 2009, and has been used since for gout treatment.

Vinca alkaloids are a class of over 80 different types of alkaloids extracted from *Vinca minor*, a viny ornamental plant that was described by P. Dioscorides mentioned in the same book as a medicinal plant useful for various symptoms. In 1948, R. Noble of Western Ontario University showed that extracts of *V. rosea* widely used as a folk remedy for diabetes caused hematopenia, from which he predicted its potential as an anticancer drug and showed that it is similar to mustard gas. In 1958, Noble successfully purified vinblastine, the effective component, after a long trial period [3]. Around the same time, G.H. Svoboda et al. from Eli Lilly, were screening for potential diabetes medicines from *V. rosea*, and in 1959, found that an extract fraction demonstrated anticancer effects in an animal model for leukemia [4]. They successfully purified the responsible substance in this fraction in 1962, resulting in the isolation of vincristine, another vinca alkaloid [5].

Subsequently, the functional mechanism of vinblastine and vincristine was studied. In 1960, C.G. Palmer et al. of Indiana University observed that vinblastine arrested the cell cycle at metaphase during cell division in a manner similar to colchicine [6]. Thereafter, a group of researchers observed abnormalities in spindle fiber formation, and K.G. Bensch et al. of Stanford University and R. Marantz et al. of Albert Einstein College of Medicine discovered in 1969 that vinblastine and vincristine bind tubulin, the main constituent protein of the microtubules of spindle fibers [7, 8]. In 1976, R.J. Owellen et al. of Johns Hopkins University showed that the binding of vinblastine to tubulin inhibited the polymerization of microtubules [9], and in 1977, R.W. Tucker of Sidney Farber Cancer Institute revealed that suppression of spindle fiber formation by vinblastine in cells correlated with its cytotoxicity (Fig. 6.3) [10].

Although the structures of vinblastine and vincristine are the same except for the methyl group and the formyl group bound to the indole ring structure, respectively, they have distinct anticancer activities. Vinblastine primarily had potent effects on germ cell cancers, with relatively severe toxicities, whereas vincristine was effective in the treatment of pediatric solid tumors such as Wilms' Tumor, or neuroblastoma, with relatively milder toxicities. Vinblastine and vincristine were approved by the FDA as anticancer drugs in 1961 and 1963, respectively, and are being used currently.

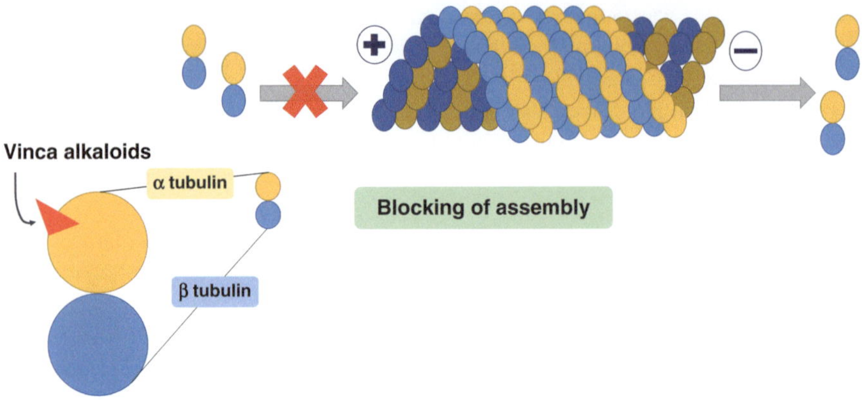

Fig. 6.3 Mechanism of action of vinca alkaloid. α-tubulin and β-tubulin form a head-to-tail polymerization, leading to cylindrical microtubules. Microtubule is formed from binding between alternating tubulin monomers that polymerize in a line, in which an α subunit is exposed at one end and a β subunit is exposed at the other. The exposed α and β ends are referred to as the (−) and (+) ends, respectively. Polymerization occurs at the (+) end, where vinca alkaloids bind to β-tubulin. Although vinca alkaloids do not participate in microtubule breakdown, they can inhibit formation of new microtubules

6.1.1.2 Vinorelbine

After the success of vinblastine and vincristine, Eli Lilly Company and other research groups screened additional vinca alkaloids and synthesized novel derivatives of the two existing drugs, in order to develop anticancer drugs with decreased neurotoxicities. P. Potier group of the Centre National de la Recherche Scientifique in France synthesized a derivative of vinblastine, vinorelbine, which bound to tubulin more strongly and had a higher hydrophobicity [11].

Since vinblastine non-selectively functions not only against microtubules during mitosis, but also against microtubules responsible for transport in the axons of neurons, it caused peripheral neuropathy, among other severe side effects. In contrast, vinorelbine preferentially targets microtubules involved in mitosis, reducing neuropathy [12]. In addition, it was observed that systemic distribution of vinorelbine was specifically concentrated in the lung; hence, vinorelbine produced excellent treatment results in clinical trials with lung cancer patients. It was approved by the FDA as a treatment for advanced non-small cell lung cancer in 1994 [13, 14]. Moreover, vinorelbine was also approved as an anticancer drug for metastatic breast cancer, and is currently being used widely in the treatment of metastatic lung cancer and breast cancer.

6.1.2 Macrolide: Eribulin

In 1985, D. Uemura et al. of Shizuoka University in Japan discovered halichondrin B in *Halichondria okadai*, a sea sponge living in the coast of Japan through a drug screening protocol using mouse tumor models. Halichondrin B belongs to the polyether macrolide class, and demonstrated a potent anticancer effect (Fig. 6.4) [15]. In

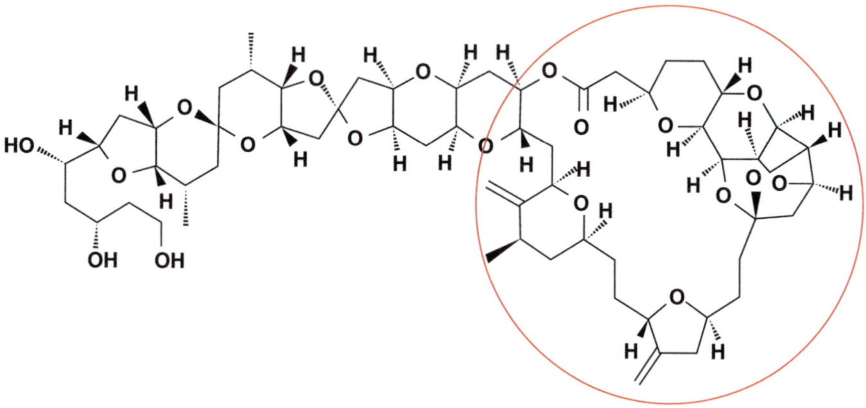

Fig. 6.4 Molecular structure of halichondrin B. The parts marked in *red* were used for the development of eribulin

1991, the E. Hamel research group of the U.S. National Cancer Institute found that halichondrin B bound to tubulin, similar to vinca alkaloids, and inhibited microtubule formation [16].

Halichondrin B had stronger activity than the vinca alkaloids. However, since halichondrin B was present in sea sponges in extremely low amounts, only 300 mg of halichondrin B was isolated from one ton of sea sponges. Therefore, Y. Kishi of Harvard University who was interested in the strong activity of halichondrin B, succeeded in total synthesis of halichondrin B in 1992 [17]. Nevertheless, mass production was not easy owing to its molecular weight, which is as high as about 1,110 MW. In 1997, Y. Kishi group identified the essential core region of halichondrin B's structure responsible for its anticancer activity, and then conducted a collaboration study with Eisai, a Japanese pharmaceutical company, to develop structurally simplified derivatives [18]. As a result, in 2001, B.A. Littlefield et al. of Eisai Institute and Kishi group successfully developed eribulin, a macrocyclic ketone compound, via the synthesis of various derivatives with improved efficacy. Eribulin had excellent anticancer activity, and was thus able to undergo active clinical trials [19]. Then, it was found that compared to the control group, the median overall survival of the group treated with eribulin was prolonged to 13.1 months from 10.6 months in a clinical trial with metastatic breast cancer patients. Objective response rate was also high; therefore, eribulin was finally approved by the FDA as an anticancer drug for metastatic breast cancer in 2010 [20].

6.1.3 *Taxane*

6.1.3.1 Paclitaxel (Taxol)

M.E. Wall et al. of the Research Triangle Institute of North Carolina University in the United States participated in the NCI plant-screening program from the mid-1950s, wherein they investigated the anticancer effects of plants collected by the

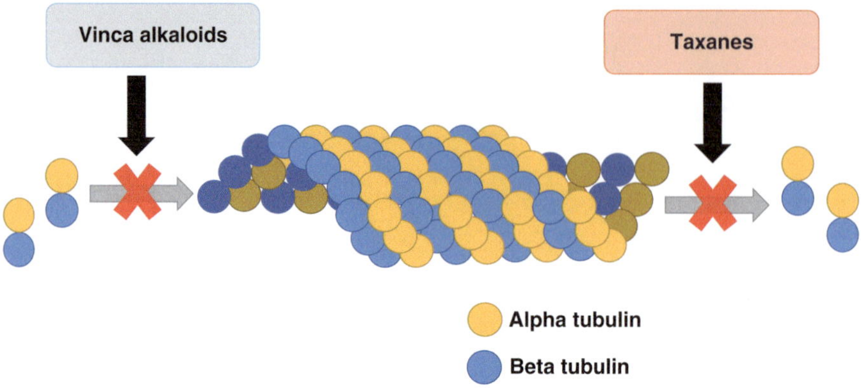

Fig. 6.5 Mechanism of action of paclitaxel. Vinca alkaloids and taxanes are anti-microtubule compounds that both block the normal function of microtubules, but they have opposite effects of action. Vinca alkaloids inhibit the formation of microtubules to interfere with cancer cell growth. However, taxanes stabilize microtubules and interfere with their breakdown, suppressing cell proliferation and inducing apoptosis

United States Department of Agriculture. In 1967, they discovered paclitaxel (named taxol when initially discovered), another anticancer drug found in the bark extracts of the Pacific yew (*Taxus brevifolia*), which also bound to tubulins [21]. However, paclitaxel was present at an extremely low amount in the extracts, and its isolation process was very complicated. Other significant problems included its low solubility, which caused problems during intravenous injection, and relatively low anticancer effects in various murine leukemia tumor models [22]. Thus, the NCI ceased the development of taxol as an anticancer drug.

Afterwards, paclitaxel was later revealed to have a new anticancer mechanism. D.A. Fuchs and R.K. Johnson of the NCI studied the effects of paclitaxel on cells in 1978, and found that paclitaxel arrested the cell cycle of cancer cells at metaphase during cell division [23]. Therefore, paclitaxel was predicted to have a similar mechanism as the vinca alkaloids. However, in 1979, S.B. Horwitz of Albert Einstein College of Medicine revealed that paclitaxel inhibits breakdown of spindle fiber microtubules, resulting in the arrest of cell division. This is opposite to the mode of action of vincristine, which suppresses microtubule formation and inhibits the growth of cancer cells (Fig. 6.5) [24].

Because paclitaxel was found to have a new anticancer mechanism, the NCI implemented a clinical trial to develop it as a novel anticancer drug. The phase I clinical trial found that paclitaxel had few side effects, and excellent anticancer efficacy; hence, an active clinical trial was performed against various cancers. The Johns Hopkins Oncology Center conducted phase II clinical trial for 4 years, and found clear treatment effects on ovarian cancer in 1989 [25]. However, the sample was insufficient for a phase III clinical trial; therefore, the NCI performed the clinical trial after establishing a paclitaxel supply contract with Bristol-Myers Squibb (BMS). The resulting trial confirmed its treatment effects on ovarian cancer, and paclitaxel was approved by the FDA in 1992 as an anticancer drug for ovarian cancer. Later on, additional clinical trials confirmed the efficacy of paclitaxel on various solid cancers including breast cancer, stomach cancer, lung cancer, bladder cancer, and Kaposi's sarcoma, and it was approved as a treatment for these various carcinomas. Currently, paclitaxel is one of the most widely administered anticancer drugs worldwide.

The bark of yew tree trunks was known to mostly contain paclitaxel. However, G. Strobel, a botanist, and A. Stierle, a chemist, of Montana State University revealed that paclitaxel was actually synthesized by *Nodulisporium sylviforme*, a commensal fungus of yew trees in 1993 [26]. Since 1994, paclitaxel has mostly been produced through the fermentation of plant cells developed by BMS.

6.1.3.2 Docetaxel

Since paclitaxel was produced only in small amounts from the bark of rare pacific yew trees through a complex purification process, a number of studies in 1980s developed various methods to yield paclitaxel in excellent quantities. In 1984, the P. Potier group of the Centre National de la Recherche Scientifique in France was successful in extracting 10-deacetylbaccatin, an inactive precursor of taxane, on a large scale from the leaves of European yew (*Taxus baccata*) [27]. They then conducted a study to develop derivatives with the same activity to paclitaxel using this material. They screened various taxane derivatives obtained from 10-deacetylbaccatin III using the semisynthetic method coupled with tubulin binding assay, and finally developed docetaxel in 1989, which binds to tubulin two-fold more strongly than paclitaxel [28]. Docetaxel is advantageous because it is more soluble in an aqueous solution than paclitaxel, and has superior effects in various kinds of animal cancer models [29]. Docetaxel was approved by the FDA as a breast cancer drug in 1996 after clinical trials. In addition, docetaxel has been widely used for the treatment of lung cancer, stomach cancer, head and neck cancer, ovarian cancer, and prostate cancer, based on clinical trials.

6.1.3.3 Cabazitaxel

Despite the improved treatment effects of paclitaxel and docetaxel, they had limitations. A study on the metabolism of these drugs discovered that these anticancer drugs, after being absorbed into cells, were pumped out again by p-glycoprotein, losing their anticancer activities [30]. In 2000, in order to develop a new drug that could overcome this disadvantage, Sanofi-Aventis developed cabazitaxel, which has a low binding capacity to p-glycoprotein and a high permeability across the blood–brain barrier [31].

This drug was produced via a semisynthetic method from a diastereomer of 10-deacetyl baccatin III that was extracted from yew leaves (similar to docetaxel), and was observed to have higher cytotoxicity toward cultured cancer cells than docetaxel [31]. The curable effects of cabazitaxel on metastatic prostate cancer (metastatic castration-resistant prostate cancer, CRPC), an incurable cancer, was confirmed by clinical trial, and thus was approved by the FDA as a treatment for metastatic prostate cancer in 2010 [32].

6.1.4 Ixabepilone

After the success of paclitaxel and docetaxel, new types of drugs with improved solubility that could evade the resistance mechanism were screened, resulting in the discovery of epothilone A and B, two antifungal drugs from the culture medium of *Sorangium cellulosum*, myxobacteria, by the Merck Institute in 1992. In 1995, D.M. Bollag et al. of the same institute discovered that epothilone A and B bind to tubulin in a manner similar to paclitaxel [33].

This drug belongs to the polyketide macrolide class, has a different structure from taxanes, and demonstrates cytotoxicity against cells resistant to paclitaxel. However, use of epothilone A and B as anticancer drugs was limited owing to their instability during drug metabolism. Thus, F.Y. Lee et al. of Bristol-Myers Squibb synthesized and developed derivatives in an attempt to enhance their stability. Of these approximately 300 types of synthesized derivatives, ixabepilone was observed to have marked resistance to degradation by esterase in the body [34]. Developed in 2001, ixabepilone had a structure wherein the lactone ring of epothilone B was substituted for a lactam ring. It showed excellent anticancer effects in an animal xenograft model. Since ixabepilone was confirmed to have an effect against metastatic breast cancer in the clinical trial performed afterward, it was registered as an FDA-approved drug in 2007 [35].

6.1.5 Podophyllotoxins: Topoisomerase II Inhibitors

Podophyllotoxin derivatives such as etoposide and teniposide function as topoisomerase II inhibitors and exhibit anticancer effects, while the anthracycline class of antibiotics including actinomycin D, daunorubicin, and doxorubicin, have similar anticancer mechanisms (Fig. 6.6).

6.1.5.1 Etoposide and Teniposide

Podophyllotoxin is a plant-derived drug with a long history of use in cancer treatment. “Leech Book of Bald”, a book on medicinal plants that was written in early 900 s during the medieval times states that cancer was treated with the roots of chervil, which are rich in podophyllotoxin. In addition, in 1861 R. Bentley reported the successful treatment of verruca with podophyllin resin from *Podophyllum peltatum*. V. Podwyssotski isolated podophyllotoxin, a non-glycosidic compound, from the roots of podophyllum for the first time in 1880. In 1946, M. Sullivan of WM. Beaumont General Hospital in Texas observed that the treatment of condyloma acuminatum, a kind of venereal disease, with podophyllin arrested the cells at metaphase during cell division, in a manner similar to colchicine [36]. Podophyllin and podophyllotoxin were investigated in animal cancer models in 1950 and were found to be very toxic; they were not able to advance to the clinical trial stage at that time.

Sandoz (currently, Novartis AG), a Swiss pharmaceutical company, focused on the physiological efficacy of various glycosides from vegetables, had been studying

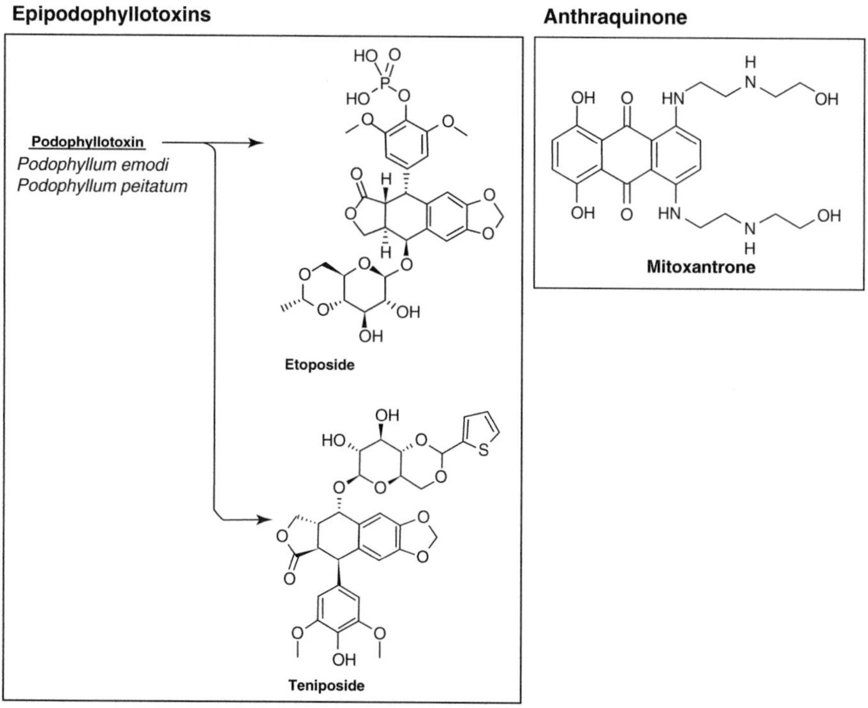

Fig. 6.6 Structure of topoisomerase II inhibitors and the process of their development

the glycoside extracts of podophyllum since the 1950s. H. Stahelin and A. von Wartburg et al. developed a new extraction method, and in 1954, discovered novel podophyllotoxin glycoside compounds with reduced toxicity from the roots of *P. peltatum*. However, they also found that their anticancer efficacy became weaker than non-glycosidic compound. Thus, they developed semisynthetic derivatives with reduced toxicity and increased anticancer efficacy by modifying the podophyllotoxin glycoside [37]. As a result, in 1964 they produced 4′-demethylepipodophyllotoxin benzylidene glucoside, a compound with reduced bone marrow toxicity and obvious anticancer effects in the L-1210 tumor model; in 1970, they developed thiophene-2-aldehyde (teniposide) after further modifications [38]. Von Wartburg and Kuhn developed another derivative, etoposide by reacting 4′-demethylepipodophyllotoxin benzylidene glucoside with acetaldehyde in 1971, which could be taken orally [39].

The molecular mechanisms of the anticancer effects of these drugs were reported in the 1980s. In 1976, J.D. Loike and S.B. Horwitz of the Albert Einstein College of Medicine found that podophyllotoxin exerted its cytotoxicity by directly acting on tubulins to stop cell growth at metaphase during cell division, whereas etoposide and teniposide did not act on tubulin and instead uniquely induced DNA cleavage, leading to cell death [40]. Based on these studies, in 1984 L.F. Liu group of Johns Hopkins Medical School found that etoposide and teniposide directly suppressed topoisomerase II, which controls DNA torsional stress (Fig. 6.7) [41].

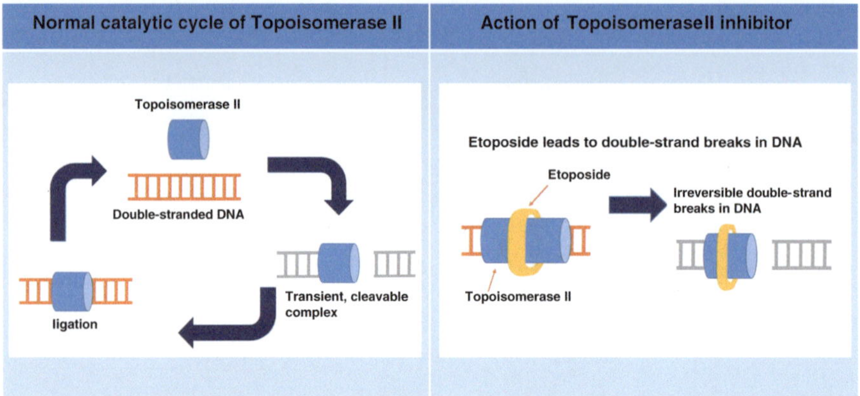

Fig. 6.7 Mechanism of action for topoisomerase II inhibitors. Topoisomerase II cleaves double-stranded DNA during the process of DNA replication and stabilizes DNA by reducing torsional stress before rejoining cut ends. However, in phases S–G2 of the cell cycle, when the inhibitor etoposide forms a complex with topoisomerase II, rejoining of DNA ends after cutting is inhibited, leading to DNA damage and suppression of cell division

Clinical trials for both etoposide and teniposide were implemented in 1971, and approved by the FDA; etoposide was approved for treatment of testicular cancer and non-small cell lung cancer in 1983, whereas teniposide was approved for intractable childhood ALL in 1992. These two drugs are currently used clinically.

6.1.6 Camptothecins: Topoisomerase I Inhibitors

6.1.6.1 Topotecan and Irinotecan

Camptothecin is an alkaloid extracted from *Camptotheca acuminate*, a plant used as an anticancer drug in traditional Chinese medicine. M.E. Wall et al. of the Research Triangle Institute, who also discovered paclitaxel, discovered camptothecin as another candidate compound for anticancer treatment in 1966 [42]. Camptothecin was found to have potent bladder toxicity during its clinical trial, halting further clinical investigation. However, research on its functional mechanism continued. The L.F. Liu group of Johns Hopkins Medical School, who identified the suppression of DNA topoisomerase II as etoposide's functional mechanism, also found that camptothecin directly suppressed DNA topoisomerase I, another enzyme that controls DNA supercoiling (Fig. 6.8) [43].

Inspired by this finding, W. Kingsbury et al. of GlaxoSmithKline developed topotecan in 1991, which is a derivative with reduced toxicity [44]. In addition, S. Sawada et al. of the Yakult Institute for Microbiological Research in Japan developed irinotecan, a prodrug of camptothecin in 1991 [45]. Once irinotecan is absorbed into the body, it is activated via metabolism to strongly inhibit DNA topoisomerase I. The FDA approved topotecan for metastatic ovarian cancer, and irinotecan for metastatic colorectal cancer in 1996. Furthermore, they were approved for

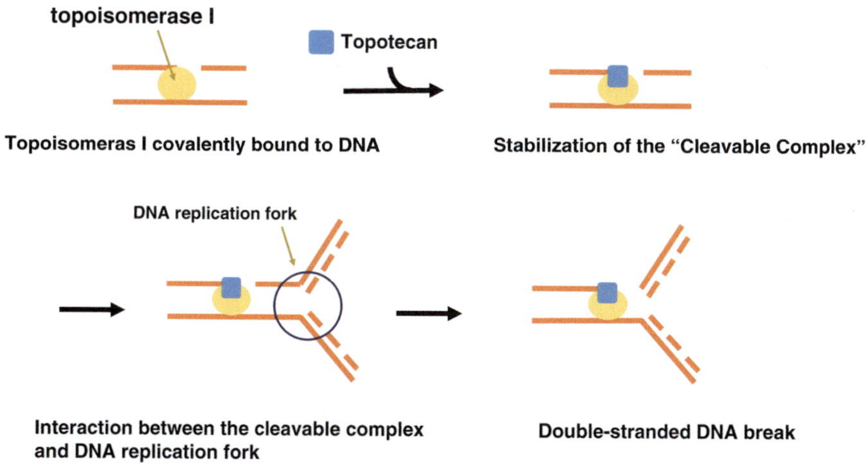

Fig. 6.8 Mechanism of action for topoisomerase I inhibitors. Topoisomerase I binds to double-stranded DNA during the process of DNA replication and splits DNA into single strands, stabilizing DNA by reducing torsional stress. Subsequently, ligation is performed by topoisomerase I. However, topoisomerase I inhibitors such as topotecan and irinotecan inhibit DNA religation; therefore, when dividing cells reach the start of replication, the double-strands are cleaved, which ultimately induces apoptosis

stomach cancer, lung cancer, and glioblastoma based on further clinical trial results, and now are in use clinically.

6.1.7 Omacetaxine Mepesuccinate (Homoharringtonine, HHT)

Omacetaxine mepesuccinate is a semisynthetic derivative of cephalotaxine, a type of alkaloid extracted from Japanese plum-yew (*Cephalotaxus harringtonia*) belonging to taxaceae. Seeds of the Japanese plum-yew were used for the treatment of dry cough and sputum in traditional Chinese medicine. The Chinese government requested scientists to develop new drugs from the traditional Chinese medicine during the Cultural Revolution, whereupon researchers in the Fukien region found that alkaloids extracted from *C. fortune* had anticancer effects in 1970 [46].

In 1972, R.G. Powell et al. of the Northern Regional Research Laboratory located in Illinois, USA, also reported the extraction of five alkaloids, namely, cephalotaxine, harringtonine (HT), homoharringtonine (HHT), isoharringtonine (IHT), and deoxyharringtonine (dHT) from *C. harringtonia*, of which HHT had the strongest anticancer effect in an animal model using P388 leukemia cells [47].

M.T. Huang of Albert Einstein University discovered in 1975 that homoharringtonine strongly suppressed protein synthesis, while other researchers further elucidated that its mechanism was related to elongation step of protein synthesis [48]. HHT binds to the A (acceptor) site of 60S ribosome and suppresses the binding of aminoacyl-tRNA, inhibiting the synthesis of proteins required for the proliferation of cancer cells.

The Shanghai Institute of Materia Medica conducted clinical trials with a mixture of harringtonine and homoharringtonine that were partially purified from *C. fortuneii*, and reported their treatment effects against acute myeloid leukemia and chronic myeloid leukemia in 1977 [49]. In 1984, the Phase I clinical trial performed with a highly purified homoharringtonine and led by the NCI in the US showed an excellent clinical efficacy in non-lymphocytic leukemia, particularly in chronic myeloid leukemia [50]. However, since homoharringtonine was present in the cephalotaxus alkaloids at low concentrations, clinical trials were stopped owing to difficulty in maintaining an adequate drug supply.

Instead, various research groups investigated synthesis methods, and J. P. Robin et al. of Oncopharm in France developed a mass production method in 1999 for highly purified homoharringtonine using cephalotaxine, a compound that was present in cephalotaxus alkaloids in abundance but had no anticancer activity. Nevertheless, since imatinib had markedly superior effects in the treatment of chronic myeloid leukemia during that time, homoharringtonine was on the verge of disappearance without attracting any attention as an anticancer drug. However, as there were reports of chronic myeloid leukemia patients who showed resistance to imatinib, there was renewed focus on homoharringtonine by researchers of the M.D. Anderson Cancer Center of Texas.

R. Chen et al. of the M.D. Anderson Cancer Center found that homoharringtonine suppressed the translation of Bcr-Abl mRNA in 2006 [51], and R. Tang et al. of Universite' Pierre et Marie Curie also revealed that homoharringtonine suppressed translation of Mcl-1, a tumor protein that is deeply correlated with chronic myeloid leukemia (Fig. 6.9) [52].

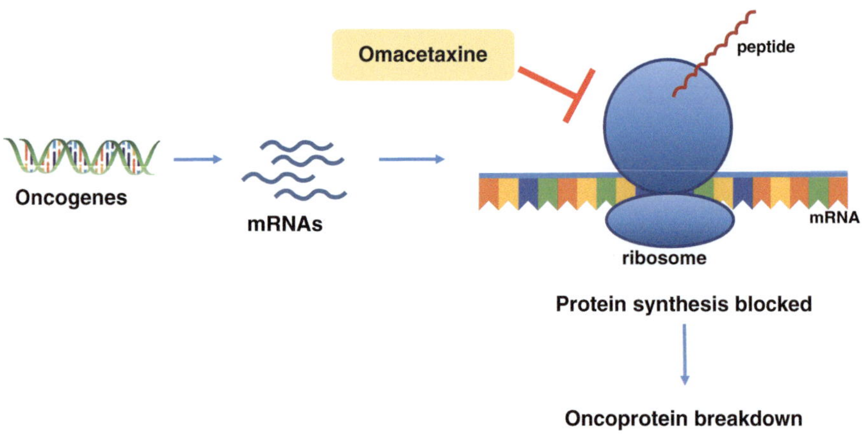

Fig. 6.9 Anticancer mechanism of omacetaxine. Omacetaxine (homoharringtonine) binds to the A-site on ribosomes and inhibits protein synthesis, resulting in reduced concentration of proteins with a short half-life, such as Bcr-Abl (which is related to the development of chronic myeloid leukemia), leading to cell death. Similarly, the anticancer effect of omacetaxine is known to occur as the result of inhibiting the synthesis of oncoproteins, including Mcl-1 and Myc, which are important regulators of cell survival and proliferation in cancer cells, respectively

Then, J. Cortes et al. of the M.D. Anderson Cancer Center conducted a clinical trial with chronic myeloid leukemia patients who were resistant to Bcr-Abl kinase inhibitors such as imatinib, wherein they observed that homoharringtonine had effects not only on patients with the imatinib-resistant Bcr-Abl mutant, but also on chronic myeloid leukemia patients with a Bcr-Abl T315I mutation who were resistant to the 2nd generation Bcr-Abl inhibitors [53]; thus homorringtonine was approved by the FDA as a medicine for chronic myeloid leukemia in 2012.

6.2 Anticancer Antibiotics

Anticancer antibiotics are antibiotics extracted from soil microorganisms that have anticancer activities. They range from compounds that were developed from actinomycin D by S. Waksman to antibiotics in the anthracycline group, including daunorubicin, doxorubicin, epirubicin, and idarubicin, as well as mithramycin and bleomycin. Many are now in clinical use. Most of them were isolated from various *Streptomyces* species, and inserted between DNA bases to cause DNA damage for their anticancer effects.

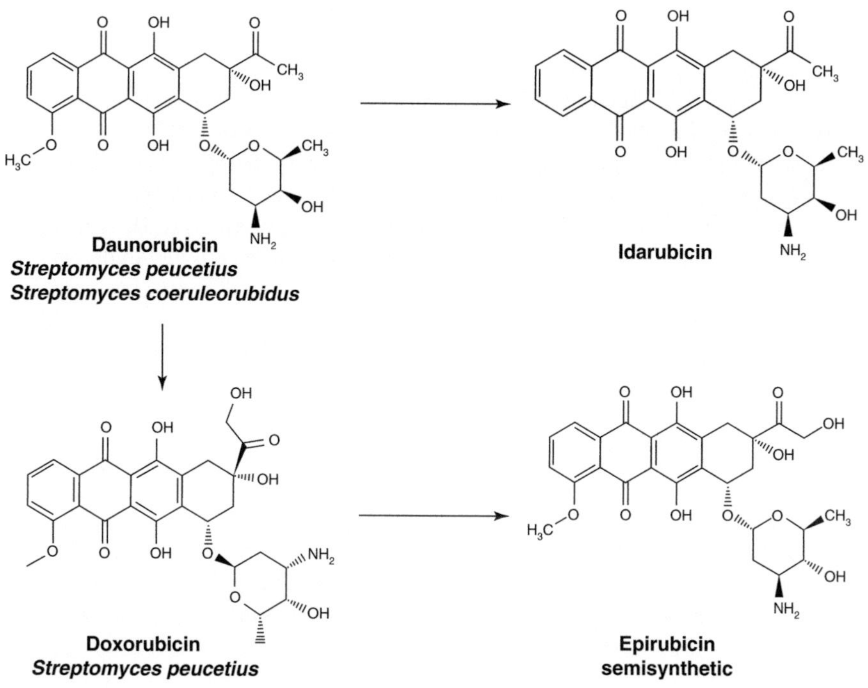

Fig. 6.10 Types of anthracycline and the process of their development

6.2.1 Actinomycin D (Dactinomycin)

Since the discovery of penicillin from blue mold (*Penicillium glaucum*) by A. Fleming in 1928, antibiotics have become an essential drug group in chemotherapy. Although antibiotics were defined as bioactive substances that kill bacteria, their application was gradually extended to other diseases and they were applied to cancer treatments from the 1950s. S. Waksman, a microbiologist of Rutgers College who first used the term "antibiotics" in 1942, discovered not only streptomycin, a tuberculosis medication, but also other various antibiotics including actinomycin, streptothricin, neomycin, and candicidin from *Streptomyces* (the richest source for antibiotics development), for which he was awarded the Nobel Prize in physiology or medicine in 1952.

S. Farber of Harvard Medical School identified the potential use of aminopterin and methotrexate of the antimetabolite group for anticancer chemotherapy, and focused on antibiotics to screen for novel anticancer drugs in 1954. He investigated the anticancer effects of about 20 types of antibiotics that Waksman had previously discovered, in mouse leukemia models, of which actinomycin D (dactinomycin) was observed to have the most potent anticancer efficacy in mouse cancer models. Actinomycin D belongs to the chromopeptide class of antibiotics that Waksman discovered in *Streptomyces chrysomallus* in 1954 [54]. Farber failed to obtain clear results from the first clinical trial with childhood leukemia patients, but did observe outstanding effects on Wilms' Tumor, a rare carcinoma, by investigating the anticancer effects of this drug in other carcinoma patients, which led to the expansion of anticancer chemotherapy to treatment of solid cancers [55].

H. M. Sobell and S. C. Jain of Rochester University discovered that the phenoxazone chromophore of actinomycin D intercalated the backbones of CpG dinucleotides of DNA via hydrophobic interactions by using X-ray crytallography analysis in 1972; other researchers reported that actinomycin D either suppressed DNA-mediated RNA polymerase, or inhibited the function of topoisomerase II, which induced double-strand DNA breakage [56, 57]. Based on aforementioned findings, actinomycin D obtained FDA approval as a treatment for Wilms' Tumor, rhabdomyosarcoma, and genital cancer in 1964, and is currently in use.

6.2.2 Anthracycline

Anthracycline group contain the highest number of drugs among antibiotic anticancer drugs, including such drugs as daunorubicin, doxorubicin, epirubicin, and idarubicin. Moreover, synthetic compounds such as mitoxantrone and valrubicin that were developed in an attempt to improve the efficacy of antibiotics in the anthracycline group demonstrate anticancer effects with similar functional mechanisms. These anticancer drugs commonly function as topoisomerase II inhibitors to cause DNA damage, which results in the suppression of cancer cell growth and the induction of apoptosis.

6.2.2.1 Daunorubicin (Daunomycin)

The history of the use of anthracyclines as antibiotic anticancer drugs dates back to when two research groups discovered daunorubicin around the same time in 1963. A. Grelin et al. of Farmitalia Research Laboratories in Italy discovered that *Streptomyces peucetius* isolated in Apulia region yielded antibiotics with a ruby color that had high cancer suppression efficacy in a mouse cancer model [58]. M. Dubost et al. of Rhône Poulenc in France discovered the same compound from *Streptomyces caeruleorubidus* around the same time; hence, the two groups named this antibiotic "daunorubicin" after the name of the discovered region (Dauni, the name of the Apulia region in Roman times) and its color [59].

The structure of daunorubicin comprises a daunosamine sugar bound to the anthraquinone mother nucleus with a hydrophobic surface structure. W.J. Pigram of King's College in the UK found that anthraquinone penetrated into DNA bases via hydrophobic interactions through X-ray crytallography analysis in 1972 [60]. A. Di Marco et al. of the National Cancer Institute in Italy reported suppression of DNA and RNA synthesis by insertion of anthracycline into them in 1975. Following this study, many studies were performed on the anticancer mechanisms of the anthracycline group, including daunorubicin, with various mechanisms uncovered. Ultimately, daunorubicin's major effect was found to be owing to the suppression of activity by topoisomerase II after insertion into DNA. In 1984, the L.F. Liu group of Johns Hopkins Medical School revealed that doxorubicin, an anthracycline drug, directly suppressed topoisomerase II [61]. They discovered that once anthracycline bound to topoisomerase II, topoisomerase II would cleave DNA, and the end of the cleaved DNA would be fixed to topoisomerase II via a covalent bond. The DNA was blocked from re-ligation, causing cell death (Fig. 6.11). It was also reported that anthracycline induced reactive oxygen species, which caused damage to various cell components such as DNA, proteins, and lipids, resulting in further anticancer effects.

Daunorubicin was observed to have effects on various kinds of hematopoietic malignancies in animal experiments, and clinical efficacy of daunorubicin were confirmed by clinical trials on patients with acute lymphocytic leukemia in 1966 and acute myeloid leukemia in 1969 [62, 63]. Based on these results, daunorubicin was approved by the FDA as an anticancer drug for acute myeloid leukemia and acute lymphocytic leukemia in 1979, and is still used widely.

6.2.2.2 Doxorubicin (Adriamycin)

Since severe cardiotoxicity was observed during daunorubicin treatment, studies were conducted to develop drugs with reduced toxicity. In 1969, F. Arcamone et al. of the Farmitalia Institute discovered doxorubicin, which is 14-hydroxy daunorubicin, from a mutant of *S. peucetius*. The compound had similar cardiotoxicity and a much stronger activity [64]. Doxorubicin is also called adriamycin, because it was first collected from a bacterial strain in the soil at the coast of the Adriatic sea in Southern Italy.

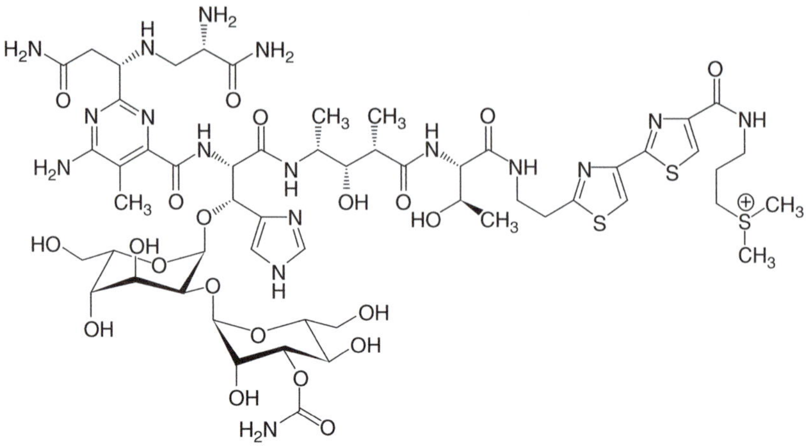

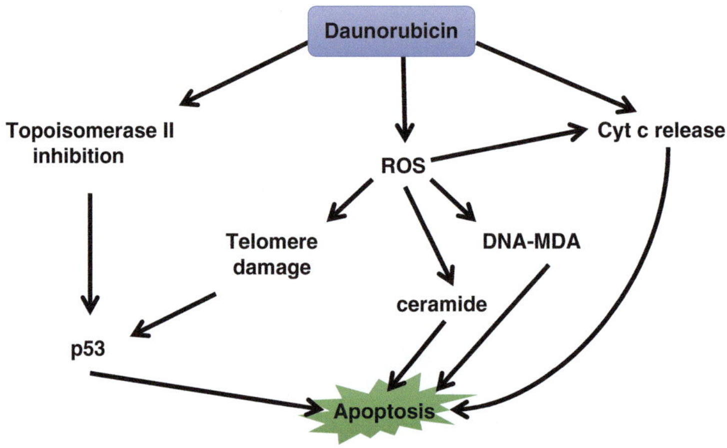

Fig. 6.11 Mechanism of action for anthracycline. When daunorubicin is inserted between DNA bases, DNA is damaged via topoisomerase and apoptosis occurs. p53 plays an important role in the response to DNA damamge and apoptosis. Daunorubicin is also known to induce apopotosis by damaging DNA and the cell membrane through the formation of free radicals

Doxorubicin demonstrated effects not only against leukemia, the main target of daunomycin, but also against solid cancers. A. Di Marco et al. of the National Cancer Institute in Italy first observed its effects in murine solid cancer models [65], based on which G. Bonadonna et al. of the same institute performed clinical trials in patients with various carcinomas, resulting in the confirmation of its effects on a wide variety of cancers including leukemia, Hodgkin lymphoma, bladder cancer, breast cancer, stomach cancer, ovarian cancer, thyroid cancer, soft tissue sarcoma, and osteosarcoma. In addition, other researchers observed its effects on solid cancers [66]. Doxorubicin was approved by FDA as an anticancer drug in 1974, and is still used widely.

6.2.2.3 Epirubicin and Idarubicin

The success of daunorubicin and doxorubicin promoted the synthesis of various derivatives. F. Arcamone et al. of the Farmitalia Institute developed two improved drugs in 1975: epirubicin was an epimer with a 4′-hydroxyl group on the sugar of doxorubicin, and idarubicin had reduced toxicity owing to the removal of the methoxyl group on the aromatic ring of daunorubicin [67]. The anticancer effects of epirubicin were similar to doxorubicin, while its cardiotoxicity was low. Idarubicin, unlike daunorubicin or doxorubicin, could be administered orally, and its anticancer activity was similar to doxorubicin [68]. Thus, idarubicin and epirubicin obtained FDA approval for treatment of acute myeloid leukemia in adults in 1990 and for breast cancer in 1999, respectively.

6.2.2.4 Anthracenedione: Mitoxantrone (Dihydroxyanthracenedione, DHAD)

Mitoxantrone was developed by studies aiming to improve the cardiotoxicity of daunorubicin and doxorubicin. The C.C. Cheng group of the Midwest Research Institute in Missouri, US, developed mitoxantrone in 1978. Mitoxantrone is a synthetic drug developed by removing the sugar group [69], based on the report that sugar on doxorubicin correlated with cardiotoxicity. Although mitoxantrone improved the irreversible cardiotoxicity of doxorubicin, its application in the treatment of carcinomas was mostly limited [70]. In 1987, it was approved by the FDA as a medicine for acute non-lymphocytic leukemia. Similar to anthracycline, mitoxantrone inserts into DNA base pairs, inhibits DNA synthesis and DNA repair, and inhibits topoisomerase II [71].

6.2.2.5 Valrubicin

In 1974, M. Israel of Sidney Farber Cancer Institute developed valrubicin (N-trifluoroacetyladriamycin-14-valerate), a derivative of doxorubicin with reduced toxicity [72]. The trifluoroacetyl group is bound to the amino group of glycoside on doxorubicin in this drug, and a hydrocarbon ester composed of 5 carbons was attached to carbon number 14 to facilitate cell penetration. In collaboration with E. Frei, M. Israel observed that valrubicin had superior anticancer effects and decreased toxicities in animal cancer models when compared with doxorubicin [73]. Valrubicin was predicted to exert its cytotoxicity through the suppression of topoisomerase II, although its functional mechanism has not yet fully elucidated. Clinical trials on valrubicin were led by the Dana-Farber Cancer Institute [74], and FDA approved it as a medicine for incurable bladder cancer resistant to BCG-treatment in 1998. However, it is rarely used at present.

6.2.3 *Mithramycin (Plicamycin)*

In 1953, W.E. Grundy and J.C. Sylvester et al. discovered mithramycin, a new antibiotic in the polyketide class from *S. plicatus* that suppressed the growth of gram positive bacteria [75]. In 1962, K.V. Rao et al. reported the anticancer effects of mithramycin in an animal adenocarcinoma model for the first time [76]. J.H. Brown et al. reported in 1965 that this drug had excellent antitumor effects against testicular cancer [77]. Later on, a clinical trial was performed with patients with malignant testicular cancer, and the FDA approved this drug for malignant testicular cancer in 1970. However, since mithramycin was found to have adverse reactions including fatal thrombocytopenia and hemorrhage [78], its production was ceased after 2000. Thereafter, mithramycin treatment of testicular cancer was replaced by platinum-based regimen. Although mithramycin was predicted to interact with DNA, details of its functional mechanism remain unknown.

6.2.4 *Bleomycin*

H. Umezawa, a microbiologist of the Institute of Microbial Chemistry in Japan who discovered kanamycin, a tuberculosis medicine in 1956, began studying antibiotics with anticancer effects in 1953. He discovered phleomycin from a culture medium of *S. verticillus* in 1956. The drug had a strong anticancer effect in an animal cancer models. However, it was clinically infeasible due to its marked nephrotoxicity [79]. Afterwards, he developed a new purification method in 1966, yielding bleomycin, a glycopeptidic antibiotic that had almost no kidney toxicity [80].

Umezawa studied the metabolism of bleomycin in the body and its distribution in tissues, and found that it was rapidly hydrolyzed in most tissues except in the skin and lung, resulting in few adverse reactions, including less bone marrow toxicity. He also predicted that cancers derived from the skin and lung (mostly carcinomas) could be effectively treated with bleomycin because these tissues had low hydrolyzing activities [81]. In 1982, the Umezawa group developed a complete chemical synthesis method for the mass production of bleomycin [82].

In 1978, A.D. D'Andrea and W.A. Haseltine of Harvard Medical School studied the molecular mechanism of bleomycin, and found that bleomycin formed free radicals after insertion into DNA, which induced DNA cleavage (Fig. 6.12) [83]. Bleomycin was approved by the FDA as a treatment for Hodgkin's lymphoma, head and neck cancer, cervical cancer, and genital cancer in 1973 following clinical trials. Later, bleo-

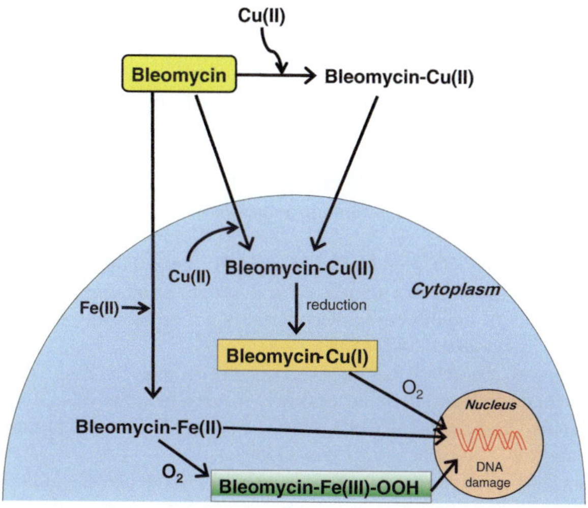

Fig. 6.12 Mechanism of action for bleomycin. Bleomycin binds with the transition metal Fe (*II*) before gaining oxygen to form active bleomycin-Fe (*III*)-OOH. In another reaction, bleomycin binds with Cu (*II*) before being reduced to form bleomycin-Cu (*I*), which becomes active bleomycin by reacting with oxygen. Activated bleomycin causes DNA damage, which leads to apoptosis

mycin was also found to have excellent effects in the treatment of testicular cancer. It has been mostly used for the treatment of Hodgkin's lymphoma and testicular cancer.

References

1. Lits FJ (1934) Contribution a l'étude des réactions cellulaires provoquées par la colchicine. Compt rend Soc de biol 115:1421
2. Dustin AP (1934) Contribution a l'étude de l'action des poisons caryoclasiques sur les tumeurs animales; action delacoichicine sur le sarcome greffé, type Crocker, de la souris. Bull Acad roy de med de Belgique 14:487
3. Noble RL, Beer CT, Cutts JH (1958) Role of chance observations in chemotherapy: Vinca rosea. Ann NY Acad Sci 76:882–894
4. Neuss N, Gorman M, Svoboda GH et al (1959) Vinca alkaloids. III.1 characterization of leurosine and vinca leukoblastine, new alkaloids from Vinca rosea Linn. J Am Chem Soc 81:4754–4755
5. Svoboda GH, Johnson IS, Gorman M, Neuss N (1962) Current status of research on the alkaloids of *Vinca rosea* Linn. (*Catharanthus roseus* G. Don). J Pharm Sci 51:707–720
6. Palmer CG, Livengood D, Warren AK, Simpson PJ, Johnson IS (1960) The action of vincaleukoblastine on mitosis in vitro. Exp Cell Res 20:198–201
7. Bensch KG, Marantz R, Wisniewski H, Shelanski ML (1969) Induction in vitro of microtubular crystals by vinca alkaloids. Science 165:495–496
8. Marantz R, Ventilla M, Shelanski ML (1969) Vinblastine-induced precipitation of microtubule protein. Science 165:498–499
9. Owellen RJ, Hartke CA, Dickerson RM, Hains FO (1976) Inhibition of tubulin-microtubule polymerization by drugs of the vinca alkaloid class. Cancer Res 36:1499–1502
10. Tucker RW, Owellen RJ, Harris SB (1977) Correlation of cytotoxicity and mitotic spindle dissolution by vinblastine in mammalian cells. Cancer Res 37:4346–4351
11. Mangeney P, Andriamialisoa RZ, Lallemand JY, Langlois N, Langlois Y, Potier P (1979) 5′-Noranhydrovinblastine. Prototype of a new class of vinblastine derivatives. Tetrahedron 35:2175–2179
12. Binet S, Fellous A, Lataste H, Krikorian A, Couzinier JP, Meniniger V (1989) In situ analysis of the action of Navelbine on microtubules using immunofluorescence. Semin Oncol 16(Suppl 4):5–8

13. Leveque D, Quoix E, Dumont P, Massard G, Hentz JG, Charloux A, Jehl F (1993) Pulmonary distribution of vinorelbine in patients with non small cell lung cancer. Cancer Chemother Pharmacol 33:176–178
14. The Elderly Lung Cancer Vinorelbine Italian Study (ELVIS) Group (1999) Effects of vinorelbine on quality of life and survival of elderly patients with advanced non-small cell lung cancer. J Natl Cancer Inst 91:66–72
15. Uemura D, Takahashi K, Yamamoto T, Katayama C, Tanaka J, Okumura Y, Hirata Y (1985) Norhalichondrin A: an antitumor polyether macrolide from a marine sponge. J Am Chem Soc 107:4796–4798
16. Bai RL, Paull KD, Herald CL, Malspeis L, Pettit GR, Hamel E (1991) Halichondrin B and homohalichondrin B, marine natural products binding in the vinca domain of tubulin. Discovery of tubulin-based mechanism of action by analysis of differential cytotoxicity data. J Biol Chem 266:15882–15889
17. Aicher TD, Buszek KR, Fang FG, Forsyth CJ, Jung SH, Kishi Y et al (1992) Total synthesis of halichondrin B and norhalichondrin B. J Am Chem Soc 114:3162–3164
18. Stamos DP, Sean SC, Kishi Y (1997) New synthetic route to the C.14-C.38 segment of halichondrins. J Org Chem 62:7552–7553
19. Towle MJ, Salvato KA, Budrow J, Wels BF, Kuznetsov G, Aalfs KK, Welsh S et al (2001) In vitro and in vivo anticancer activities of synthetic macrocyclic ketone analogues of halichondrin B. Cancer Res 61:1013–1021
20. Twelves C, Cortes J, Vahdat LT, Wanders J, Akerele C, Kaufman PA (2010) Phase III trials of eribulin mesylate (E7389) in extensively pretreated patients with locally recurrent or metastatic breast cancer. Clin Breast Cancer 10:160–163
21. Wall ME, Wani MC (1967) Recent progress in plant anti-tumor agents. 153rd National Meeting of the American Chemical Society
22. Wani MC, Taylor HL, Wall ME, Coggon P, McPhail AT (1971) Plant antitumor agents, VI: the isolation and structure of taxol, a novel antileukemic and antitumor agent from *Taxus brevifolia*. J Am Chem Soc 93:2325–2327
23. Fuchs DA, Johnson RK (1978) Cytologic evidence that taxol, an antineoplastic agent from *Taxus brevifolia*, acts as a mitotic spindle poison. Cancer Treat Rep 62:1219–1222
24. Schiff PB, Fant J, Horwitz SB (1979) Promotion of microtubule assembly in vitro by taxol. Nature 22:665–667
25. McGuire WP, Rowinsky EK, Rosenshein NB, Grumbine FC, Ettinger DS, Armstrong DK, Donehower RC (1989) Taxol: a unique antineoplastic agent with significant activity in advanced ovarian epithelial neoplasms. Ann Intern Med 111:273–279
26. Stierle A, Strobel G, Stierle D (1993) Taxol and taxane production by *Taxomyces andreanae*, an endophytic fungus of pacific yew. Science 260:214–216
27. Senilh V, Blechert S, Colin M, Guenard D, Picot F, Potier P, Varenne P (1984) Mise en evidence de nouveaux analogues du taxol, extraits de *Taxus baccata*. J Nat Prod 47:131–137
28. Mangatal L, Adeline MT, Guenard D, Gueritte-Voegelein F, Potier P (1989) Application of the vicinal oxyamination reaction with asymmetric induction to the hemisynthesis of taxol and analogues. Tetrahedron 45:4177–4190
29. Lavelle F, Fizames C, Gueritte-Voegelein F, Guenard D, Potier P (1989) Experimental properties of RP 56976, a taxol derivative. Proc Am Assoc Cancer Res 30:2254
30. Lockhart AC, Tirona RG, Kim RB (2003) Pharmacogenetics of ATP-binding cassette transporters in cancer and chemotherapy. Mol Cancer Ther 2:685–698
31. Sanofi-aventis (2000) XRP6258 investigator's brochure. Antony (France): Sanofi-aventis
32. De Bono JS et al (2010) Cabazitaxel or mitoxantrone with prednisone in patients with metastatic castration resistant prostate cancer (mCRPC) previously treated with docetaxel: final results of a multinational phase III trial (TROPIC). J Clin Oncol 28(Suppl 15):4508
33. Bollag DM, McQueney PA, Zhu J, Hensens O, Koupal L, Liesch J, Goetz M, Lazarides E, Woods CM (1995) Epothilones, a new class of microtubule-stabilizing agents with a taxol-like mechanism of action. Cancer Res 55:2325–2333
34. Lee FY, Borzilleri R, Fairchild CR, Kim SH, Long BH, Reventos-Suarez C, Vite GD, Rose WC, Kramer RA (2001) BMS-247550: a novel epothilone analog with a mode of action similar to paclitaxel but possessing superior antitumor efficacy. Clin Cancer Res 7:1429–1437

35. Vahdat LT et al (2007) Phase III trial of ixabepilone plus capecitabine compared to capecitabine alone in patients with metastatic breast cancer (MBC) previously treated or resistant to an anthracycline and resistant to taxanes. J Clin Oncol 25:18S
36. King LS, Sullivan M (1946) The similarity of the effect of podophyllin and colchicine and their use in the treatment of condylomata acuminata. Science 104:244–245
37. Emmenegger H, Stahelin H, Rutschmann J, Renz J, von Wartburg A (1961) On the chemistry and pharmacology of podophyllum glucoside and its derivatives. Drug Res 11:327–333
38. Stahelin H (1970) 4′-Demethyl-epipodophyllotoxin thenylidene glucoside (VM 26), a podophyllum compound with a new mechanism of action. Eur J Cancer 6:303–311
39. Keller-Julsen C, Kuhn M, von Wartburg A, Stahelin H (1971) Mitosis-inhibiting natural products. 24. Synthesis and antimitotic activity of glycosidic lignan derivatives related to podophyllotoxin. J Med Chem 14:936–940
40. Loike JD, Horwitz SB (1976) Effects of podophyllotoxin and VP-16-213 on microtubule assembly in vitro and nucleoside transport in HeLa cells. Biochemistry 15:5435–5443
41. Ross W, Rowe T, Glisson B, Yalowich J, Liu L (1984) Role of topoisomerase II in mediating epipodophyllotoxin-induced DNA cleavage. Cancer Res 44:5857–5860
42. Wall ME, Wani MC, Cook CE, Palmer KH, McPhail AT, Sim GA (1966) Plant antitumor agents. I. The isolation and structure of camptothecin, a novel alkaloidal leukemia and tumor inhibitor from *Camptotheca acuminata*. J Am Chem Soc 88:3888–3890
43. Hsiang YH, Hertzberg R, Hecht S, Liu L (1985) Camptothecin induces protein-linked DNA breaks via mammalian DNA topoisomerase I. J Biol Chem 260:14873–14878
44. Kingsbury WD, Boehm JC, Jakas DR et al (1991) Synthesis of water-soluble (aminoalkyl)camptothecin analogs: inhibition of topoisomerase I and antitumor activity. J Med Chem 34:98–107
45. Sawada S, Okajima S, Aiyama R et al (1991) Synthesis and antitumor activity of 20(S)-camptothecin derivatives: carbamate-linked, water-soluble derivatives of 7-ethyl-10-hydroxycamptothecin. Chem Pharm Bull 39:1446–1450
46. No Authors Listed (1976) Cephalotaxine esters in the treatment of acute leukemia. A preliminary clinical assessment. Chin Med J 2:263–272
47. Powell RG, Weisleder D, Smith CR Jr (1972) Antitumor alkaloids for Cephalataxus harringtonia: structure and activity. J Pharm Sci 61:1227–1230
48. Huang MT (1975) Harringtonine, an inhibitor of initiation of protein biosynthesis. Mol Pharmacol 11:511–519
49. No Authors Listed (1977) Harringtonine in acute leukemias. Clinical analysis of 31 cases. Chin Med J 3:319–324
50. Legha SS, Keating M, Picket S, Ajani JA, Ewer M, Bodey GP (1984) Phase I clinical investigation of homoharringtonine. Cancer Treat Rep 68:1085–1091
51. Chen R, Gandhi V, Plunkett WA (2006) Sequential blockade strategy for the design of combination therapies to overcome oncogene addiction in chronic myelogenous leukemia. Cancer Res 66:10959–10966
52. Tang R, Faussat AM, Majdak P, Marzac C, Dubrulle S, Marjanovic Z, Legrand O, Marie JP (2006) Semisynthetic homoharringtonine induces apoptosis via inhibition of protein synthesis and triggers rapid myeloid cell leukemia-1 down-regulation in myeloid leukemia cells. Mol Cancer Ther 5:723–731
53. Cortes J, Khoury HJ, Corm S et al (2008) Safety and efficacy of subcutaneous (SC) omacetaxine mepesuccinate in imatinib (IM)-resistant chronic myeloid leukemia (CML) patients with the T315I mutation-results of an ongoing multicenter phase 2/3 study. Blood (ASH Annual Meeting Abstracts) 112:3239
54. Manaker RA, Gregory FJ, Vining LC, Waksman SA (1955) Actinomycin: III. The properties of a new actinomycin. Antibiotics Ann 1954–1955:853–857
55. Farber S, D'Angio G, Evans A, Mitus A (1960) Clinical studies of actinomycin D with special reference to Wilms' tumor in children. Ann NY Acad Sci 89:421–425
56. Sobell HM, Jain SC (1972) Stereochemistry of actinomycin binding to DNA: II. Detailed molecular model of actinomycin-DNA complex and its implications. J Mole Biol 68:21–28
57. Ross WE, Bradley MO (1981) DNA double-stranded breaks in mammalian cells after exposure to intercalating agents. Biochem Biophys Acta 654:129–134

58. Grelin A, Spella C, Di Marco A, Canevazzi G (1963) Descrizione e classificazione di un attionamicette (Streptomyces Peucetius sp nova) produltore di un sostanza ad attivite antitumorale; La daunomicina. Giorn Microbio 11:109–118
59. Dubost M, Gauter P, Maral R et al (1963) Un nouvel antibiotique a proprieties cytostatique. La rubidomycine. CR Acad Sci Paris 257:1813–1815
60. Pigram WJ, Fuller W, Hamilton LD (1972) Stereochemistry of intercalation: interaction of daunomycin with DNA. Nature New Biol 235:17–19
61. Tewey KM, Rowe TC, Yang L et al (1984) Adriamycin-induced DNA damage mediated by mammalian DNA topoisomerase II. Science 226:466–468
62. Jacquillat C, Tanzer J, Boiron M et al (1966) Rubidomycin: a new agent active in the treatment of acute lymphoblastic leukemia. Lancet 288:27–28
63. Boiron M, Jacquillat C, Weil M et al (1969) Daunorubicin in the treatment of acute myelocytic leukemia. Lancet 293:330–333
64. Arcamone F, Cassinelli G, Fantini G et al (1969) Adriamycin, 14-hydroxydaunomycin, a new antitumor antibiotic from *S. peucetius* var. *caesius*. Biotechnol Bioeng 11:1101–1110
65. Di Marco A, Gaetani M, Scarpinato B (1969) Adriamycin (NSC-123,127): a new antibiotic with antitumor activity. Cancer Chemother Rep 53:33–37
66. Bonadonna G, Monfardini S, DeLena M, Fossati-Bellani F (1969) Clinical evaluation of Adriamycin, a new antitumor antibiotic. Br Med J 3:503–506
67. Arcamone F, Penco S, Vigevani A et al (1975) Synthesis and antitumor properties of new glycosides of daunomycinone and adriamycinone. J Med Chem 18:703–707
68. Arcamone F, Bernardi L, Giardino P et al (1976) Synthesis and antitumor activity of 4-demethoxydaunorubicin, 4-demethoxy-7,9-diepidaunorubicin, and their beta anomers. Cancer Treat Rep 60:829–834
69. Zee-Cheng RKY, Cheng CC (1978) Antineoplastic agents. Structure-activity relationship study of bis(substituted aminoalkylamino)anthraquinones. J Med Chem 21:291–294
70. Savaraj N, Lu K, Manuel V, Loo TL (1982) Pharmacology of mitoxantrone in cancer patients. Cancer Chemother Pharmacol 8:113–117
71. Crespi MD, Ivanier SE, Genovese J, Baldi A (1986) Mitoxantrone affects topoisomerase activities in human breast cancer cells. Biochem Biophys Res Commun 136:521–528
72. Israel M, Tinter SK, Lazarus H, Brown B, Modest EJ (1974) Adriamycin derivatives: preparation and antitumor evaluation. Abstracts. 11th Intern Cancer Congress 4:752–753
73. Israel M, Modest EJ, Frei E III (1975) N-Trifluoroacetyladriamycin-14-valerate, an analog with greater experimental antitumor activity and less toxicity than Adriamycin. Cancer Res 35:1365–1368
74. Markman M, Homesley H, Norberts DA et al (1996) Phase I trial of intraperitoneal AD 32 in gynecologic malignancies. Gynecol Onco 61:90–93
75. Grundy WE, Goldstein AW, Rickher JC, Hanes ME, Warren HB, Sylvester JC (1953) Aureolic acid, a new antibiotic. I Microbiological studies. Antimicrob Chemother 3:1215–1221
76. Rao KV, Cullen WP, Sobin BA (1962) A new antibiotic with antitumor properties. Antibiot Chemother 12:182–186
77. Brown IH, Kennedy BJ (1965) Mithramycin in the treatment of disseminated testicular neoplasma. New Engl J Med 272:111–118
78. Curreri AR, Ansfield FJ (1960) Mithramycin-human toxicology and preliminary therapeutic investigations. Cancer Chemother Rep 8:18–22
79. Maeda K, Kosaka H, Yagishita K, Umezawa H (1956) A new antibiotic, phleomycin. J Antibiot 9:82–85
80. Umezawa H, Maeda K, Takeuchi T, Okami Y (1966) New antibiotics bleomycins A and B. J Antibiot 19:200–209
81. Umezawa H, Takeuchi T, Hori S, Sawa T, Ishizuka M, Ichikawa T, Komai T (1972) Studies on the mechanism of antitumor effect of bleomycin on squamous cell carcinoma. J Antibiot 25:409–420
82. Takita T, Umezawa Y, Saito S, Morishima H, Naganawa H, Umezawa H, Tsuchiya T et al (1982) Total synthesis of bleomycin A2. Tetrahedron Lett 23:521–524
83. D'Andrea AD, Haseltine WA (1978) Sequence specific cleavage of DNA by the antitumour antibiotics neocarzinostatin and bleomycin. Proc Natl Acad Sci 75:3608–3612

Chapter 7
Immunotherapeutic Anticancer Drugs and Other Miscellaneous Anticancer Drugs

Immunotherapeutic anticancer agents eliminate cancer cells by acting on the immune system and activating the immune response against cancer cells. This class of drugs includes cytokines such as INF-α and IL-2, nonspecific immune stimulants BCG and levamisole, and recently developed anti-CTLA-4 monoclonal antibody ipilumumab.

Other miscellaneous anticancer agents developed as clinical drugs include photodynamic therapeutic agents, asparaginase, arsenic trioxide, and hydroxyurea (Fig. 7.1).

7.1 Immunotherapeutic Anticancer Drugs

At the end of the nineteenth century, W. Coley of New York's Memorial Hospital pioneered the development of anticancer immunotherapy. Coley observed tumor shrinkage in a patient who had an ulcer with erysipelas due to streptococcal infection accompanying the tumor, and proposed the hypothesis that cancer could be treated

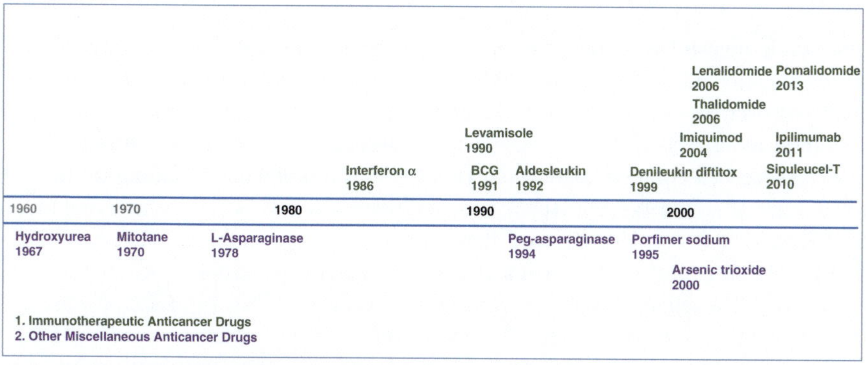

Fig. 7.1 Types of immunotherapeutic and other anticancer agents, as well as a chronology of their development

K.-W. Kim et al., *Cancer Drug Discovery*, DOI 10.1007/978-94-024-0844-7_7

by the immune system or by an inflammatory response. To test this hypothesis, in 1893, Coley conducted an experiment by inoculating *Streptococcus pyogenes* and *Serratia marcescens* into cancer patients and reported that the size of tumor decreased in patients due to a strong inflammatory response following the bacterial infection [1]. This study later led to the discovery of lipopolysaccharide (LPS), which is an endotoxin produced by bacteria, and LPS from various bacteria have been screened as anticancer agents. Further, in 1975, E.A. Carswell et al. at the Memorial Sloan-Kettering Cancer Center observed that TNF-α, produced by innate immune cells in response to LPS, induces necrosis of cancer tissues [2]. Thus, Coley's study became the starting point for the development of immunotherapeutic anticancer agents that can treat cancer through enhancement of immunity, using the innate immune response as well as the adaptive immune response involving antibodies or T cells.

Currently, immunotherapeutic anticancer agents in clinical use include cytokines such as interferon-α and IL-2, nonspecific immuno-stimulants such as BCG and levamisole, as well as sipuleucel-T (a dendritic cell based therapeutic agent that enhances prostate cancer-specific cell-mediated immunity), and ipilimumab (a monoclonal antibody against CTLA, which inhibits the activation of cytotoxic T lymphocytes). Such immunotherapeutic anticancer agents are currently being actively developed along with targeted anticancer agents.

7.1.1 Cytokines

Cytokines that regulate the activity of immune cells were the first immunotherapeutic anticancer drugs to be developed. A variety of cytokines have since been discovered and their anticancer effects were examined. However, the only cytokines currently approved for clinical uses are interferon-α (IFN- α) and interleukin-2 (IL-2).

7.1.1.1 Interferon-α

In 1954, while investigating the efficacy of smallpox vaccines at the University of Tokyo, Y. Nagano and Y. Kojima injected UV-inactivated smallpox virus into rabbit skin and prepared an extract of the infected tissues after a certain period of time. They studied the effect of this extract on the proliferation of smallpox virus and found that there is a component in this extract which inhibits the proliferation of smallpox virus [3]. In 1957, A. Isaacs and J. Lindenmann working at the British Medical Research Council discovered that infecting the egg amnion with inactivated influenza virus produced a substance that inhibited the proliferation of the live influenza virus, this active substance was named "interferon (IFN)" [4]. Later, it was observed that interferon synthesized following infection with various pathogens such as bacteria, parasites as well as viruses, inhibits not only their proliferation but also the growth of various host cells, including host immune cells. This led to investigations of IFN as a potential anticancer agent.

In humans, interferons are divided into three classes (IFN-α, IFN-β, IFN-γ). Since more than 20 distinct IFN genes have been identified, purification of a single pure interferon and the discovery of their genes took a long time. In 1979, S. Pestka's group at the Roche Institute of Molecular Biology in New Jersey purified human INF-α and reported a partial sequence of its amino acids [5]. In 1980, Pestka's group identified the cDNA and its sequence, and succeeded in producing IFN-α2, a recombinant protein [6]. In the same year, C. Weissmann's group at the Institute of Molecular Life Sciences located in Zurich, Switzerland, discovered that IFN-α is a product of multiple genes (humans possess 12 *IFN-α* genes), and succeeded in producing IFN-α2b recombinant protein in collaboration with Schering-Plough Ltd [7].

Later, clinical trials with IFN-α2a and IFN-α2b were conducted in various cancers, and the FDA approved these two drugs as therapeutic agents for hairy cell leukemia in 1986. Therefore, these were the first cytokine-derived anticancer agents to be developed for clinical use [8]. As cytokines, interferons bind to receptors on target cells, activating JAK-1 and TYK2 tyrosine protein kinases, which in turn induce translocation of the transcription factor STAT1 into the nucleus, where it initiates transcription of more than 100 different genes. As a result, interferons regulate various cellular functions such as cell proliferation, death, differentiation, and motility, as well as physiological processes such as the infection suppression response and angiogenesis.

Owing to the complexity of effects regulated by interferons, delineating the molecular mechanisms responsible for the anticancer effects exhibited by interferons took a long time. It is hypothesized that interferon induced increased expression of MHC class I proteins in cancer cells facilitates the destruction of cancer cells by NK cells and cytotoxic T cells. In addition, interferon increased expression of MHC class II proteins in hematopoietic cells such as dendritic cells and macrophages, which activate cancer cell-specific helper T cells, thereby exerting anticancer effects [9, 10]. Furthermore, various factors such as protein kinase R (PKR), promyelocytic leukemia (PML), RAP46/Bag-1, phospholipid scramblase, the apoptosis inducer APO2L/TRAIL, and Fas ligand are also known to mediate the anticancer effects of interferons (Fig. 7.2).

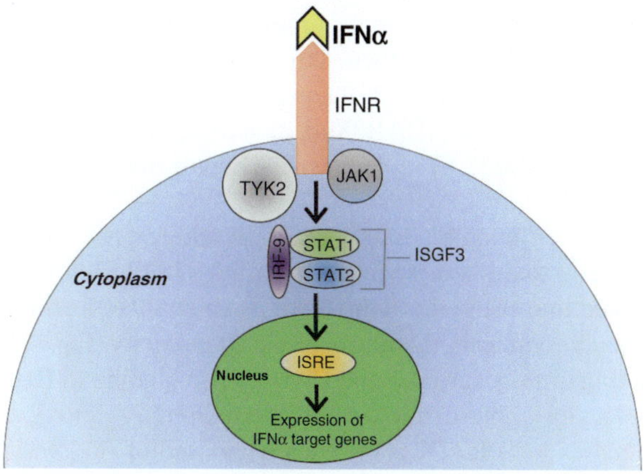

Fig. 7.2 Anticancer mechanism of interferon-α. Interferon-α (*IFNα*) binds to receptors on the membrane of target cells. Subsequently, protein kinases such as JAK-1 and TYK-2 are activated, and interferon-stimulated gene factor 3 (*ISGF3*) is formed from STAT1, STAT2, and IRF-9. ISGF3 moves into the nucleus and binds to interferon-sensitive response elements (*ISRE*) on DNA, inducing expression of various genes and causing a range of responses, such as suppression of cell growth, induction of apoptosis, modulation of cell motility, and regulation of angiogenesis

7.1.1.2 IL-2 (Interleukin-2, Aldesleukin)

IL-2 was the second cytokine-derived anticancer drug to be developed. In 1965, L. Lowenstein's group and L. MacLean's group at McGill University in Canada independently discovered that the culture medium from leukocytes contained a substance that induced proliferation of T lymphocytes [11, 12]. In 1983, K.A. Smith at Dartmouth University purified this active substance IL-2, using an antibody that neutralizes its activity, and determined its N-terminal amino acid sequence [13]. Immediately afterwards, T. Taniguchi et al. at the Japanese Foundation for Cancer Research identified the cDNA sequence of IL-2. Thus, mass production of IL-2 recombinant proteins became possible [14]. Later, S.A. Rosenberg et al. at the NCI conducted various clinical trials to treat cancer in different tissues using IL-2 by inducing T lymphocyte proliferation [15]. As IL-2 was effective in the treatment of metastatic renal carcinoma and melanoma, it was approved by the FDA as a therapeutic agent for these cancers [16]. Even today, IL-2 is an important treatment option for these cancers.

The anticancer mechanisms of IL-2 are proposed to be mediated by the activation of immune cells, especially cytotoxic T-lymphocytes (CTLs) and unlike interferons there is no direct toxic effect on the cancer cells. While IL-2 is known to activate lymphokine-activated killer (LAK) cells and monocytes that kill cancer cells, promote proliferation of T cells stimulated by antigens, and increase cytotoxicity of T lymphocytes and natural killer (NK) cells *in vitro*, the exact mechanisms of IL-2-mediated anticancer effects *in vivo* are not completely understood.

7.1.2 Denileukin Diftitox (DAB389IL2)

IL-2R comprises three kinds of membrane proteins – CD25 (α chain), CD122 (β chain), and CD132 (γ chain) – and these three proteins combined have a high binding affinity for IL-2. In 1987, D.P. Willams et al. at Boston University developed to produce denileukin diftitox (DAB389IL2), a toxic protein that can bind to the IL-2 receptor (IL-2Rα, CD25), by replacing the receptor-binding site of diphtheria toxin with IL-2 [17].

The toxin is endocytosed upon binding with IL-2R and reaches the acidic vesicles. Here, the diphtheria toxin is dissociated from DAB389IL2 by an enzymatic reaction and is released into the cytoplasm where it inhibits the functions of ribosomes involved in protein synthesis, thereby exerting cytotoxicity (Fig. 7.3). IL-2Rα alone has a low binding affinity for IL-2 and DAB389IL2 binding to IL-2Rα alone does not trigger endocytosis, but denileukin diftitox exhibits cytotoxicity specifically against cells that express IL-2R complexes composed of IL-2Rα/β/γ, which have high IL-2 binding affinity.

Since the expression of IL-2R trimeric complexes was reported in cutaneous T-cell lymphoma, the anticancer effect of (DAB389IL2) was investigated mainly in cutaneous T-cell lymphoma [18, 19]. Later, a therapeutic effect of DAB389IL2 was

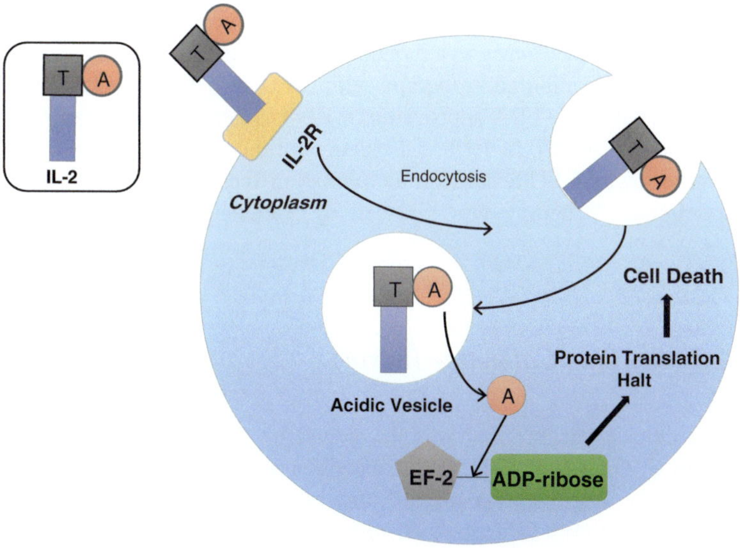

Fig. 7.3 Anticancer mechanism of denileukin diftitox (*DAB389IL2*). Denileukin diftitox protein is a drug formed from a fusion of the membrane translocation domain (*T*) of toxin A from diphtheria toxin (*DT*) with human IL-2. When denileukin diftitox binds to the interleukin-2 (IL-2) receptor (IL-2R) and is endocytosed in an acidic vesicle, the drug undergoes structural changes due to the acidic environment, causing the toxic part (*A*) of DT to separate and move into the cytoplasm. DTA causes ADP-ribosylation of elongation factor 2 (EF2) on ribosomes, interfering with protein synthesis and killing cancer cells

observed in cutaneous T-cell lymphoma, and the FDA approved it as a therapeutic agent for cutaneous T-cell lymphoma in 1999.

Further, preliminary experiments with denileukin diftitox in ovarian and renal cancers have shown an increase in immune function by activation of cytotoxic T cells [20].

7.1.3 Levamisole

Levamisole, a derivative of imidazothiazole, was developed as an anthelmintic by A.H.M. Raeymaekers et al. at Janssen Inc. in Belgium in 1966 [21]. In 1971, G. Renoux and M. Renoux at the Laborotoire d'Immunologie in France observed that levamisole as a vaccine adjuvant enhances immune function upon bacterial vaccine inoculation, and found that this occurs by stimulation of the cellular immune system [22]. Later, to investigate the efficacy of levamisole in treating cancer by immunostimulant, they injected levamisole into a mouse model transplanted with a highly metastatic Lewis lung cancer cells and found that it effectively inhibited growth of the primary cancer as well as the onset of secondary metastatic cancer [23]. Based on these results, clinical trials of levamisole were conducted in various cancers. In a clinical trial in colorectal cancer patients supported by the U.S. NCI, levamisole did not show an efficacy as a monotherapy, but an efficacy was observed when it was used as a combination therapy with 5-FU in patients with stage III colorectal cancer. Hence, the FDA approved it in 1990 as a stage III colorectal cancer therapeutic agent [24, 25]. In 1998, 5-FU/leucovorin combination therapy was found to be superior to 5-FU/levamisole combination therapy. Therefore, 5-FU/levamisole combination therapy was replaced by 5-FU/leucovorin combination therapy.

7.1.4 BCG (Bacillus Calmette-Guérin)

BCG is a tuberculosis vaccine that was developed by the French physiologists A. Calmette and C. Guérin in 1906, and it has been used to prevent tuberculosis since 1921. From the mycobacteria species, they chose to culture *Mycobacterium bovis*, rather than the highly infectious *M. tuberculosis*, on a potato slice soaked with bile and glycerol thereby reducing its toxicity to develop it as a vaccine. In 1924, P.A. Lewis and D. Loomis at the Rockefeller Institute for Medical Research discovered that compared to inoculation with other infectious pathogens, *Mycobacterium tuberculosis* inoculation into a guinea pig induced a strong humoral immune response, the delayed hypersensitivity reaction [26]. Such an enhancement of the immune response was later reported to inhibit proliferation of other infectious pathogens and exhibit an inhibitory effect on cancer in animal implantation tumor models. B. Zbar and H.J. Rapp at the NCI focused on these findings in the 1970s and initiated a comprehensive study using a guinea pig model with tumor implantation in order to develop BCG as a new anticancer agent [27]. They reported that BCG inoculation is highly effective for treatment of skin cancer providing a scientific rationale for clinical development of BCG in cancer. The therapeutic effect of BCG was further investigated in patients with various cancers, and in 1976, A. Morales et al. at Queen's University in Canada reported a remarkable therapeutic efficacy of BCG in bladder cancer when directly injected into the bladder (intravesical injection) [28]. Through clinical results in bladder cancer [29], BCG was finally approved by the FDA as a therapeutic agent for bladder cancer in 1991, and is still used clinically.

The precise mechanism of action of BCG in the treatment of bladder cancer has not been determined. However, it is proposed that when BCG is injected around the tumor lesion, uroepithelial cells around that region recognize BCG as an external antigen and secrete cytokines such as IL-1, IL-6, IL-8, TNF-α, and granulocyte-macrophage colony stimulating factor (GM-CSF), which recruit various immune cells. Among these immune cells, dendritic cells and macrophages facilitate the differentiation of $CD4^{+}$T cells into Type 1 helper T cells (Th) 1 through increased expression of MHC class II as well as presentation of bladder cancer antigens. This response via the Th 1 immune system mainly increases the secretion of IFN-γ, IL-2, and IL-12 and activates various kinds of cellular immunity ultimately resulting in

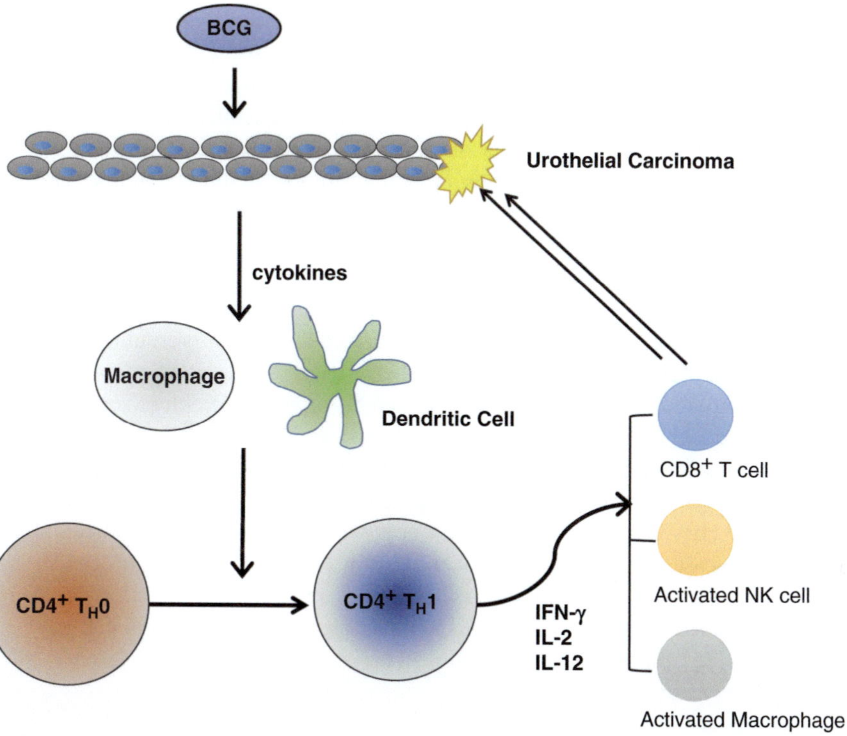

Fig. 7.4 Anticancer mechanism of BCG. When BCG binds to urothelial cells, cytokines and chemokines are secreted, inducing recruitment and activation of immune cells. Activated dendritic cells and macrophages then cause differentiation of $CD4^+$T cells into helper T (*Th*) 1 cells, which amplify the immune response. Secreted IFN-γ, IL-2, and IL-12 activate immune cells to attack and eliminate bladder cancer cells

the elimination of bladder cancer cells (Fig. 7.4). In addition, activated neutrophils secrete tumor necrosis factor-related apoptosis-induced ligand (TRAIL), which is known to play an important role in the destruction of bladder cancer cells.

7.1.5 Imiquimod

Imiquimod (R-837 or S-26308), an immunoregulatory drug of the imidazoquinoline class, was developed by R.L. Miller et al. in 1985 at 3 M Pharmaceuticals (U.S.A) as a drug inhibiting the proliferation of Herpes simplex virus (HSV) [30]. In 1988, C.J. Harrison et al. at the Cincinnati Children's Hospital Medical Center investigated the mechanisms of imiquimod-mediated inhibition of HSV proliferation. They discovered that the drug inhibits HSV proliferation by acting on immunity- and inflammation-related cells inside the body; thereby increasing the expression of INF-α as opposed to a direct effect on viral proliferation [31]. M.J. Reiter et al. at

3 M Pharmaceuticals reported in 1994 that imiquimod enhances the innate immune response by inducing the expression of not only INF-α but also cytokines such as TNF-α and IL-6 that are involved in the innate immune response [32].

Based on these studies, Y.A. Sidky et al. at the Medical College of Wisconsin investigated the anticancer effect using the innate immune response enhanced by imiquimod in animal models with implantation of various solid tumor cell lines and demonstrated the anticancer activity of imiquimod. In 1992, it was reported that the anticancer effect of imiquimod is mainly mediated via increased INF-α expression upon imiquimod administration [33].

In 2002, H. Hemmi et al. at Osaka University in Japan demonstrated that imiquimod binds to toll-like receptor7 (TLR7) on the surface of antigen-presenting cells, such as dendritic cells and macrophages, and induces the expression of pro-inflammatory cytokines such as INF-α, TNF-α, and IL-12 and chemokines such IL-8 [34]. Since INF-α and IL-12 enhance the Th1 cell-mediated immune response, is now also known to exert its anticancer effect by enhancing the adaptive immune response.

Later, clinical trials demonstrated a therapeutic effect of imiquimod in genital warts caused by HPV infection and the FDA approved imiquimod as a therapeutic agent for this disease in 1997. Its anticancer effect was also studied in skin cancer not associated with viral infection, and a therapeutic effect was observed in basal cell carcinoma. Therefore, it was approved as a therapeutic agent for basal cell carcinoma in 2004 [35], and is currently in clinical use.

7.1.6 Ipilimumab

Ipilimumab is a humanized antibody against CTLA-4: a cytotoxic T lymphocyte inhibitory antigen. It was developed as a therapeutic antibody by Bristol-Myers Squibb Inc. Cytotoxic T lymphocytes (CTLs) are known to recognize and destroy cancer cells. When tumor specific antigens are presented to CTLs by dendritic cells, CTLs recognize the antigens through T cell receptors (TCRs), become activated, and consequently attack cancer cells expressing these antigens. However, J.P. Allison et al. at UC Berkeley found that this activation could be inhibited upon binding of CTL cell membrane protein CTLA-4 with the B-7 membrane protein of the antigen-presenting cells (Fig. 7.5) [36]. In 1996, using an animal model of colorectal cancer, the same group observed that treatment with antibodies against CTLA-4 blocks the CTL inhibitory function of CTLA-4, allowing constant CTL activation, thereby exerting a profound therapeutic effect in colorectal cancer [37]. Later, the therapeutic effects of CTLA-4 antibodies were verified in various animal cancer models and T. Keler et al. at Medarex Inc. (a daughter company of Bristol-Myers Squibb) developed ipilimumab as a complete humanized monoclonal antibody in collaboration with J.P. Allison in 1999 [38].

Clinical trials of ipilimumab were conducted with a focus on melanoma because the cancer-specific CTLs [tumor-infiltrating lymphocytes (TIL)] are frequently found in melanoma [39]. A clinical trial using ipilimumab was conducted on patients with metastatic melanoma and had received standard chemotherapy with dacarbazine. The results showed an increase in overall survival by 3.6 months [40]; ipilimumab was therefore approved as a therapeutic agent for malignant melanoma in 2011.

7.1.7 *Sipuleucel-T*

Dendreon, a biotech company in the U.S. developed a method to produce Sipuleucel-T, a dendritic cell that can activate T cells with cytotoxicity against prostate cancer cells, in 2000 [41]. When dendritic cells are isolated from the patients' blood and treated with a genetically engineered surface antigen of prostate cancer cells, PA2024 which is prostatic acid phosphatase (PAP) and GM-CSF fusion protein, the dendritic cells engulf these proteins and present a segment of PAP as an antigen on their surface. When these activated dendritic cells are injected into patients with prostate cancer, cytotoxic T lymphocytes ($CD8^+$ T cell) that respond to PAP are produced and these T cells destroy prostate cancer cells specifically (Fig. 7.6) [41]. After large-scale clinical trials were conducted on prostate cancer patients confirming the therapeutic effect of Sipuleucel-T [42], the FDA approved it as a therapeutic agent for metastatic prostate cancer in 2010.

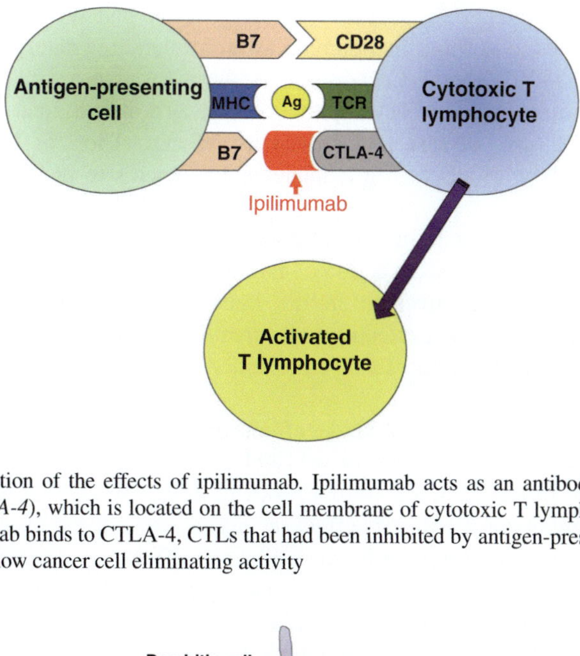

Fig. 7.5 Depiction of the effects of ipilimumab. Ipilimumab acts as an antibody against CTL antigen-4 (*CTLA-4*), which is located on the cell membrane of cytotoxic T lymphocytes (*CTLs*). When ipilimumab binds to CTLA-4, CTLs that had been inhibited by antigen-presenting cells are activated and show cancer cell eliminating activity

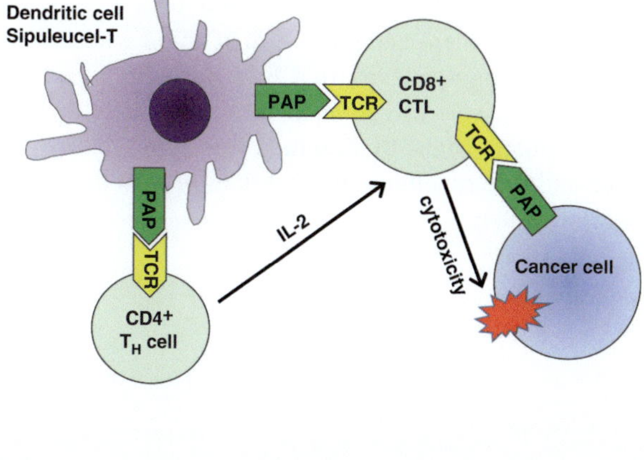

Fig. 7.6 Depiction of sipuleucel-T's actions. When $CD4^+$Th cells are activated by sipuleucel-T dendritic cells, they secrete interleukin-2 (*IL-2*), which promotes proliferation of PAP-specific $CD8^+$Tc cells. $CD8^+$Tc cells recognize PAP expressed on the surface of prostate cancer cells and attack these cells

7.1.8 Thalidomide

Thalidomide is a derivative of glutamic acid. W. Kunz at Chemie Grunenthal Inc. in Germany discovered it as a non-peptide byproduct of the process of developing peptide antibiotics in 1953. His colleague H. Keller noticed that its structure was similar to the sedative glutethimide and investigated whether thalidomide produced similar effects. He discovered that it produced an antiemetic and hypnotic effect. Thalidomide was subsequently approved as a therapeutic agent for morning sickness (hyperemesis gravidarum) in pregnant women [43]. However, since more than 10,000 infants were reportedly born with deformities, including phocomelia, from pregnant women who had taken this drug, thalidomide became one of the most notorious drugs in history and its use was prohibited in the early 1960s.

In 1965, J. Sheskin at the Hadassah University in Israel prescribed thalidomide to treat sleep disorder due to pain in a patient with Hansen's disease and observed that the erythema due to Hansen's disease was cured in this patient. This observation facilitated studies to develop thalidomide as an immune-regulatory and anti-inflammatory drug [44]. Celgene Corporation, a pharmaceutical company in the U.S., led a major clinical study to develop thalidomide as a drug to treat erythema in patients with Hansen's disease and proved its efficacy. Thus, in 1998 FDA approved thalidomide with strict drug management protocols to prevent adverse effects of the drug [45].

A study by E.P. Sampaio et al. in 1991 at Rockefeller University determined the mechanism of the anti-inflammatory action of thalidomide by inhibiting the expression of TNF-α, a cytokine involved in the induction of inflammation [46]. Thalidomide was also found to be effective in the treatment of autoimmune diseases such as rheumatoid arthritis, Behçet's disease, and systemic lupus erythematosus (SLE) (Fig. 7.7).

A study was performed on the anticancer effects of thalidomide by R. D'Amato and J. Folkman at Harvard University in 1994 [47]. They proposed that the deformities caused by thalidomide were a result of defective angiogenesis during the development and evaluated its effect on angiogenesis using animal models. They observed that along with an inhibitory effect on cancer growth thalidomide remarkably suppressed tumor angiogenesis. This led to various studies on the anticancer potential of thalidomide. B. Barlogie's group at the University of Arkansas, in collaboration with J. Folkman, conducted a study using thalidomide mediated inhibition of angiogenesis to treat multiple myeloma with profound angiogenesis. In 1999, Barlogie's group was the first to report that thalidomide was effective in treating multiple myeloma [48]. Following additional clinical trials, thalidomide was approved by the FDA as a therapeutic agent for multiple myeloma in combination with dexamethasone in 2006, and is still in clinical use.

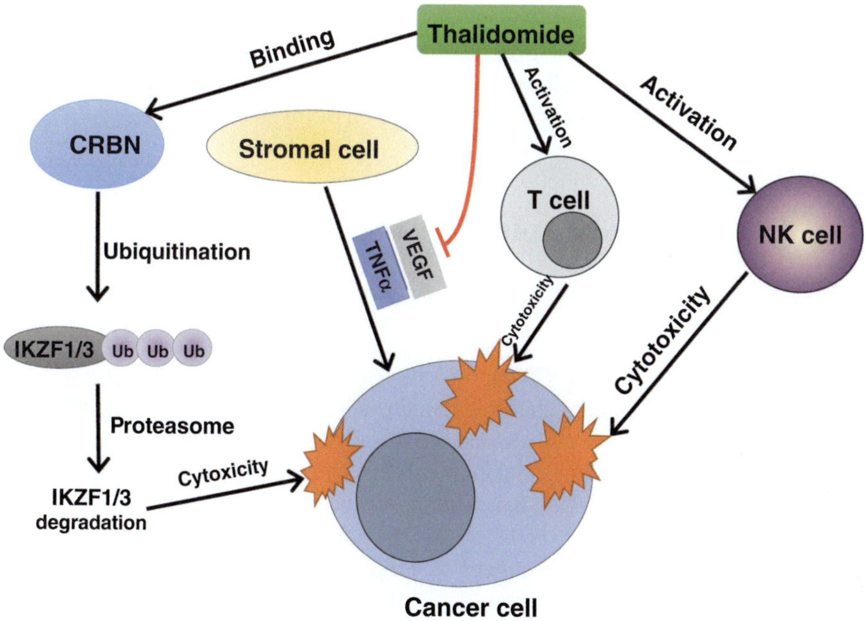

Fig. 7.7 Anticancer mechanism of thalidomide. Thalidomide blocks angiogenesis by inhibiting the expression of VEGF and TNF-α secreted by stromal cells surrounding cancer cells and induces cytotoxic T cells and NK cells to kill multiple myeloma cells. By binding cereblon (*CRBN*) in multiple myeloma cells, thalidomide promotes degradation of Ikaros family zinc finger protein 1 (*IKZF1*) and IKZF3 transcription factors through ubiquitination. Degradation of IKZF1 and IKZF3 regulates the transcriptional activity of several molecules related to the immune system and causes apoptosis in cancer cells

7.1.9 Lenalidomide and Pomalidomide

After discovering the superiority of thalidomide as an anti-inflammatory and anticancer drug, Celgene Inc. conducted a study on second-generation thalidomide derivatives that exhibit improved efficacy and less toxicity. G.W. Muller et al. synthesized various derivatives from thalidomide and EM-12, an analogue of thalidomide and verified their effects on the inhibition of TNF-α expression in peripheral blood mononuclear cells (PBMCs) induced by LPS. They discovered that two of the derivatives, pomalidomide and lenalidomide with an amino group conjugated to the fourth carbon of the phthaloyl ring, exhibited better efficacy compared to other derivatives [49]. These drugs showed a 50,000-fold higher inhibitory effect on the expression of TNF-α compared to thalidomide. After clinical trials in various diseases, including myeloma, lenalidomide and pomalidomide were FDA-approved as therapeutic agents for multiple myeloma in 2006 and 2013, respectively [50, 51]. In 2014,

J. Krönke et al. at the Brigham and Women's Hospital studied the molecular mechanisms of action of these drugs in multiple myeloma and discovered that lenalidomide binds to the E3 ubiquitin ligase complex and facilitates the degradation of IKZF1 and IKZF3, important transcription factors for proliferation of myeloma cells [52].

7.2 Other Miscellaneous Anticancer Drugs

7.2.1 Mitotane (o,p-Dichlorodiphenyldichloroethane)

Mitotane is a derivative of DDT (dichlorodiphenyltrichloroethane) and is a para isomer of DDD (dichlorodiphenyldichloroethane), which was used as a pesticide along with DDT. In 1949, A.A. Nelson and G. Woodard reported that DDD injection to dogs triggered adrenal cortical damage [53]. The major component responsible for this damage to the adrenal gland was determined to be mitotane. D.M. Bergenstal et al. at the NCI predicted that the adrenal cortical specific action of mitotane could be applied in treatment of adrenocortical carcinoma. In 1959, after injecting mitotane in cancer patients, they reported a therapeutic effect in adrenocortical carcinoma [54]. Since the therapeutic effect of mitotane was confirmed by major clinical trials in patients with adrenocortical carcinoma, it was approved by FDA in 1970 and is still in clinical use. Although the anticancer mechanism of mitotane is not clearly known, it is postulated that o,p-DDA [1,1-(o,p-dichlorodiphenyl) acetic acid] produced by the action of an unidentified drug metabolic enzyme abundant in the adrenal cortex acts as a free radical and disrupts mitochondrial function, leading to cytotoxicity [55].

7.2.2 Asparaginase

Asparaginase is an enzyme that metabolizes asparagine into aspartic acid and ammonia. It exerts an anticancer effect by inhibiting the production of proteins necessary for the proliferation of cancer cells. In 1953, J.G. Kidd's group at the New York Hospital-Cornell Medical Center observed that injecting the serum of guinea pig into a murine leukemia model alleviated lymphocytic leukemia [56]. This phenomenon was not reproducible on injecting horse or rabbit serum. Therefore, they proposed that a specific anticancer substance is present in the serum of guinea pig. In 1963, D. Broome at the same institute came across a report from 1922 that guinea pig serum contains higher amount of asparaginase compared to the sera of other animals. This along with the finding from 1956 by R.E. Neuman and T.A. McCoy at the Samuel Roberts Noble Foundation Research Institute in Oklahoma that asparagine is required in the culture of Walker Carcinosarcoma 256 cells helped D. Broome to establish that the anticancer substance in the serum of guinea pig could be asparaginase [57, 58].

However, there were practical difficulties in obtaining asparaginase from the serum of guinea pigs to treat patients. To isolate asparaginase enough for treating a single leukemia patient, serum from 4,000 guinea pigs was needed each day. In 1964, L.T. Mashburn and J.C. Wriston at the Memorial Sloan-Kettering Cancer Center reported that L-asparaginase purified from *E. coli* culture medium has an anticancer effect; this allowed mass production of L-asparaginase [59]. Although normal lymphocytes, other normal tissues, and cancer cells can all synthesize L-asparagine, acute lymphoblastic leukemia (ALL) cells specifically synthesize low amounts of L-asparagine, which leads to a selective toxicity for ALL cells upon L-asparaginase treatment. Hence, major clinical trials using L-asparaginase were conducted in ALL patients, and it was approved by the FDA as a therapeutic agent for ALL in 1978.

However, due to the xenogenous nature of L-asparaginase produced by *E. coli*, it generally induced an immune hypersensitive reaction during the treatment. Therefore, further studies were conducted to overcome this adverse effect. In 1978, Y. Ashihara et al. at the Tokyo Institute of Technology observed that Peg-asparaginase, in which polyethylene glycol (PEG) was conjugated to L-asparaginase lowered immune stimulation and weakened the hypersensitive response [60]. Studies investigating the drug metabolism of Peg-asparaginase elucidated that the drug half-life was also markedly extended and it was predicted to be an anticancer agent with improved efficacy and fewer toxicities over L-asparaginase. After clinical trials in ALL patients, Peg-asparaginase was approved by the FDA as a therapeutic agent for ALL in 1994.

In 1968, H.E. Wade et al. at the Microbiological Research Establishment in England studied the activity of asparaginases from more than 200 species of bacteria and discovered a significantly higher activity of asparaginases from the culture medium of a plant pathogenic bacterium, *Erwinia chrysanthemi* [61]. Cross reactivity of the immune response was not observed between the asparaginase produced by *E. chrysanthemi* and the asparaginase produced by *E. coli*. Therefore, it was approved by the FDA as a therapeutic agent for ALL patients who exhibited a hypersensitive reaction to asparaginase produced from *E. coli*.

7.2.3 Porfimer Sodium: Photodynamic Therapy (PDT)

In photodynamic anticancer therapy, irradiation with specific wavelengths activates the chemicals injected into patients. These chemicals generate reactive oxygen species, subsequently destroying cancer cells. In 1900, O. Raabe at the University of Munich in Germany reported that acridine added to the culture medium of paramecia killed them in a light-dependent manner [62]. His advisor, H. von Tappeiner found that oxygen was involved in this process and proposed the term photodynamic therapy for the first time. In 1903, Tappeiner reported that applying eosin to patients with skin cancer and irradiating white light alleviated the symptoms of skin cancer, thereby introducing photodynamic therapy as a treatment for cancer [63].

The drugs that are most frequently used for the study of photodynamic therapy are porphyrin compounds. The well-known porphyrin: protoporphyrin binds to iron and forms heme, which is a major component of hemoglobin in erythrocytes. In 1911, W. Hausmann at Universität Wien first reported that hematoporphyrin formed on exposing erythrocytes to acid killed erythrocytes and paramecia in a light-dependent manner [64]. In 1913, F. Meyer-Betz at the University of Munich injected hematoporphyrin to himself and observed that it showed phototoxicity when exposed to sunlight [65]. Later, in 1942, H. Auler and G. Banzer in Berlin reported that hematoporphyrin specifically accumulated in tumor tissues in cancer patients [66]. In 1961, R. Lipson and his colleagues at the University of Minnesota produced a haematoporphyrin derivative (HPD) by adding sulfuric acid and acetic acid to hematoporphyrin and injected it into cancer patients. As a result, it was observed that HPD accumulated in cancer tissues with significantly higher sensitivity than hematoporphyrin, and it was proposed for application in cancer diagnosis [67]. Later, studies on the therapeutic effect of HPD in cancer were conducted in animal models, and T.J. Dougherty et al. at the Roswell Park Cancer Institute in New York observed in 1975 that when HPD was injected in mice with breast cancer and the mice were irradiated with red light, the cancer was completely eradicated [68]. Around the same time, J.F. Kelly et al. at St. Mary's Hospital in London reported excellent therapeutic effects of HPD in a bladder cancer model [69]. In 1956, J.F. Kelly et al. conducted clinical trials in bladder cancer patients and observed a therapeutic effect of HPD in cancer. Later, clinical trials were conducted in various cancers, and the FDA approved Porfimer sodium as a therapeutic agent for esophageal cancer in 1995. However, it is currently rarely used due to the development of concurrent chemoradiotherapy.

7.2.4 Arsenic Trioxide

Use of arsenic trioxide as a drug has a long history. Shinnongbonchogyeong (AD 250; also known as Shennong Bencao Jing, or the Herbal Classic of Shennong), published during the Han dynasty in China, mentions the use of arsenic trioxide as a therapeutic agent for chill, anemia, ulcer, extermination of insects, and tumors. The Compendium of Materia Medica published in China around AD 1590 mentions that it was used for treatment of chronic ulcers and cervical lymphadenopathy. In the West, Ibn Sina from the Persian Empire in the eleventh century mentions arsenic trioxide as a therapeutic agent for cancer, and Paracelsus from Switzerland, who established the basis for toxicology in the sixteenth century, also mentioned it as a therapeutic agent for cancer, ulcers, and wounds.

In the eighteenth century, T. Fowler from England made Fowler's solution, which is arsenic trioxide dissolved in potassium bicarbonate solution, and reported its effect in diseases such as malaria, headache, and fever. In 1865, H. Lissauer from Breslau, Germany, used Fowler's solution for cancer treatment and reported that it cured acute leukemia [70]. Fowler's solution was widely used as a therapeutic agent for leukemia until the introduction of chemotherapy in the 1940s.

In China in the 1970s when using Western medicine became difficult due to the Cultural Revolution, there were attempts to develop alternative drugs from traditional therapy. Treatment of leukemia with arsenic trioxide was attempted by T.D. Zhang et al. at the Harbin University. They reported in 1981 that it especially had a superior therapeutic effect in acute promyelocytic leukemia (APL) [71]. Arsenic trioxide was registered as the first anticancer drug in China. Later, S.L. Soignet et al. at the Memorial Sloan-Kettering Cancer Center in the U.S. conducted clinical trials using arsenic trioxide in APL patients [72]. In a clinical trial on APL patients who did not respond to all-*trans* retinoic acid (ATRA) treatment or whose APL relapsed after treatment, arsenic trioxide was highly effective with a complete remission in more than 85 % cases, and it was approved by the FDA in 2000 [73]. Currently, arsenic trioxide is used in APL when there is resistance against all-*trans* retinoic acid treatment.

Although the anticancer mechanisms of arsenic trioxide in APL have not been fully understood, J. Zhu et al. at Shanghai Second Medical University suggested in 1997 that arsenic trioxide generates free radicals and induces oxidative stress, which decreases the stability of PML-RARα protein, an oncogenic fusion protein commonly observed in APL, resulting in tumor cell death (Fig. 7.8) [74].

7.2.5 *Hydroxyurea (Hydroxycarbamide)*

Hydroxyurea was first synthesized by W.F.C. Dresler at the Rostock University in Germany in 1869 [75]. In 1928, F. Rosenthal et al. at the Breslau University in Germany discovered that hydroxyurea inhibited growth of leukocytes in the bone marrow of rabbits [76]. Based on these findings, various research groups conducted studies to develop hydroxyurea as a new anticancer agent in the 1960s, and

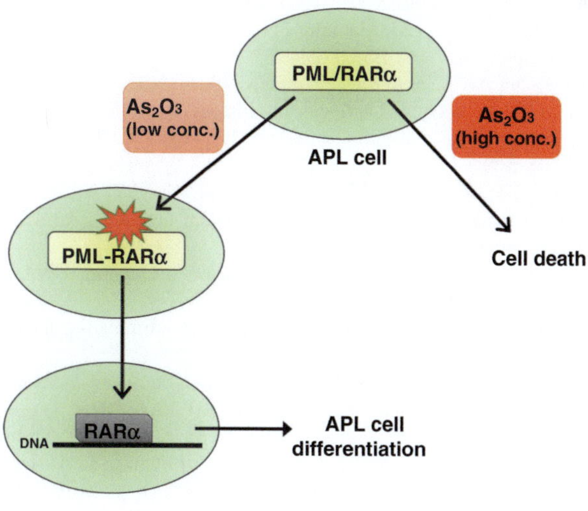

Fig. 7.8 Arsenic trioxide mechanism of action. At low concentrations, arsenic trioxide (As_2O_3) binds to PML and promotes degradation of the PML-RARα (retinoic acid receptor α) complex, inducing differentiation of immature APL cells. At high concentrations, AS_2O_3 induces death of APL cells directly

B. Stearns et al. at the Squibb Institute observed an anticancer effect of hydroxyurea in an animal leukemia model [77]. Further, clinical trials were conducted in various kinds of cancer, and B.J. Kennedy et al. at the University of Minnesota Medical Center reported superior efficacy of hydroxyurea in chronic myeloid leukemia (CML) in 1966 [78]. It was therefore approved by the FDA as a therapeutic agent for myeloproliferative disorder in 1967. Since then, hydroxyurea has been actively used for the treatment of chronic myeloid leukemia (CML) such as polycythemia vera (PV) and essential thrombocythemia.

Studies on its mechanism of action conducted around the same time showed that hydroxyurea binds to ribonucleotide reductase and inhibits the formation of deoxyribonucleotides from ribonucleotides, which disrupts DNA synthesis during the S phase, thereby exerting an anticancer effect [79, 80].

References

1. Coley WB (1893) The treatment of malignant tumors by repeated inoculations of erysipelas, with a report of ten original cases. Am J Med Sci 105:487–511
2. Carswell EA, Old LJ, Kassel RL, Green S, Fiore N, Williamson B (1975) An endotoxin – induced serum factor that causes necrosis of tumors. Proc Natl Acad Sci 72:3666–3670
3. Nagano Y, Kojima Y (1954) Pouvoir immunisant du virus vaccinal inactivé par des rayons ultraviolets. CR Seans Soc Biol Fil 148:1700–1702
4. Isaacs A, Lindenmann J (1957) Virus interference. I. The interferon. Proc R Soc Lond B Biol Sci 147:258–267
5. Rubinstein M, Rubinstein S, Familletti PC, Miller RS, Waldman AA, Pestka S (1979) Human leukocyte interferon: production, purification to homogeneity and initial characterization. Proc Natl Acad Sci 76:640–644
6. Maeda S, McCandliss R, Gross M, Sloma A, Familletti PC, Tabor JM, Evinger M, Levy WP, Pestka S (1980) Construction and identification of bacterial plasmids containing nucleotide sequence for human leukocyte interferon. Proc Natl Acad Sci 77:7010–7013
7. Streuli M, Nagata S, Weissmann C (1980) At least three human type alpha interferons: structure of alpha 2. Science 209:1343–1347
8. Quesada JR, Hersh EM, Manning J et al (1986) Treatment of hairy cell leukemia with recombinant alpha-interferon Blood 68:493–497
9. Imai K, Ng AK, Glassy MC, Ferrone S (1981) Differential effect of interferon on the expression of tumor-associated antigens and histocompatibility antigens on human melanoma cells: relationship to susceptibility to immune lysis mediated by monoclonal antibodies. J Immunol 127:505–509
10. Basham TY, Bourgeade MF, Creasey AA, Merigan TC (1982) Interferon increases HLA synthesis in melanoma cells: interferon-resistant and sensitive cell lines. Proc Natl Acad Sci 79:3265–3269
11. Kasakura S, Lowenstein L (1965) A factor stimulating DNA synthesis derived from the medium of leukocyte cultures. Nature 208:794–795
12. Gordon J, MacLean LD (1965) A lymphocyte-stimulating factor produced *in vitro*. Nature 208:795–796
13. Smith KA, Favata MF, Oroszlan S (1983) Production and characterization of monoclonal antibodies to human interleukin 2. J Immunol 131:1808–1815
14. Taniguchi T, Matsui H, Fujita T, Takaoka C, Kashima N, Yoshimoto R, Hamuro J (1983) Structure and expression of a cloned cDNA for human interleukin-2. Nature 302:305–310
15. Rosenberg SA, Lotze MT, Muul LM et al (1985) Observations on the systemic administration of autologous lymphokine activated killer cells and recombinant interleukin-2 to patients with metastatic cancer. N Engl J Med 313:1485–1492

16. Weiss GR, Margolin KA, Aronson FR et al (1992) A randomized phase II trial of continuous infusion interleukin-2 or bolus injection interleukin-2 plus lymphokine-activated killer cells for advanced renal cell carcinoma. J Clin Oncol 10:275–281
17. Williams DP, Parker K, Bacha P, Bishai W, Borowski M, Genbauffe F, Strom TB, Murphy JR (1987) Diphtheria toxin receptor binding domain substitution with interleukin-2: genetic construction and properties of a diphtheria toxin-related interleukin-2 fusion protein. Protein Eng 1:493–498
18. Nakase K, Kita K, Nasu K et al (1994) Differential expression of interleukin-2 receptors (alpha and beta chain) in mature lymphoid neoplasms. Am J Hematol 46:179–183
19. Olsen E, Duvic M, Frankel A et al (2001) Pivotal phase III trial of two dose levels of denileukin diftitox for the treatment of cutaneous T-cell lymphoma. J Clin Oncol 19:376–388
20. Attia P, Maker AV, Haworth LR, Rogers-Freezer L, Rosenberg SA (2005) Inability of a fusion protein of IL-2 and diphtheria toxin (Denileukin Diftitox, DAB389IL-2, ONTAK) to eliminate regulatory T lymphocytes in patients with melanoma. J Immunother 28:582–592
21. Raeymaekers AHM, Allewijn FTN, Vandenberk J et al (1966) Novel broad-spectrum anthelmintics. Tetramisole and related derivatives of 6-arylimidazo [2,1-b]thiazole. J Med Chem 9:545–549
22. Renoux G, Renoux M (1971) Immunostimulating effect of an imidotiiazole in the immunization of mice against Brucella abortus infection. C R Acad Sci Hebd Seances Acad Sci 272:349–350
23. Renoux G, Renoux M (1972) Levamisole inhibits and cures a solid malignant tumour and its pulmonary metastases in mice. Nat New Biol 240:217–218
24. Moertel CG, Fleming TR, Macdonald JS et al (1990) Levamisole and fluorouracil for adjuvant therapy of resected colon carcinoma. N Engl J Med 322:352–358
25. Laurie JA, Moertel CG, Fleming TR et al (1989) Surgical adjuvant therapy of large-bowel carcinoma: an evaluation of levamisole and the combination of levamisole and fluorouracil. J Clin Oncol 7:1447–1456
26. Lewis PA, Loomis D (1924) Allergic irritability. The formation of antisheep hemiolytic amboceptor in the normal and tuberculous guinea pig. J Exp Med 40:503–515
27. Zbar B, Bernstein ID, Rapp HJ (1971) Suppression of tumor growth at the site of infection with living Bacillus Calmette-Guérin. J Natl Cancer Inst 46:831–839
28. Morales A, Eidinger D, Bruce AW (1976) Intracavitary Bacillus Calmette-Guerin in the treatment of superficial bladder tumors. J Urol 116:180–183
29. Lamm DL, Blumenstein BA, Crawford ED et al (1991) A randomized trial of intravesical doxorubicin and immunotherapy with bacille Calmette-Guérin for transitional cell carcinoma of the bladder. N Engl J Med 325:1205–1209
30. Miller RL, Imberston LM, Reiter MJ, Schwartzmiller DS, Pecore SE, Gerster JF (1985) Inhibition of herpes simplex virus infections in a guinea pig model by S-26308. Abstracts of the 25th ASM Interscience Conference on Antimicrobial Agents and Chemotherapy. p. 235
31. Harrison CJ, Jenski L, Voychehovski T, Bernstein DI (1988) Modification of immunological responses and clinical disease during topical R-837 treatment of genital HSV-2 infection. Antiviral Res 10:209–223
32. Reiter MJ, Testerman TL, Miller RL, Weeks CE, Tomai MA (1994) Cytokine induction in mice by the immunomodulator imiquimod. J Leukoc Biol 55:234–240
33. Sidky YA, Borden EC, Weeks GE, Reiter MJ, Hatcher JE, Bryan GT (1992) Inhibition of murine tumor growth by an interferon – inducing imidazoquinolinamine. Cancer Res 52: 3528–3533
34. Hemmi H, Kaisho T, Takeuchi O et al (2002) Small anti-viral compounds activate immune cells via the TLR7 Myd88-dependent signaling pathway. Nat Immunol 3:196–200
35. Schulze HJ, Cribier B, Requena L et al (2005) Imiquimod 5% cream for the treatment of superficial basal cell carcinoma: results from a randomized vehicle-controlled phase III study in Europe. Br J Dermatol 152:939–947
36. Krummel MF, Allison JP (1995) CD28 and CTLA-4 have opposing effects on the response of T cells to stimulation. J Exp Med 182:459–465
37. Leach D, Krummel M, Allison JP (1996) Enhancement of antitumor immunity by CTLA-4 blockade. Science 271:1734–1736

38. Keler T, Halk E, Vitale L et al (2003) Activity and safety of CTLA-4 blockade combined with vaccines in cynomolgus macaques. J Immunol 171:6251–6259
39. Muul LM, Spiess PJ, Director EP, Rosenberg SA (1987) Identification of specific cytolytic immune responses against autologous tumor in humans bearing malignant melanoma. J Immunol 138:989–995
40. Hodi FS, O'Day SJ, Medermitt DF et al (2010) Improved survival with ipilimumab in patients with metastatic melanoma. N Engl J Med 363:711–723
41. Small EJ, Fratesi P, Reese DM, Strang G, Laus R, Peshwa MV, Valone FH (2000) Immunotherapy of hormone-refractory prostate cancer with antigen-loaded dendritic cells. J Clin Oncol 18:3894–3903
42. Small EJ, Schellhammer PF, Higano CS et al (2006) Placebo-controlled phase III trial of immunologic therapy with sipuleucel-T (APC8015) in patients with metastatic, asymptomatic hormone refractory prostate cancer. J Clin Oncol 24:3089–3094
43. King W, Keller H, Muckter H (1956) N-Phthalylglutaminsaure-imid. Experimentelle Untersuchungen an einem neuen synthetischen Produktmit sedativen Eigenschaften. Arzneimittelforschurg 6:426–442
44. Sheskin J (1965) Thalidomide in the treatment of lepra reactions. Clin Pharmacol Ther 6:303–306
45. Calderon P, Anzilotti M, Phelps R (1997) Thalidomide in dermatology. New indications for an old drug. Int J Dermatol 36:881–886
46. Sampaio EP, Sarno EN, Galilly R, Cohn ZA, Kaplan G (1991) Thalidomide selectively inhibits tumor necrosis factor alpha production by stimulated human monocytes. J Exp Med 173: 699–703
47. D'Amato RJ, Loughan MS, Flynn E, Folkman J (1994) Thalidomide is an inhibitor of angiogenesis. Proc Natl Acad Sci 91:4082–4085
48. Singhal S, Mehta J, Desikan R et al (1999) Antitumor activity of thalidomide in refractory multiple myeloma. N Engl J Med 341:1565–1571
49. Muller GW, Chen R, Huang SY et al (1999) Amino-substituted thalidomide analogs, potent inhibitors of TNF-alpha production. Bioorg Med Chem Lett 9:1625–1630
50. Weber DM, Chen C, Niesvizky R et al (2006) Lenalidomide plus high-dose dexamethasone provides improved overall survival compared to high-dose dexamethasone alone for relapsed or refractory multiple myeloma (MM): results of a North American phase III study (MM-009). J Clin Oncol (Meeting Abstracts) 24:7521
51. San Miguel J, Weisel K, Moreau P et al (2013) Pomalidomide plus lowdose dexamethasone versus high-dose dexamethasone alone for patients with relapsed and refractory multiple myeloma (MM-003): a randomised, open-label, phase 3 trial. Lancet Oncol 14:1055–1066
52. Krönke J, Udeshi ND, Narla A, Grauman P et al (2014) Lenalidomide causes selective degradation of IKZF1 and IKZF3 in multiple myeloma cells. Science 343:301–305
53. Nelson AA, Woodard G (1949) Severe adrenal cortical atrophy (cytotoxic) and hepatic damage produced in dogs by feeding 2,2-bis(parachlorophenyl)-1,1-dichloroethane (DDD or TDE). Arch Pathol 48:387–393
54. Bergenstal DM, Lipsett MB, Moy RH, Hertz R (1959) Regression of adrenal cancer and suppression of adrenal function in men by o, p'-DDD. Trans Am Phys 72:341–350
55. Andersen A, Warren DJ, Nome O, Vesterhus L, Slordal L (1995) A high-pressure liquid chromatographic method for measuring mitotane [1,1-(o,p'-dichlorodiphenyl)- 2,2-dichloroethane] and its metabolite 1,1-(o, p'-dichlorodiphenyl)-2,2- dichloroethene in plasma. Ther Drug Monit 17:526–531
56. Kidd JG (1953) Regression of transplanted lymphomas induced *in vivo* by means of normal guinea pig serum. I. Course of transplanted cancers of various kinds in mice and rats given guinea pig serum, horse serum, or rabbit serum. J Exp Med 98:565–582
57. Broome JD (1961) Evidence that the L-asparaginase activity of guinea pig serum is responsible for its antilymphoma effects. Nature 191:1114–1115
58. Broome JD (1963) Evidence that the L-asparaginase of guinea pig serum is respnsible for its antilymhpoma effects. I. Properties of the L-asparaginase of guinea pig serum in relation to those of the antilymphoma substance. J Exp Med 118:99–120

59. Mashburn LT, Wriston JC Jr (1964) Tumor inhibitory effect of L-asparaginase from *Escherichia coli*. Arch Biochem Biophys 105:450–453
60. Ashihara Y, Kono T, Yamazaki S, Inada Y (1978) Modification of *E. coli* L-asparaginase with polyethylene glycol: disappearance of binding ability to anti-asparaginase serum. Biochem Biophys Res Commun 83:385–391
61. Wade HE, Elsworth R, Herbert E et al (1968) A new L-asparaginase with antitumor activity. Lancet 2:776–777
62. Raabe O (1900) Uber die Wirkung fluoreszierender Stoffe auf Infusorien. Zeitung Biol 39:524–526
63. von Tappeiner H, Jesionek A (1903) Therapeutische versuche mit fluoreszierenden stoffen. Muench Med Wochenschr 47:2042–2044
64. Hausmann W (1911) Die sensiblisierende Wirkung des Hematoporphyrins. Biochem Zeitung 30:276–316
65. Meyer-Betz F (1913) Untersuchungen uber die biologische photodynamische Wirkung des Hematoporphyrins und anderer Derivative des Blut und Galenafarbstoffs. Dtsch Arch Klin 112:476–503
66. Auler H, Banzer G (1942) Untersuchungen uber die Rolle der Porphyrine bei geschwulstkranken Menschen und Tieren. Z Krebsforsch 53:65–68
67. Lipson RL, Baldes EJ, Olsen AM (1961) The use of an derivative of hematoporphyrin in tumor detection. J Natl Cancer Inst 26:1–11
68. Dougherty TJ, Grindey GB, Fiel R, Weishaupt KR, Boyle DG (1975) Photoradiation therapy. II Cure of animal tumors with hematoporphyrin and light. J Natl Cancer Inst 55:115–121
69. Kelly JF, Snell ME, Berenbaum MC (1975) Photodynamic destruction of human bladder carcinoma. Br J Cancer 31:237–244
70. Lissauer H (1865) Zwei fälle von leucaemie. Berl Klin Wochenschr 2:403–404
71. Zhang TD, Sun HD, Hu HX (1981) Treatment of acute promyelocytic leukemia with Ailing number one combination therapy: a study of 73 cases. Heilongjiang J Tradit Chin Med 4:40–44
72. Soignet SL, Maslak P, Wang ZG et al (1998) Complete remission after treatment of acute promyelocytic leukemia with arsenic trioxide. N Engl J Med 339:1341–1348
73. Soignet SL, Frankel S, Douer D, Tallman M et al (2001) United States multicenter study of arsenic trioxide in relapsed acute promyelocytic leukemia. J Clin Oncol 19:3852–3860
74. Zhu J, Koken MH, Quignon F et al (1997) Arsenic-induced PML targeting onto nuclear bodies: implications for the treatment of acute promyelocytic leukemia. Proc Natl Acad Sci 94:3978–3983
75. Dresler WFC, Stein R (1869) Ueber den Hydroxylharnstoff. Justus Liebigs Ann Chem Pharmacol 150:242–252
76. Rosenthal F, Wislicki L, Kollek L (1928) Uber die beziehungen von schwersten blutgiften zu abbauprodukten des eiweisses. Klin Wochenschr 7:972–977
77. Stearns B, Losee KA, Bernstein J (1963) Hydroxyurea: a new type of potential antitumor agent. J Med Chem 6:201
78. Kennedy BJ, Yarbro JW (1966) Metabolic and therapeutic effects of hydroxyurea in chronic myeloid leukemia. JAMA 195:1038–1043
79. Young CW, Hodas S (1964) Hydroxyurea: inhibitory effect on DNA metabolism. Science 146:1172–1174
80. Krakoff IH, Brown NC, Reichard P (1968) Inhibition of ribonucleoside diphosphate reductase by hydroxyurea. Cancer Res 28:1559–1565

Chapter 8
Hormonal Anticancer Drugs

Paul Ehrlich, a pioneer in chemotherapy, experienced many failures while developing anticancer chemotherapy due to the indiscriminate toxicity of chemotherapy drugs. In 1915, based on his experience, he stressed on the importance of understanding the biological difference between normal cells and cancer cells for the development of a cancer-specific magic bullet. This suggestion was realized with the invention of targeted anticancer agents after decades of basic research in the field of cancer biology. Another example of an anticancer drug that was successfully developed after understanding the biological characteristics of a specific cancer is the hormonal anticancer drug.

The observation that removal of the testes of prostate cancer patients and ovaries of breast cancer patients alleviated the cancers themselves led to the discovery of hormonal anticancer drugs. Further studies reported that hormones such as testosterone and estrogen, which are secreted by the testis and ovaries, are related to the development of prostate and breast cancer, respectively. These discoveries led to the development of anticancer agents from synthetic compounds or other hormones that regulate the production of these sex hormones (Fig. 8.1).

8.1 Hormonal Anti-prostate-Cancer Drugs

The discovery that testosterone aggravates prostate cancer was based on the findings that prostate development was modulated by the endocrine system of the testicles. In 1786, J. Hunter, a Scottish surgeon and pioneer of modern surgery, discovered that the size of the testis and prostate of animals concurrently changed depending on the season. He also observed prostate shrinkage in animals whose testicles had been removed. This led to the hypothesis that testis regulates prostate development. In 1893, W.J. White, a surgeon in Philadelphia, performed orchiectomy on a dog and found that it led to changes in the anatomical structure of its prostate, degeneration of the prostate gland tissue and surrounding muscle tissue, and a decrease in prostate weight [1].

K.-W. Kim et al., *Cancer Drug Discovery*, DOI 10.1007/978-94-024-0844-7_8

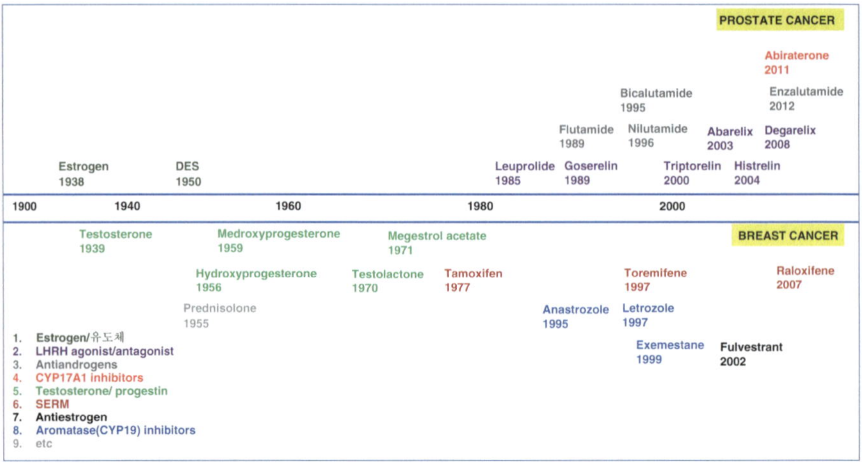

Fig. 8.1 Types of hormonal anticancer agent and a chronology of their development

C.B. Huggins of the University of Chicago performed a study on how testosterone secreted from the testicles accelerated the growth of the prostate cancer and used orchiectomy or estrogen administration to inhibit this process. In 1939, Huggins studied the physiological phenomena of a canine prostate and its prostatic fluid secretion when he observed that testis removal decreased prostatic fluid secretion and prostate size. After assuming that this phenomenon was due to the decrease in testosterone levels by orchiectomy, he administered testosterone to the dog and observed contrary results in the prostate. In addition, when estrogen was administered to a normal dog, the effects were similar to those of orchiectomy, which led to the assumption that estrogen exerts anti-testosterone effects [2].

Based on these results, in 1940, Huggins investigated the effects of orchiectomy and estrogen administration on the spontaneous development of prostate cancer in a dog. He discovered that the development of prostate cancer was significantly inhibited [3]. This discovery led to the hypothesis that prostate cancer cells cannot survive independently, and their development is dependent on the hormones of the host, similar to the development of normal prostate cells. In 1941, Huggins conducted a clinical trial to see if these effects also occur in humans. He found that diethylstilbestrol (DES), a form of synthetic estrogen, inhibited testosterone synthesis and acted as a chemical castration agent, alleviating the symptoms of prostate cancer over a period of several months [4, 5]. After such therapeutic effects were discovered, in 1950, the FDA approved DES for the treatment of prostate cancer, following its FDA approval in 1941 for the alleviation of post-menopausal symptoms and treatment of congestion of the mammary glands. Huggins received the Nobel Prize in Physiology or Medicine in 1966 for his contribution to prostate cancer treatment using castration and DES. The use of DES for prostate cancer treatment was the first attempt to use a selective agent rather than a non-selective cytotoxic agent for cancer treatment.

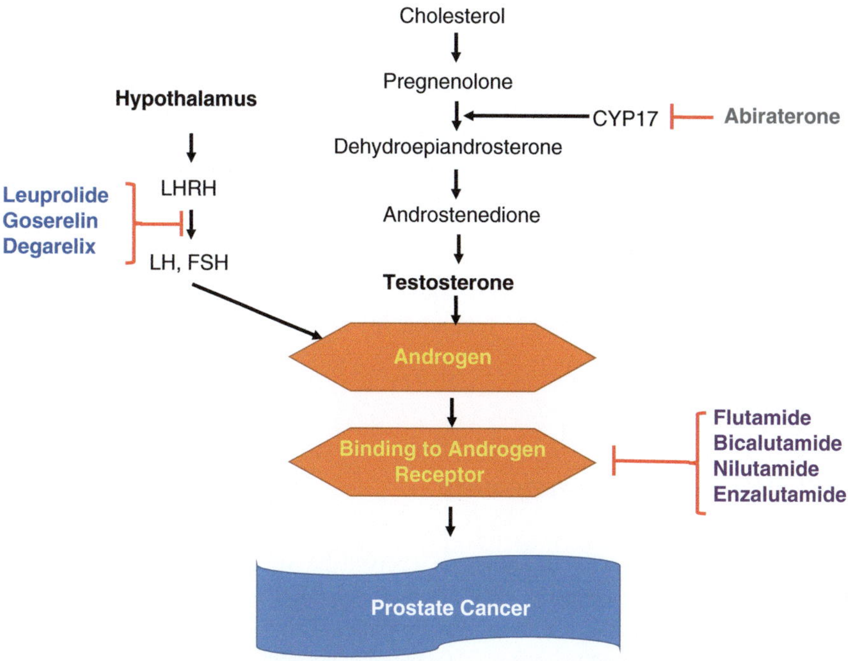

Fig. 8.2 Hormonal anticancer agents used in the treatment of prostate cancer

Later, various strategies were developed to inhibit androgen action. The principles behind these treatments are based on the scientific discovery of the hypothalamo-pituitary-gonadal/adrenal axis, the functions of which are mediated by various hormones. First, two peptide hormones, luteinizing hormone-releasing hormone (LHRH) and corticotropin-releasing factor (CRF), are released in the hypothalamus and stimulate the pituitary gland to release luteinizing hormone (LH) and adrenocorticotropic hormone (ACTH), respectively. LH stimulates testosterone synthesis in the testis, while ACTH accelerates the production of androstenedione and dehydro-epiandrosterone in the adrenal cortex. These three steroidal hormones are absorbed by the prostate gland and transformed into androgen. The 5-α-reductase in the prostate gland cells transforms testosterone into 5α-dihydrotestosterone that acts as the main androgen. Similar to estrogen, 5α-dihydrotestosterone has been found to accelerate the development of prostate cancer cells by binding with the androgen receptor (AR).

This circuit has a feedback control system in which testosterone acts on the hypothalamus and pituitary gland to inhibit the release of LHRH and LH, and the cortisol synthesized in the adrenal cortex inhibits the production of CRF and ACTH in the hypothalamus and pituitary gland. Based on the androgen synthesis control system, various treatment methods have been developed (Fig. 8.2), including surgical removal of the testis, the site of testosterone synthesis, and the use of other medicines that inhibit the function of androgen. Among these medicines, the LHRH agonist is mainly used to treat prostate cancer.

The main principles used for the treatment of prostate cancer and the representative drugs, are as follows.

① Inhibition of testosterone production in the testis through a decrease in the LH level in the pituitary glands (LHRH agonists/antagonists: leuprolide, goserelin, and degarelix)
② Direct inhibition of androgen functions for androgen-dependent prostate cancer cells (anti-androgens: flutamide, bicalutamide, and 5-a-reductase inhibitors)
③ Inhibition of androgen precursor synthesis in the testis and adrenal cortex (abiraterone)

8.1.1 LHRH Agonists/Antagonists

A.V. Schally of Tulane University of Louisiana received the Nobel Prize in Physiology or Medicine in 1977 for discovering CRF, TRH, and LHRH released by the hypothalamus and for studying the physiological functions. In 1971, Schally extracted purified LHRH from the hypothalami of 250,000 pigs and determined its 10-amino acid sequence. He also used purified or chemically synthesized LHRH to define the hormone's function of stimulating the secretion of both LH and follicle-stimulating hormone (FSH) in the pituitary gland [6, 7]. LHRH has a high potential as a marker for diagnosing hypogonadism caused by pituitary gland disorders, thus promoting ovulation in amenorrhea patients and treating oligospermia. However, it has a short half-life of 2–4 min; therefore, efforts have been since 1971 toward screening for an LHRH agonist with a longer half-life by composing various peptides [8].

The testing of LHRH agonists in animals revealed that temporary administration increased LH and FSH secretion and sexual steroid hormone synthesis, but long-term administration caused a significant decrease in the synthesis of sexual steroid hormones, particularly testosterone [9]. After Schally observed that the inhibitory effects of LHRH agonists in testosterone synthesis were similar to those of castration, he investigated the possible use of LHRH agonists to treat prostate cancer. In 1981, triptorelin, a synthesized LHRH agonist, was first administered to rat prostate cancer models to observe the effects of LHRH agonists in the treatment of prostate cancer [10]. In 1982, Schally worked with G. Tolis of the Royal Victoria Hospital in Canada and reported an evident therapeutic effect of triptorelin on prostate cancer [11].

Subsequently, various LHRH agonists, such as leuprolide, goserelin, and histrelin, were used in clinical trials to treat prostate cancer. As studies revealed that the effects of LHRH agonists were equivalent to those of DES or castration, the FDA approved the use of leuprolide, goserelin, triptorelin, and histrelin as anticancer drugs in 1985, 1989, 2000, and 2004, respectively. LHRH antagonists have also been developed for prostate cancer, with the FDA approving abarelix and degarelix in 2003 and 2008, respectively.

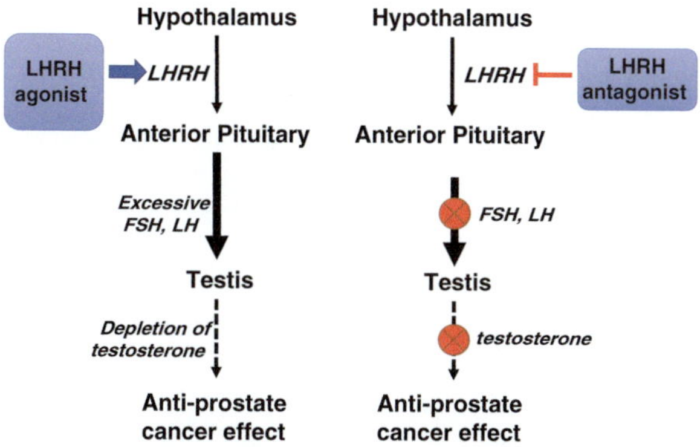

Fig. 8.3 Mechanism of action for luteinizing hormone-releasing hormone (LHRH) agonists and antagonists. LHRH agonists act on the anterior pituitary to promote secretion of adrenocorticotropic hormone (ACTH) and luteinizing hormone (LH), leading to depletion of these hormones in the pituitary gland. As a result, the testes become unable to produce testosterone, soon resulting in decrease of the supply of testosterone to the prostate gland, which acts as an anti-prostate cancer mechanism. Conversely, LHRH antagonists act on the anterior pituitary to inhibit production of FSH and LH, inhibiting prostate cancer by blocking immediate testosterone production

LHRH agonists are more stable than LHRH, and therefore, can increase testosterone concentration to 140–160 % within the first few days. However, their long-term administration disturbs the feedback system of androgen synthesis, reducing testosterone synthesis to near-depletion levels and eventually inhibiting the development of prostate cancer cells. On the other hand, LHRH antagonists consistently inhibit testosterone synthesis without an initial increase in the testosterone concentration (Fig. 8.3).

8.1.2 Anti-androgens

8.1.2.1 First-Generation Anti-androgens: Flutamide, Bicalutamide, and Nilutamide

In 1968, S. Liao of the University of Chicago observed that when radiolabeled testosterone was administered to a rat, the testosterone accumulated specifically in the prostate tissue. An analysis of the metabolites of radiolabeled testosterone accumulated in the prostate showed that 5α-dihydrotestosterone (5α-DHT), which is the most effective androgen, was stably detected in the nucleus. The centrifugal sedimentation method was used to determine 5α-DHT attached to which nuclear components. The results revealed that 5α-DHT formed a complex with the protein strongly associated with chromatin. Based on these results, he hypothesized that testosterone is converted into 5α-DHT in the prostate cells, binds to the androgen receptors (ARs) in the nucleus, and functions in a manner similar to that of steroid

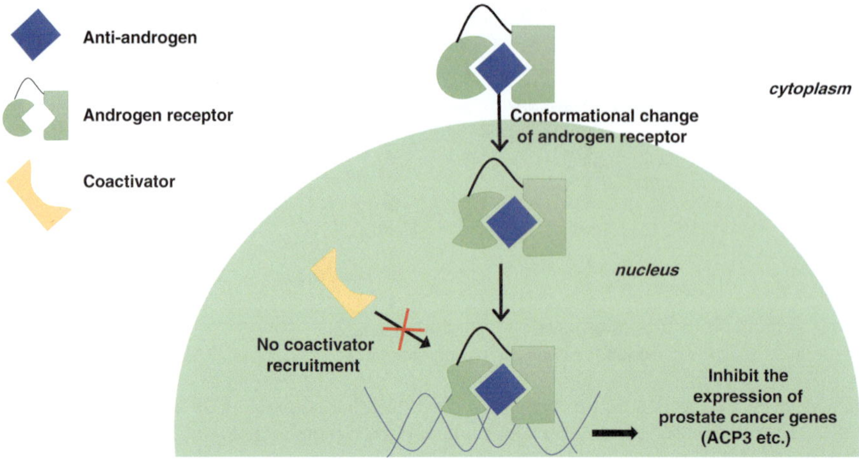

Fig. 8.4 Mechanism of action for antiandrogen. When antiandrogens bind to androgen receptors, they induce structural changes in the receptors, after which the antiandrogen-androgen receptor complex moves into the nucleus, where it binds to DNA. Because the structure of the androgen receptor after binding to antiandrogens is not the activated receptor, but is instead a different, inactivated form, it cannot bind with the coactivators required for expression of prostate cancer genes

hormones by regulating gene expression [12]. Furthermore, these findings accelerated the development of anti-androgen drugs that treat prostate cancer by disrupting the binding between androgen and AR.

In 1972, R.O. Neri, a researcher at Schering Corporation observed the therapeutic effects of flutamide, which was discovered as a non-steroidal anti-androgen, on the benign prostate hyperplasia of a dog [13]. In 1974, Liao investigated the mechanisms of flutamide and discovered that it acts as an anti-androgen by competitively disrupting the binding of 5α-DHT and AR (Fig. 8.4) [14]. In 1989, after clinical trials, the FDA approved flutamide as the first anti-androgen treatment for prostate cancer. Since then, much effort has been made to improve the safety of the drug, and pharmaceutical companies have developed other non-steroidal anti-androgen drugs, such as bicalutamide (AstraZeneca) in 1995 and nilutamide (Sanofi-Aventis) in 1996, which has been approved by the FDA as drugs for prostate cancer.

However, anti-androgen treatment alone has weaker therapeutic effects compared to DES, orchiectomy, or LHRH agonists. As a result, anti-androgens are used along with LHRH agonists to alleviate the initial overreactions of LHRH agonists. Anti-androgen treatment alone is used with limitations to maintain the quality of life (i.e., the sex life and psychological stability) of individuals with terminal-stage prostate cancer.

8.1.2.2 Second-Generation Anti-androgen: Enzalutamide

Based on the three-dimensional structure analyses of ARs, C. Sawyers of the Sloan-Kettering Cancer Center and M. Jung of the University of California, Los Angeles, in 2009 developed a second-generation agent, enzalutamide, whose

AR-binding affinity is more than five times greater than that of the existing first-generation AR antagonist, bicalutamide [15]. Unlike the first-generation AR antagonists, enzalutamide suppresses nuclear translocation of AR and strongly inhibits the functions by disrupting the binding to DNA and its co-activators [16]. Enzalutamide was tested in a clinical trial against malignant prostate cancers that either showed a high expression of ARs or showed resistance to surgical or chemical castration due to mutation. The drug extended the overall survival by a median of 4.6 months in comparison to the placebo group, which led to approval by the FDA in 2012 for metastatic, castration-resistant prostate cancers [17, 18].

8.1.3 CYP17A1 Inhibitor: Abiraterone

Other types of anticancer drugs that treat prostate cancer by disrupting androgen functions have also been developed since 2000. These drugs do not act directly on the AR, but lower the androgen concentration in the body by inhibiting 17-α-hydroxylase/C17,20 lyase (CYP17A1), an enzyme that changes androgen precursors into androgens. CYP17 changes pregnenolone and progesterone into their 17-α-hydroxy derivatives and cleaves the side chain through its lyase activity, leading to the production of androgen precursors, such as dehydroepiandrosterone (DHEA) and androstenedione.

In 1979, J. Heeres of Janssen Pharmaceuticals discovered ketoconazole, an imidazole antifungal medication. Further research on its mechanism revealed that ketoconazole inhibited steroid synthesis pathway in a fungus [19]. In 1983, A. Pont at Stanford University discovered that ketoconazole disrupted androgen synthesis by inhibiting CYP17 in the adrenal glands of vertebrates; ketoconazole was then presented as a new drug for the treatment of prostate cancer [20, 21]. However, the therapeutic efficacy of ketoconazole was minimal, and its specificity was not high enough; it also showed potentially serious side effects. Thus, further research was carried out to address these shortcomings [22].

In 1994, M. Jarman and S.E. Barrie of the Institute of Cancer Research in the United Kingdom analyzed the structure of CYP17 and developed a pyridyl steroid medication called "abiraterone," which had higher specificity than ketoconazole and irreversibly inhibited CYP17 (Fig. 8.5) [23]. In animal studies, abiraterone lowered the serum testosterone concentration to 0.1 nM and increased the serum LH concentration by three- or fourfold without any side effects such as corticosterone synthesis inhibition, which is common with ketoconazole. These results showed that the effects of abiraterone were specific to CYP17. Further clinical trials showed that the drug increased the median overall survival rate by 4.6 months compared to placebo in malignant prostate cancer patients who showed tolerance to surgical or chemical castration treatment. As a result, the FDA approved abiraterone in 2011 as a medicine for metastatic, castration-resistant prostate cancers [24].

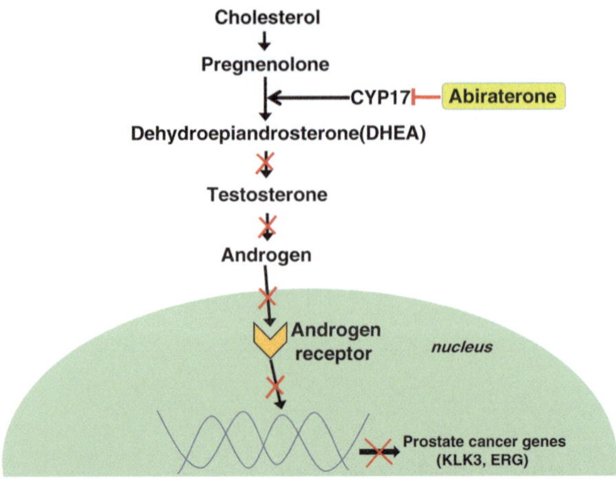

Fig. 8.5 Anticancer mechanism of abiraterone. Abiraterone acetate inhibits CYP17-dependent synthesis of DHEA, suppressing synthesis of adrenal androgen, testosterone, and estrogen, as well as synthesis of androgen in prostate cancer cells. The decrease in androgen receptor (AR) ligand abundance exerts an anticancer effect by suppressing transcription of AR-regulated genes, including prostate specific antigen (PSA) and ETS-related gene (ERG)

8.2 Hormonal Anti-breast-Cancer Drugs

Breast cancer is another hormone-dependent cancer. In the late 1890s, the Scottish surgeon G. Beatson learned from local herdsmen that removing the ovaries of cows increased milk secretion. He assumed that this was possible because the ovaries control the physiological actions of the breasts. Thus, he investigated the possibility of oophorectomy as a breast cancer treatment. He discovered that removing the ovaries of breast cancer patients alleviated their cancer-related symptoms [25]. Since then, many surgeons have performed oophorectomy on breast cancer patients, and in one-third of such patients, therapeutic effects have been reported [26].

Estrogen, a sex hormone synthesized in the ovaries that controls the physiological actions of the breasts, was first discovered in 1923 by E.A. Doisy at St. Louis University. He was the first to discover estrogen activity in ovarian follicle extracts and provided the basis for the research on the mechanism and treatment of breast cancer [27]. Doisy then proceeded to separate the three physiologically important estrogens: estrone (E1), estriol (E3), and estradiol (E2), in that order. In 1936, A. Lacassagne of the Radium Institute in France administered estrogen to female mice for a long period of time to investigate the hormonal actions of estrogen on breast cancer. He discovered that the incidence of breast cancer increased and proposed the regulation of the estrogen activity for breast cancer treatment [28]. As the relationship between the hormonal actions of estrogen and breast cancer progression became known, various treatments, from oophorectomy to removal of other estrogen-modulating organs such as the adrenal gland or pituitary gland, were widely performed until the 1960s.

E. Jensen of the University of Chicago clarified the mechanism of action of estrogen. In 1962, he used radioisotope-labeled estrogen to investigate its distribution. He found estrogen accumulation in the uterus, vagina, and anterior pituitary gland [29]. He continued his research on the identification of estrogen receptors (ERs) and finally discovered ER in 1968 [30]. An investigation of the distribution of estrogen in breast cancer patients showed the accumulation of estrogen in the cancer tissues of some patients. This led to the assumption that these tissues contained receptors that modulated the actions of estrogen, and that such receptors were related to the therapeutic effects of oophorectomy [31].

8.2.1 Selective Estrogen Receptor Modulator (SERM)

8.2.1.1 Tamoxifen: First-Generation SERM

Estrogen inhibits FSH, which stimulates follicle maturation and delays ovulation. This principle was the basis of research in the late 1950s to develop synthetic estrogen analogues into female contraceptives. The American Pharmaceutical Company Searle developed the first female contraceptive called "Enovid" in 1960. A. Walpole and D. Richardson at ICI Pharmaceuticals in the UK then developed new female contraceptives by synthesizing derivatives from triphenylethylene chemicals that had effects similar to those of estrogen. In 1967, they discovered tamoxifen, which inhibited ovulation in rats [32]. However, further investigation showed that tamoxifen had the opposite effect in humans, i.e., it promoted ovulation.

Walpole and Jensen focused on the relationship between estrogen and breast cancer and hypothesized that if tamoxifen, which has been shown to exert anti-estrogen effects on ovulation, had chemical castration effects similar to those of oophorectomy, it would also aid in breast cancer suppression. In 1971, Walpole and oncologist M. Cole investigated the therapeutic efficacy of tamoxifen through clinical trials and found that some breast cancer patients experienced definite alleviation of symptoms [33]. In 1976, the biochemist V.C. Jordan, using isotopic labeling, discovered that tamoxifen strongly inhibited breast cancers with ERs, but did not have any effect on ER-negative breast cancers [34].

After several clinical trials, the FDA finally approved tamoxifen for the treatment of metastatic breast cancers. In 1986, B. Fisher of the Allegheny University of the Health Sciences in Pittsburgh conducted a clinical trial using tamoxifen as an adjuvant therapy in breast cancer patients. In the trial, the tamoxifen group showed a 55 % lower recurrence rate compared to the control group after three years [35]. In 1990, the FDA also approved tamoxifen as an adjuvant for breast cancer patients with no lymph node metastasis. Tamoxifen is still widely used in clinical practice.

Since tamoxifen showed minimal side effects even after long-term administration, B. Fisher also investigated the preventive effects in women at a high risk of breast cancer. He examined the breast cancer incidence rates after 5 years of tamoxifen use and found that the tamoxifen group had 50 % lower incidence than the

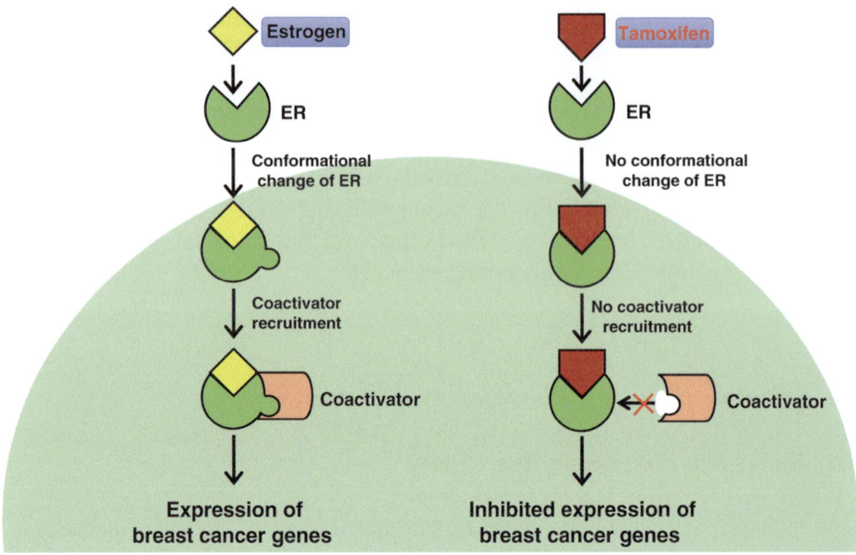

Fig. 8.6 Mechanism of action for tamoxifen. Tamoxifen binds to estrogen receptors (ERs) in competition with estrogen. When tamoxifen binds to ERs, it does not induce a structural change and thus, impairs binding of coactivators. When ERs are not bound to coactivators, they cannot induce ER-dependent gene expression. Thus, tamoxifen produces an anticancer effect by inhibiting expression of breast cancer-related genes

placebo group. After he reported such results in 1998, the FDA approved the use of the drug as a preventive medicine for breast cancer [36].

The use of tamoxifen to treat breast cancer was the first targeted treatment based on the understanding of the interaction between oncogenic molecules of specific cancer cells and drugs that specifically target such molecules. This helped reduce the toxicities often observed with chemotherapeutic agents and greatly influenced future developments of molecule-targeted anticancer therapies (Fig. 8.6).

8.2.1.2 Second-Generation SERM

In 1987, V.C. Jordan of the University of Leeds in the UK observed that while tamoxifen inhibited ERs in the breasts and uterus, it acted similar to the action of estrogen in the bones and during the metabolism of blood lipids [37]. He later called medicines with such tissue-specific activation effects "selective estrogen receptor modulators (SERMs)." Even though tamoxifen very effectively treated breast cancer, further studies revealed side effects, such as endometrioma or formation of a thrombus, with its long-term administration. Second-generation SERMs with reduced side effects were developed in the late 1980s [38].

Toremifene

The first FDA-approved second-generation SERM was toremifene, which was developed by a Finnish pharmaceutical company Farmos in 1986 [39]. Toremifene was an analogue of tamoxifen and showed effects similar to SERM, such as inhibition of ERs in the breasts and estrogen action by aiding receptor activation in the bones and blood lipid metabolism. However, lower estrogen activity was observed in the uterus compared to tamoxifen, with improved safety [39].

In clinical trials on terminal breast cancer patients past menopause, toremifene showed therapeutic effects on cancers, similar to those of tamoxifen [40]. High doses of toremifene were also observed to alleviate symptoms in terminal breast cancer patients who developed resistance to tamoxifen. This led to the approval of toremifene by the FDA in 1997 as a therapeutic option for metastatic breast cancers [41].

Raloxifene

Raloxifene is a second-generation SERM that was developed by C.D. Jones of Eli Lilly and Company in 1984. It is a benzothiophene medicine with a chemical structure different from that of non-steroidal triphenylethylene compounds such as tamoxifen and toremifene. This second-generation SERM was discovered during the search for new compounds that could overcome the limitations of tamoxifen, such as its weak estrogen agonist activity and strong antagonist activity, and loss of activity after its conversion into another isomer in the body [42]. Raloxifene was more effective than tamoxifen in inhibiting the proliferation of uterine tissues caused by estradiol in rats and strongly inhibited cancer growth in rat breast cancer models. Based on these results, Eli Lilly and Company attempted to develop raloxifene as a therapeutic option for tamoxifen-resistant metastatic breast cancers, but failed to show therapeutic effects unlike those observed with tamoxifen. Raloxifene was clinically tested for osteoporosis treatment [43, 44]. Eli Lilly and Company then investigated the preventive effects of raloxifene on breast cancer in subjects in an osteoporosis clinical trial. The results in 2001 showed that raloxifene reduced the incidence of invasive breast cancer by 86 % [45]. Further clinical trials that compared raloxifene with tamoxifen showed that raloxifene had similar preventive effects and lower risks of side effects, such as the formation of thrombus, cataract, or endometrioma [46]. Thus, the FDA approved it in 2007 as a preventive medicine for breast cancer.

8.2.2 Anti-estrogen: Fulvestrant

Tamoxifen and second-generation SERMs show anti-estrogen activities in certain tissues such the breasts, and may cause endometrioma in the uterus, where estrogen is activated. As a result, compounds that act as anti-estrogen agents even in the uterus were developed. Many such compounds have been synthesized, but fulvestrant, which A.E. Wakeling and J. Bowler of ICI developed in 1988, is the only compound that is clinically used [47].

Based on previous study results that suggest that the addition of long side-chains to the C7 of estradiol did not affect its binding ability to ERs, Wakeling discovered a 7α-alkyl estradiol analogue called "fulvestrant." Fulvestrant inhibited the expression of the progesterone receptor (PR) by estradiol in the uterine tissues of rats, and its long-term use caused uterine tissue degeneration, which was also observed in oophorectomies. In addition, administering fulvestrant to carcinogen-induced animal breast cancer models showed strong breast cancer growth inhibition [47]. This implied that fulvestrant acted effectively as an anti-estrogen agent.

In 1993, S. Dauvois of ICI studied the molecular mechanism of fulvestrant and reported that while its binding affinity to ERs is similar to that of tamoxifen, it specifically disrupted the complex formation of estrogen with ERs and nuclear translocation of ERs [48]. Dauvois also observed that fulvestrant accelerated the rapid degradation of ER proteins (Fig. 8.7) [49].

These results suggested the potential use of fulvestrant as an anticancer agent superior to tamoxifen. To confirm this, related clinical trials were conducted.

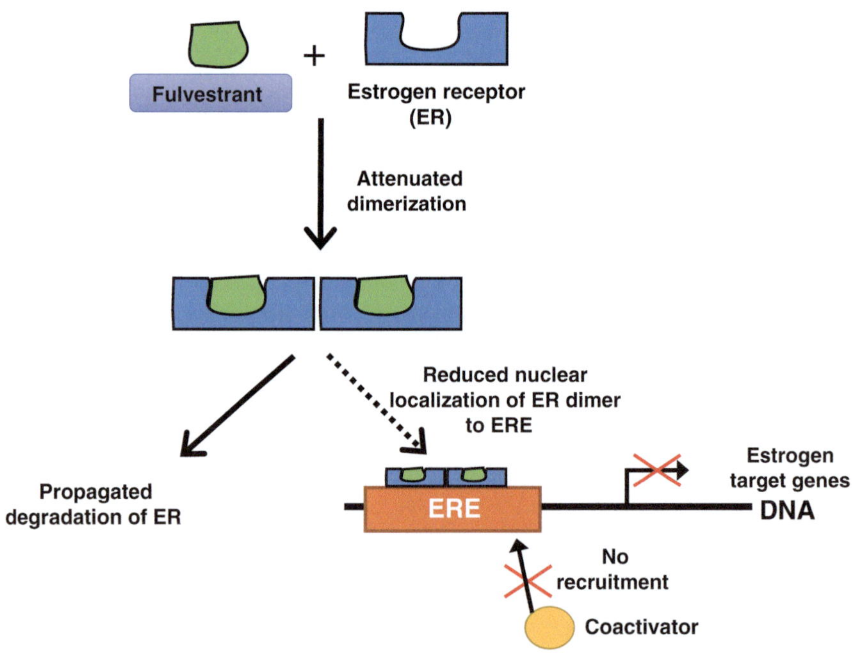

Fig. 8.7 Mechanism of action for fulvestrant. Fulvestrant competes with estrogen at estrogen receptors (ERs). Because ERs bound to fulvestrant are less able to form dimers, rapid ER degradation and decreased movement of dimers into the nucleus occur. The small numbers of dimers that move into the nucleus bind to estrogen response elements (ERE), but cannot bind to coactivators; thus, transcription of estrogen-targeted oncogenes is suppressed

Fulvestrant showed therapeutic efficacies similar to those of anastrozole, an aromatase inhibitor, in tamoxifen-resistant metastatic breast cancer patients. This led to FDA approved in 2002 [50]. The biochemical characteristics of this drug are different from those of tamoxifen, which can be used concurrently with other treatments. Fulvestrant is currently used in clinical practice.

8.2.3 Aromatase (CYP29) Inhibitors

Other drugs that treat breast cancers by disrupting the actions of estrogen have also been developed. Rather than acting directly on the ER, these drugs inhibit aromatase, which transforms the precursor androgen into estrogen, and lowers the estrogen concentration in the body. In 1959, K.J. Ryan of Harvard University discovered the aromatase activity in microsomal vesicles from the human placenta that changed 19-carbon androgen into estrogen using NADPH and oxygen [51]. In 1986, S. Chen of Beckman Research Institute purified aromatase enzyme and C.T. Evans of the University of Texas cloned the gene [52, 53].

The research on aromatase inhibitors was started by investigating the side effects of aminoglutethimide, a type of anticonvulsant. In 1967, R.N. Dexter at Vanderbilt University reported that aminoglutethimide hindered the conversion of cholesterol into pregnenolone, which led to a decrease in steroid hormones, such as mineralocorticoid, glucocorticoid, and sex steroids in the adrenal glands [54]. In 1973, C.T. Griffiths and T.C. Halls at Harvard University used dexamethasone with aminoglutethimide, which inhibited steroidogenesis in the adrenal glands. They discovered that this combination alleviated breast cancer symptoms in some patients [55]. In 1974, E.A. Thompson of the University of Texas Health Science Center discovered that aminoglutethimide inhibited the activity of the aromatase obtained from microsomal vesicles in the placenta and reduced the estrogen synthesis from androstenedione [56]. Based on these results, R.J. Santen at the University of Pennsylvania in 1978, observed that aminoglutethimide acted as an aromatase inhibitor *in vivo* in breast cancer patients and greatly reduced the estrogen blood concentration in those patients. This discovery led to the development of aromatase inhibitors for breast cancer treatment [57].

However, due to the similarity of the structure of aminoglutethimide to that of glutethimide, it acted as an anticonvulsant in the nervous system. It also had low specificity, inhibiting P450scc enzymes responsible for pregnenolone from cholesterol, which led to side effects such as liver toxicity, drowsiness, skin rash, and fever. As a result, further studies were carried out for the development of safe aromatase inhibitors with high specificity.

Formestane and fadrozole were developed as second-generation aromatase inhibitors. In 1976, A.M. Brodie of the Worcester Foundation for Experimental Biology in the U.S. developed a synthetic compound called "4-hydroxyandrostenedione" (4-HOA, formestane), which was similar to androstonedione, a substrate of aromatase [58]. Formestane is an irreversible inhibitor (type II steroidal aromatase inhibitor) with improved specificity to aromatase, unlike aminoglutethimide, which is a reversible inhibitor (type I non-steroidal aromatase inhibitor). Formestane reduced the blood estrogen levels in rats by 80 % and inhibited the growth of cancer cells in animal breast cancer models [59]. Clinical trials also showed that the therapeutic efficacy of formestane was similar to that of tamoxifen [60]. Although both formestane and fadrozole were clinically effective, neither was approved as an anticancer drug.

Triazole compounds, such as anastrozole and letrozole, are type 1 aromatase inhibitors developed as third-generation aromatase inhibitors. R.E. Steele of CIBA-GEIGY discovered the non-steroidal aromatase inhibitor CGS 18320 as a second-generation aromatase inhibitor in 1987 [61]. Letrozole was evolved from CGS 18320 in collaboration with R.J. Santen in 1993 and became a third-generation aromatase inhibitor [62]. P.V. Plourde of Zeneca (a subsidiary of ICI Pharmaceuticals, currently known as AstraZeneca) developed anastrozole in 1994 [63]. Both drugs have an aromatase-inhibiting effect, which is significantly higher than that of aminoglutethimide with less side effects, such as hindrance of aldosterone or cortisol synthesis (Fig. 8.8). Clinical trials have shown that the efficacies of anastrozole and letrozole in breast cancer patients are superior to those of tamoxifen [64, 65]. Thus, the FDA approved them in 1995 and 1997, respectively, and they are still widely used.

Another third-generation aromatase inhibitor is exemestane, a formestane analogue and type II aromatase inhibitor that was developed by E. Di Salle of the Italian pharmaceutical company Farmitalia Carlo Erba [66]. Unlike formestane, which is injected intramuscularly, exemestane can be administered orally and has higher specificity and efficacy. Clinical trials have reported that its efficacy is superior to that of tamoxifen, which led to FDA approval for used as a breast cancer drug [67].

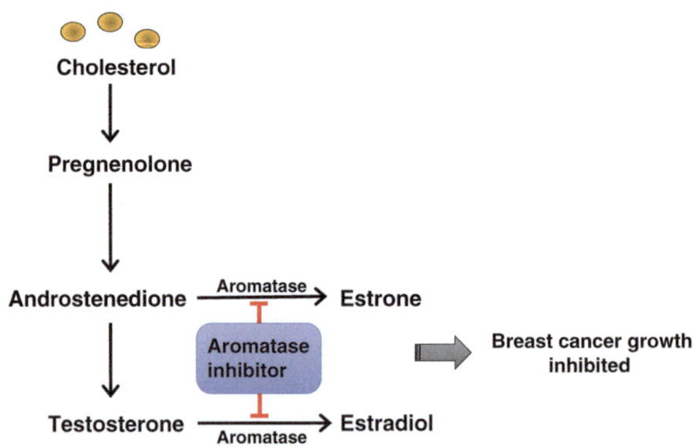

Fig. 8.8 Anticancer mechanism of aromatase inhibitors. Aromatase is responsible for converting androstenedione and testosterone produced from cholesterol into estrone and estradiol, respectively. Through inhibition of such conversion, aromatase inhibitors produce an anticancer effect by lowering the estrogen concentration within breast cancer cells.

8.3 Other Hormonal Anticancer Drugs

Other hormonal anticancer drugs are used as supplementary drugs during cancer treatment to alleviate the cancer or the side effects of chemotherapy. These drugs include corticosteroid hormones, progestogen, and somatostatin analogues.

T. Reichstein discovered corticosteroid hormones in 1944 in the adrenal cortex. Corticosteroid hormones can be classified into glucocorticoids and mineralocorticoids. Glucocorticoids, such as cortisol, can modulate the metabolism of glucose, fat, and protein or alleviate inflammation, and mineralocorticoids, such as aldosterone, can control the concentration of electrolytes. Due to their strong physiological functions, many synthesized corticosteroid hormones have been developed, some of which have been used for cancer treatment.

8.3.1 Prednisone

In 1955, A. Nobile at Schering Pharmaceuticals developed a new synthesis method for hydrocortisone, which has anti-inflammatory activity. During the synthesis process, *Corynebacterium simplex* was used for hydrolysis to remove the acetyl group attached to carbon-11 of the steroid ring. As a result, not only was the acetyl group removed, but a new double bond was also added to the steroid ring A, where prednisone and prednisolone were developed [68]. As prednisone and prednisolone had higher glucocorticoid activities than hydrocortisone but weaker mineralocorticoid activities, they were used as immunosuppressants and anti-inflammatory agents.

Prednisone and prednisolone were also used to treat adult leukemia and lymphoma and were approved by the FDA in 1955. They were further developed for the treatment of blood cancers, such as acute lymphoblastic leukemia (ALL), non-Hodgkin's lymphoma, and multiple myeloma. Prednisone was later used as a main anticancer drug in the first combination chemotherapy called VAMP (vincristine, amethopterin, mercaptopurine, and prednisone), which E. Frei and E. Freireich of NCI used in 1964 to treat acute lymphoma in children, and in 1967 in MOPP (mechlorethamine, vincristine, procarbazine, and prednisone) combination chemotherapy, which V.T. DeVita administered to successfully treat Hodgkin's lymphoma [69, 70]. These two drugs are currently being used for the treatment of various blood-borne cancers, including leukemia, lymphoma, and multiple myeloma.

8.3.2 Testolactone

In 1953, H.J. Fried at the Squibb Institute developed testolactone by fermenting progesterone using *Streptomyces zavendulae* [71]. A. Segaloff of Tulane University participated in the Breast Cancer Treatment Development Program of NCI, which was launched in 1957, during which he discovered the therapeutic effects of testolactone on progressive breast cancers in 1962, while researching on hormone therapy [72]. After several clinical trials, the FDA approved testolactone in 1970 for the treatment of breast cancer [73]. In 1975, E.A. Thompson et al. at the University of Texas Health Science Center discovered that testolactone can be used for the treatment of breast cancer by inhibiting estrogen synthesis through its aromatase-inhibiting effects [74]. However, testolactone has been replaced to formestane and exemestane and is rarely used today.

8.3.3 Progestin

Synthetic progestins (progesterone-like drugs), such as medroxyprogesterone acetate and megestrol acetate, were developed as contraceptives based on their ovulation-inhibiting effects. Medroxyprogesterone acetate is the 6-methyl analogue of acetoxyprogesterone, which the pharmaceutical companies Syntex and Upjohn developed in 1956 and used as a contraceptive. B. Ellis at the British Drug House developed megestrol acetate as an analogue of medroxyprogesterone acetate in 1960 [75]. NCI conducted clinical trials of both drugs as part of its breast cancer treatment program, and the results revealed therapeutic effects on malignant breast cancers [73]. In 1996, it was also found that megestrol acetate is effective for endometrial cancers [76]. The molecular mechanisms behind these effects have not yet been clarified, but they are assumed to lower the estrogen levels in breast cancer patients [77]. The FDA approved medroxyprogesterone acetate and megestrol acetate in 1950 and 1971, respectively. Further research revealed that these drugs alleviated appetite loss (anorexia) observed in cancer patients, due to which they have been used more as appetite boosters than as anticancer agents. They are currently being used to reduce anorexia in many metastatic cancer patients.

8.3.4 Somatostatin

In 1973, R. Guillemin's group from the Salk Institute discovered the hormone somatostatin, which is released in the hypothalamus and which inhibits the release of the growth hormone (GH) in the pituitary gland, besides determining the amino acid sequence [78]. Further studies by various research groups revealed somatostatin's inhibitory effects on the release of other peptide hormones such as insulin, glucagon, and gastrin. As the potential clinical application of somatostatin was realized, more studies on synthetic analogues were conducted to improve their short half-life. Octreotide developed by W. Bauer of Sandoz in 1982 showed therapeutic effects on neuroendocrine tumors, such as carcinoid tumors that released peptide hormones, vasoactive intestinal peptide-secreting tumors (VIPomas), and insulinomas. The FDA registered octreotide as an anticancer agent in 1987 [79–80]. In

1990, its therapeutic effects on acromegaly and gigantism caused by overproduction of growth hormones were also reported [81]. In addition to its anticancer effects, octreotide is also known to alleviate severe diarrhea accompanied by VIPomas or caused by 5-fluorouracil chemotherapy or radiation therapy.

References

1. White WJ (1892) Surgical removal of the hypertrophied prostate. Ann Surg 17:70–75
2. Huggins CB, Masina MH, Eichelberger L, Wharton JD (1939) Quantitative studies of prostatic secretion: I. Characteristics of the normal secretion; the influence of thyroid, suprarenal, and testis extirpation and androgen substitution on the prostatic output. J Exp Med 70:543–556
3. Huggins CB, Clark PJ (1940) Quantitative studies of prostatic secretion: II. The effect of castration and of estrogen injection on the hyperplastic prostate glands of dogs. J Exp Med 72: 747–762
4. Huggins C, Hodges CV (1941) Studies on prostatic cancer: I. The effect of castration, of estrogen and of androgen injection on serum phosphatases in metastatic carcinoma of the prostate. Cancer Res 1:293–297
5. Huggins C, Stephens RC, Hodges CV (1941) Studies on prostatic cancer: II. The effects of castration on advanced carcinoma of the prostate gland. Arch Surg 43:209–223
6. Schally AV, Kastin AJ, Arimura A (1971) Hypothalamic FSH and LH-regulating hormone. Structure, physiology and clinical studies. Fertil Steril 22:703–721
7. Schally AV, Arimura A, Kastin AJ, Matsuo H, Baba Y et al (1971) The gonadotropin-releasing hormone: one polypeptide regulates the secretion of luteinizing and follicle stimulating hormones. Science 173:1036–1038
8. Schally AV, Kastin AJ, Coy DH, Edward T (1976) Tyler Prize Oration – LH releasing hormone and its analogues: recent basic and clinical investigations. Internat Fertil 21:1–30
9. Vilchez-Martinez JA, Pedroza E, Arimura A, Schally AV (1979) Paradoxical effects of D-Trp6-luteinizing hormone-releasing hormone on the hypothalamic-pituitary-gonadal axis in immature female rats. Fertil Steril 31:677–682
10. Redding TW, Schally AV (1981) Inhibition of prostate tumour growth in two rat models by chronic administration of D-Trp6-LH-RH. Proc Natl Acad Sci 78:6509–6512
11. Tolis G, Ackman D, Stellos A et al (1982) Tumor growth inhibition in patients with prostatic carcinoma treated with luteinizing hormone-releasing hormone agonists. Proc Natl Acad Sci 79:1658–1662
12. Anderson KM, Liao S (1968) Selective retention of dihydrotestosterone by prostatic nuclei. Nature 219:277–279
13. Neri RO, Monahan M (1972) Effects of novel nonsteroidal antiandrogen in canine prostatic hyperplasia. Invest Urol 10:123
14. Liao S, Howell DK, Chang TM (1974) Action of a nonsteroidal antiandrogen, flutamide, on the receptor binding and nuclear retention of 5 ^{a}-dihydrotestosterone in rat ventral prostate. Endocrinology 94:1205–1209
15. Jung ME, Ouk S, Yoo D, Sawyers CL, Chen C, Tran C, Wongvipat J (2010) Structure-activity relationship for thiohydantoin androgen receptor antagonists for castration resistant prostate cancer. J Med Chem 53:2779–2796
16. Tran C, Ouk S, Clegg NJ, Chen Y, Watson PA et al (2009) Development of a second-generation antiandrogen for treatment of advanced prostate cancer. Science 324:787–790
17. Scher HI, Beer TM, Higano CS et al (2010) Antitumour activity of MDV3100 in castration-resistant prostate cancer: a phase 1–2 study. Lancet 375:1437–1446
18. Scher HI, Fizazi K, Saad F et al (2012) Increased survival with enzalutamide in prostate cancer after chemotherapy. N Engl J Med 367:1187–1197

19. Heeres J, Backx LJ, Mostmans JH, Van Cutsem J (1979) Antimycotic imidazoles. Part 4. Synthesis and antifungal activity of ketoconazole, a new potent orally active broad-spectrum antifungal agent. J Med Chem 22:1003–1005
20. Pont A, Williams PL, Azhar S, Reitz RE, Bochra C, Smith ER, Stevens DA (1982) Ketoconazole blocks testosterone synthesis. Arch Intern Med 142:2137–2140
21. Trachtenberg J, Halpern N, Pont A (1983) Ketoconazole: a novel and rapid treatment for advanced prostatic cancer. J Urol 130:152–153
22. Loose DS, Kan PB, Hirst MA, Marcus RA, Feldman D (1983) Ketoconazole blocks adrenal steroidogenesis by inhibiting cytochrome P450-dependent enzymes. J Clin Invest 71: 1495–1499
23. Barrie SE, Potter GA, Goddard PM, Haynes BP, Dowsett M, Jarman M (1994) Pharmacology of novel steroidal inhibitors of cytochrome $P450_{17a}$ (17^{a}-hydroxylase/C17-20 lyase). J Steroid Biochem Mol Biol 50:267–273
24. Fizazi K et al (2012) Abiraterone acetate for treatment of metastatic castration-resistant prostate cancer: final overall survival analysis of the COU-AA-301 randomised, double-blind, placebo-controlled phase 3 study. Lancet Oncol 13:983–992
25. Beatson CT (1896) On treatment of inoperable cases of carcinoma of the mamma: suggestions for a new method of treatment with illustrative cases. Lancet 2:162–165
26. Boyd S (1900) On oophorectomy in cancer of the breast. BMJ 2:1161–1167
27. Allen E, Doisy EA (1923) An ovarian hormone: preliminary reports on its localization, extraction and partial purification and action in test animals. JAMA 81:810–821
28. Lacassagne A (1936) Hormonal pathogenesis of adenocarcinoma of the breast. Am J Cancer 27:217–225
29. Jensen EV, Jacobson HI (1962) Basic guides to the mechanism of estrogen action. Recent Prog Horm Res 18:387–414
30. Jensen EV et al (1968) A two-step mechanism for the interaction of estradiol with rat uterus. Proc Natl Acad Sci 59:632–638
31. Jensen EV, Block GE, Smith S, Kyser K, DeSombre ER (1971) Estrogen receptors and breast cancer response to adrenalectomy. Natl Cancer Inst Monogr 34:55–70
32. Harper MJ, Walpole AL (1967) A new derivative of triphenylethylene: effect on implantation and mode of action in rats. J Reprod Fertil 13:101–119
33. Cole MP, Jones CT, Todd ID (1971) A new antioestrogenic agent in late breast cancer. An early clinical appraisal of ICI46474. Br J Cancer 25:270–275
34. Jordan VC, Jaspan T (1976) Tamoxifen as an antitumour agent: oestrogen binding as a predictive test for tumour response. J Endocrinol 68:453–460
35. Fisher B et al (1986) Adjuvant chemotherapy with and without tamoxifen in the treatment of primary breast cancer: 5-year results from the national surgical adjuvant breast and bowel project trial. J Clin Oncol 4:459–471
36. Fisher B et al (1998) Tamoxifen for prevention of breast cancer: report of the national surgical adjuvant breast and bowel project P-1 Study. J Natl Cancer Inst 90:1371–1388
37. Jordan VC, Phelps E, Lindgren JU (1987) Effects of antiestrogens on bone in castrated and intact female rats. Breast Cancer Res Treat 10:31–35
38. Tamoxifen for early breast cancer: an overview of the randomised trials. Early Breast Cancer trialists' Collaborative Group (1998) Lancet 351:1451–1467
39. Kallio S, Kangas L, Blanco G, Johansson R, Karjalainen A, Perilä M, Pippo I et al (1986) A new triphenylethylene compound, Fc-1157a. I hormonal effects. Cancer Chemother Pharmacol 17:101–108
40. Hayes DF, Van Zyl JA, Hacking A, Goedhals L, Bezwoda WR, Mailliard JA et al (1995) Randomized comparison of tamoxifen and two separate doses of toremifene in postmenopausal patients with metastatic breast cancer. J Clin Oncol 13:2556–2566
41. Vogel CL (1998) Phase II, and III clinical trials of toremifene for metastatic breast cancer. Oncology 12(Suppl 5):9–13
42. Jones CD, Jevnikar MG, Pike AJ, Peters MK, Black LJ, Thompson AR, Falcone JF, Clemens JA (1984) Structure-activity studies in a series of 3-aroyl-2-arylbenzo[b]thiophene derivatives

leading to [6-hydroxy-2-(4-hydroxyphenyl)benzo[b]thien-3-YL] [4-[2-(1-piperidinyl)ethoxy]-phenyl]methanone hydrochloride (LY156758), a remarkably effective estrogen antagonist with only minimal intrinsic estrogenicity. J Med Chem 27:1057–1066
43. Buzdar AU, Marcus C, Holmes F, Hug V, Hortobagyi G (1988) Phase II evaluation of LYL56758 in metastatic breast cancer. Oncology 45:344–345
44. Ettinger B, Black DM, Mitlak BH, Knickerbocker RK, Nickelsen T, Genant HK et al (1999) Reduction of vertebral fracture risk in postmenopausal women with osteoporosis treated with raloxifene: results from a 3-year randomized clinical trial. Multiple Outcomes of Raloxifene Evaluation (MORE) Investigators. JAMA 282:637–645
45. Cauley JA, Norton L, Lippman ME et al (2001) Continued breast cancer risk reduction in postmenopausal women treated with raloxifene: 4-year results from the MORE trial. Multiple outcomes of raloxifene evaluation. Breast Cancer Res Treat 65:125–134
46. Vogel VG, Costantino JP, Wickerham DL et al (2006) The Study of Tamoxifen and Raloxifene (STAR): report of the National Surgical Adjuvant Breast and Bowel Project P-2 Trial. JAMA 295:2727–2741
47. Wakeling AE, Bowler J (1988) Biology and mode of action of pure antioestrogens. J Steroid Biochem 30:141–147
48. Dauvois S, White R, Parker MG (1993) The antiestrogen ICI 182780 disrupts estrogen receptor nucleocytoplasmic shuttling. J Cell Sci 106:1377–1388
49. Dauvois S, Danielian PS, White R, Antiestrogen PMG, ICI (1992) 164,384 reduces cellular estrogen receptor content by increasing its turnover. Proc Natl Acad Sci 89:4037–4041
50. Osborne CK, Pippen J, Jones SE, Parker LM, Ellis M, Come S et al (2002) Double-blind, randomized trial comparing the efficacy and tolerability of fulvestrant versus anastrozole in postmenopausal women with advanced breast cancer progressing on prior endocrine therapy: results of a North American trial. J Clin Oncol 20:3386–3395
51. Ryan KJ (1959) Biological aromatization of steroids. J Biol Chem 234:268–272
52. Chen S, Shively JE, Nakajin S, Shinoda M, Hall PF (1986) Amino terminal sequence analysis of human placenta aromatase. Biochem Biophys Res Commun 135:713–719
53. Evans CT, Ledesma DB, Schulz TZ, Simpson ER, Mendelson CR (1986) Isolation and characterization of a complementary DNA specific for human aromatase-system cytochrome P-450 mRNA. Proc Natl Acad Sci 83:6387–6391
54. Dexter RN, Fishman LM, Ney RC, Liddle GW (1967) Inhibition of adrenal corticosteroid synthesis by aminoglutethimide: studies on the mechanism of action. J Clin Endocrinol 27:473–480
55. Griffiths CT, Halls TC, Saba Z, Barlow JJ, Nevinny HB (1973) Preliminary trial of aminoglutethimide in breast cancer. Cancer 32:31–37
56. Thompson EA Jr, Siiteri PK (1974) The involvement of human placental microsomal cytochrome P-450 in aromatization. J Biol Chem 249:5373–5378
57. Santen RJ, Santner S, Davis B, Veldhuis J, Samojlik E, Ruby E (1978) Aminoglutethimide inhibits extraglandular estrogen production in postmenopausal women with breast carcinoma. J Clin Endocrinol Metab 47:1257–1265
58. Brodie AM, Schwarzel WC, Brodie HJ (1976) Studies on the mechanism of estrogen biosynthesis in the rat ovary-I. J Steroid Biochem 7:787–793
59. Brodie AMH, Schwarzel WC, Shaikh A, Brodie HJ (1977) The effect of an aromatase inhibitor, 4-hydroxy-4-androstene-3,17-dione, on estrogen-dependent processes in reproduction and breast cancer. Endocrinology 100:1684–1695
60. Pérez Carrión R, Alberola Candel V, Calabresi F et al (1994) Comparison of the selective aromatase inhibitor formestane with tamoxifen as first-line hormonal therapy in postmenopausal women with advanced breast cancer. Ann Oncol 5 Suppl 7:S19–S24
61. Steele RE, Mellor LB, Sawyer WK, Wasvary JM, Browne LJ (1987) *In vitro* and *in vivo* studies demonstrating potent and selective estrogen inhibition with the nonsteroidal aromatase inhibitor CGS 16949A. Steroids 50:147–161
62. Demers LM, Lipton A, Harvey HA, Kambic KB, Grossberg H, Brady C, Santen RJ (1993) The efficacy of CGS 20267 in suppressing estrogen biosynthesis in patients with advanced stage breast cancer. J Steroid Biochem Mol Biol 44:687–691

63. Plourde PV, Dyroff M, Dukes M (1994) Arimidex: a potent and selective fourth-generation aromatase inhibitor. Breast Cancer Res Treat 30:103–111
64. Buzdar AU, Jones SE, Vogel CE, Wolter J, Plourde P, Webster A (1997) The Arimidex study group, a phase III trial comparing anastrozole (1 and 10 mg), a potent and selective aromatase inhibitor, with advanced breast carcinoma. Cancer 79:730–739
65. Ingle JN, Johnson PA, Suman VJ et al (1997) A randomized phase II trial of two dosage levels of letrozole as third-line hormonal therapy for women with metastatic breast carcinoma. Cancer 80:218–224
66. Di Salle E, Ornati G, Giudici D, Lassus M, Evans TR, Coombes RC (1992) Exemestane (FCE24304), a new steroidal aromatase inhibitor. J Stroid Biochem Mol Biol 43:137–143
67. Paridaens R, Dirix L, Lohrisch C et al (2000) Promising activity and safety of exemestane as first-line hormonal therapy in metastatic breast cancer patients: final results of an EORTC randomised phase II trial. Breast Cancer Res Treat 64:52
68. Herzog HL, Nobile A, Tolksdorf S et al (1955) New anti-arthritic steroids. Science 121:176
69. Freireich EJ, Karon M, Frei E III (1964) Quadruple combination therapy (VAMP) for acute lymphocytic leukemia of childhood. Proc Am Assoc Cancer Res 5:20
70. DeVita VT, Serpick A (1967) Combination chemotherapy in the treatment of advanced Hodgkin's disease. Proc Am Assoc Cancer Res 8:13
71. Fried HJ, Thoma RW, Klingsberg A (1953) Oxidation of steroids by microorganisms. III. Side chain degradation, ring D-cleavage and dehydrogenation in ring A. J Am Chem Soc 75: 5764–5765
72. Segaloff A, Weeth JB, Meyer KK, Rongone EL, Cunningham MEG (1962) Hormonal therapy in cancer of the breast. XIX. The effect of delta 1-testololactone on clinical course and hormonal excretion. Cancer 15:633–635
73. Goldenberg IS (1969) Clinical trial of Dl-testololactone (NSC 23759), medroxyprogesterone acetate (NSC 26386), and oxylone acetate (NSC 47438) in advanced female mammary cancer. A report of the Cooperative Breast Cancer Group. Cancer 23:109–112
74. Siiteri PK, Thompson EA (1975) Studies of human placental aromatase. J Steroid Biochem 6:317–320
75. Ellis B, Kirk DN, Petrow V, Waterhouse B, William DM (1960) Modified steroid hormones. XVII. Some 6-methyl-4,6-dienes. J Chem Soc 2828–2833
76. Lentz SS, Brady MF, Major FJ, Reid GC, Soper JT (1996) High-dose megestrol acetate in advanced or recurrent endometrial carcinoma: a Gynecologic Oncology Group Study. J Clin Oncol 14:357–361
77. Alexieva-Figusch J, Blankenstein MA, Hop WCJ, et al. (1984) Treatment of metastatic breast cancer patients with different dosages of megestrol acetate; dose relations, metabolic and endocrine effects. Eur J Cancer Clin Oncol 20:33–40
78. Brazeau P, Vale W, Burgus R, Ling N, Butcher M, Rivier J, Guillemin R (1973) Hypothalamic polypeptide that inhibits the secretion of immunoreactive pituitary growth hormone. Science 179:77–79
79. Bauer W, Briner U, Doepfner W, et al. (1982) SMS 201–995: a very potent and selective octapeptide analog of somatostatin with prolonged action. Life Sci 31:1133–1140
80. Reichlin S. Somatostatin (1987) Basic and Clinical Status. Plenum Press, New York
81. Ho KY, Weissberger AJ, Marbach P, Lazarus L (1990) Therapeutic efficacy of the somatostatin analog SMS 201–995 (Octreotide) in acromegaly. Effects of dose and frequency and long term safety. Ann Intern Med 112:173–181

Chapter 9
Molecular Targeted Anticancer Drugs

From the middle of the 1960s, combination chemotherapy was at the center of chemotherapy for cancer. Following successful treatment of various hematologic malignancies through combination chemotherapy, significant effort was aimed at utilizing such treatments in patients with solid cancers. Research into solid cancer treatment using combination chemotherapy was a core component of anticancer research programs from 1970s, but in spite of long-term, large-scale clinical trials, revolutionary results did not emerge, and the progression of anticancer chemotherapy has gradually slowed since 1980. Ultimately, in 2003, it was determined that mega-dose combination chemotherapy combined with bone marrow transplant was not superior than conventional combination chemotherapy in advanced breast cancer, and it was widely believed that cytotoxic chemotherapy had reached its limit as a treatment for solid cancer. The failure of mega-dose cytotoxic chemotherapy as a treatment for solid cancers showed researchers that a deep biological understanding of the complexity and diversity of individual types of cancer was essential for more effective cancer treatment.

A major breakthrough facilitating the development of molecular targeted agents occurred in 1976, when Varmus and Bishop discovered a proto-oncogene tyrosine kinase Src (c-Src), leading to novel research into cancer at the molecular level. The National Cancer Institute (NCI) recognized the potential of molecular cancer research and launched the Molecular Biology of Cancer Research Program in 1984 as a means of funding large-scale basic cancer research. Moreover, it was recognized that the murine leukemia model, which had a key role in screening for anticancer agents, was an insufficient method of identifying compounds with a reasonable chance of success in human clinical trials; therefore, in 1990, the NCI launched a new method of screening for anticancer drugs, which utilized 60 human cancer cell lines derived from seven different types of cancer tissues.

By early 1990, with the accumulation of knowledge about the pathogenesis and progression of cancer resulting from basic cancer research, the potential for revolutionary new anticancer treatment had become apparent. It was revealed that cancer depended on specific signaling pathway derived from specific oncogenic mutation for continued growth; moreover, it was shown that each type of cancer

K.-W. Kim et al., *Cancer Drug Discovery*, DOI 10.1007/978-94-024-0844-7_9

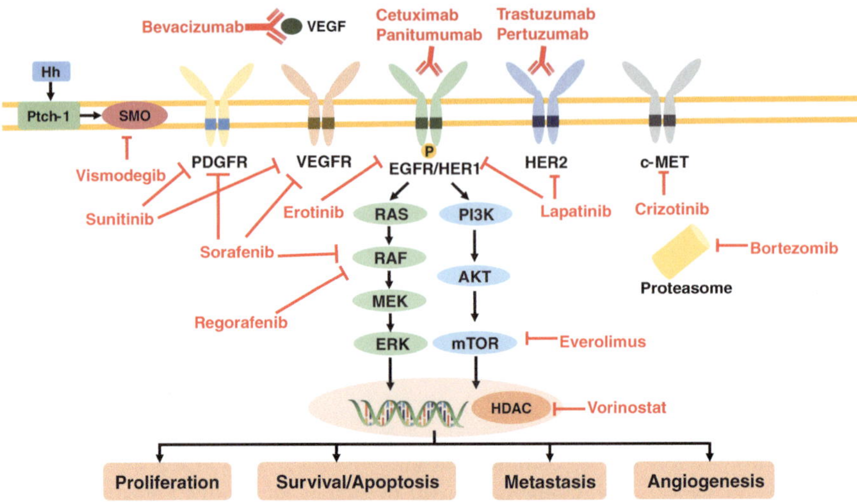

Fig. 9.1 Target proteins and intracellular signaling pathways for targeted anticancer agents

used subtly different complementary pathways for growth and metastasis. Based on these discoveries, novel molecular targeted anticancer agents began to be developed, with the goal of inactivating target molecules and cancer-specific signaling pathways.

Molecular targeted agents suppress the functions of certain proteins that play a key role during the growth and progression of cancer, thereby inhibiting cell division in certain cancers, promoting apoptosis of cancer cells, activating the immune system to destroy cancer cells, and delivering specific drugs to cancer cells. A significant advantage of molecular targeted therapy is that it is focused on specific oncogenic aberrations in cancer cells; therefore, such drugs are expected to be more selective and effective against cancer cells and have relatively fewer side effects compared to conventional cytotoxic chemotherapeutics.

Targeted agents that can bind specifically to oncoproteins are mostly developed in the form of monoclonal antibodies or small molecular compounds. Monoclonal antibodies and small molecular inhibiotrs have distinct pharmacological properties and advantages. Monoclonal antibodies cannot peneterate the cell membrane and are mostly suited to targeting proteins on the cell surface membrane. In comparison, small molecular inhibitors can cross the cell membrane and therefore mostly target intracellular proteins (Fig. 9.1). From the perspective of drug development, antibodies are generally easier, but more expensive, to develop, while small molecular inhibitors are cheaper to develop and are effective even when some oncoproteins mutated (making them undetectable to antibodies); however, the development probability for small molecular inhibitors is considerably lower than that of antibodies. Beginning with tretinoin in 1995, approximately 50 targeted anticancer agents were approved until the end of 2013, comprising the majority of recently developed anticancer drugs (Fig. 9.2).

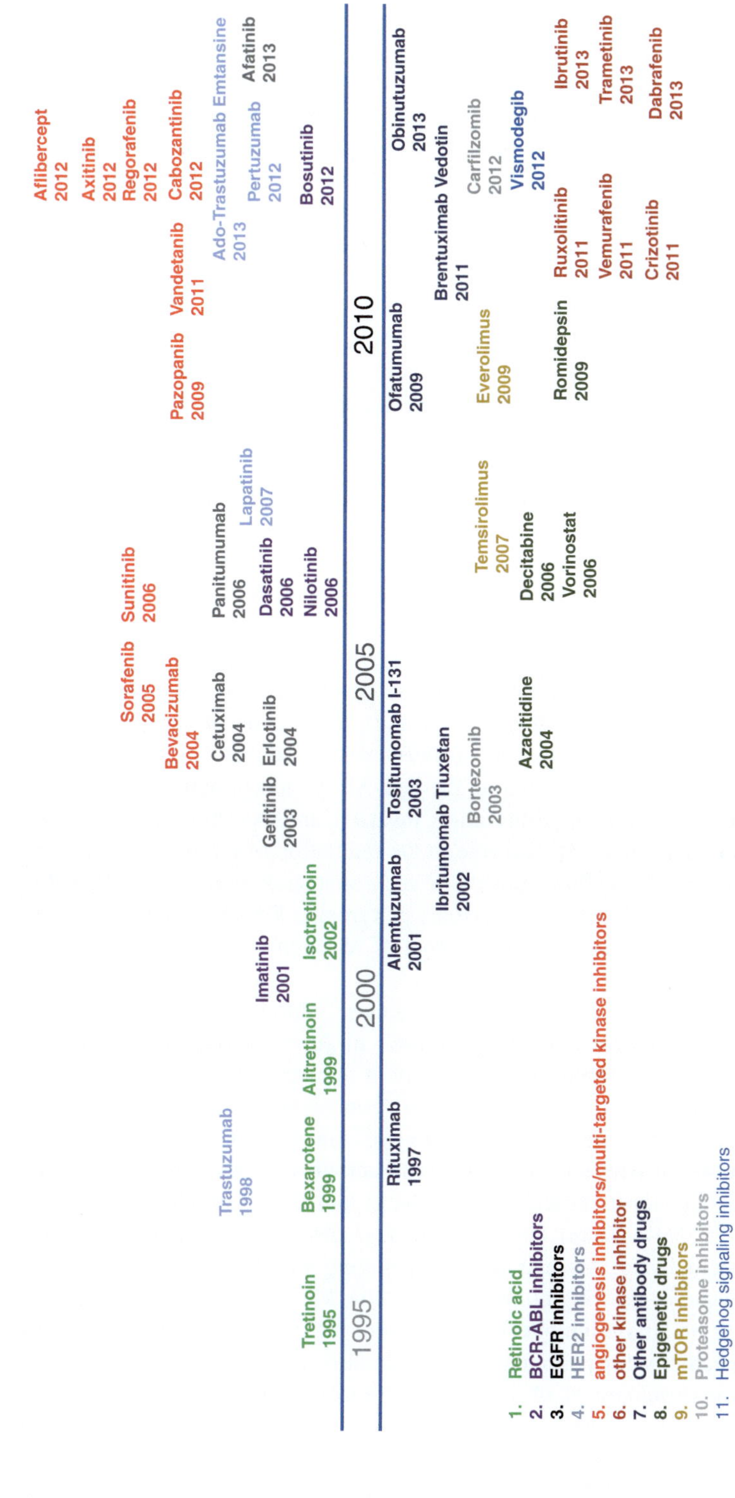

Fig. 9.2 Types of molecular targeted anticancer agents and a chronology of their development

Due to the cancer biology research over the last 40 years, a large number of genes and proteins involved in the oncogenesis have been discovered. However, oncoproteins that have been effectively targeted by cancer treatment have a very restricted set of characteristics; such proteins are mostly enzymes and have notable surface grooves where chemical reactions take place. Therefore, it is possible to inhibit the reaction occurring at a particular region of oncoprotein using small molecular inhibitor that fit the grooves. Because the majority of transcription factors and other proteins that do not have evident grooves, it is generally very difficult to suppress activity using small molecular inhibitors. The majority of enzymes that can be regulated by targeted drugs in this way are protein kinases, although proteasome components, histone deacetylases (HDAC), and DNA methyltransferases (DNMT) are also susceptible to such manipulation. Among protein kinases that can be inhibited by small molecular inhibitors, the majority are growth factor receptors or non-receptor tyrosine kinases. There are far more serine/threonine kinases than tyrosine kinases, but only a few serine/threonine kinases, including c-Raf and mitogen-activated protein kinase kinase 1 and 2 (MAP2K1/2 or MEK1/2), have been successfully targeted by anticancer agents.

Eukaryotic tyrosine kinase activity was first reported in 1980 by T. Hunter at the Salk Institute, who identified c-Src in cells from chickens and humans. Subsequently, the epidermal growth factor receptor (EGFR) and platelet-derived growth factor receptor (PDGFR) were shown to have tyrosine kinase activity. Among the 598 kinases encoded by the human genome, 90 tyrosine kinases have been identified to perform critical roles in regulating survival and proliferation of various types of cells. In terms of tumor progression, it has been established that mutation and overexpression of tyrosine kinases such as the Bcr-Abl fusion protein and EGFR in cancer cells facilitate survival, proliferation, invasion, and metastasis. Furthermore, tyrosine kinases perform the critical role in the regulation of tumor microenvironment through controling cellular processes such as angiogenesis. Because of the immense profound amount regulatory roles of tyrosine kinases in cells, tyrosine kinase inhibition has becoming a major goal of research for the development of targeted anticancer drugs.

The discovery of small molecule tyrosine kinase inhibitors was the result of a massive screening of natural compounds. In 1981, at Germany's Giessen University, H. Glossman et al. discovered that the flavonoid quercetin inhibits c-Src activity in vitro at mM concentrations. In 1983, R.L. Erikson's group at Colorado University confirmed that quercetin suppresses c-Src in vivo. However, owing to its low specificity, quercetin was also revealed to suppress the activity of serine/threonine kinases such as cAMP-dependent protein kinase (PKA) and Ca^{2+}/calmodulin-dependent protein kinase (CaMK). Later, Japanese scientists discovered natural compounds with higher specificity for tyrosine kinases, including erbstatin, genistein, and lavendustin. However, as growing numbers of tyrosine kinase were gradually discovered, these tyrosine kinase inhibitors derived from natural compounds were found to have low specificity for particular tyrosine kinases and to be unstable in vivo, which led to the development of synthetic inhibitors with higher specificity and stability.

The first study for development of synthetic tyrosine kinase inhibitors was performed by A. Levitzki at Israel's Hebrew University in the late 1980s. Using the natural substance erbstatin and itaconic acid which contain the hydroxyphenyl group found in tyrosine, as a template, he developed tyrphostin1, a benzene malononitrile with a weak inhibitory effect on serine/threonine kinases and high specificity for the EGFR, in 1988. In the following years, Levitzki's group synthesized various derivatives by altering tyrphostin1 and developed several types of tyrphostin with specificity for particular tyrosine kinases, including the insulin receptor, PDGFR, and Bcr-Abl fusion protein.

However, the drugs developed by Levitzki mostly show a limited inhibitory effect at micromolar (μM) concentrations, whereas a higher binding affinity was required for clinical applications. In addition, when the inhibitory mechanisms of these drugs were investigated, they were found to be different from those that had been expected at the start of development, with the majority of the drugs found to act as a competitive inhibitor of the binding of ATP on the ATP binding pocket, rather than tyrosine mimic on the substrate-binding domain.

Beginning in the late 1980s, pharmaceutical companies took the lead in the development of tyrosine kinase inhibitors, leading to the gradual development of drugs with higher specificity and action at nanomolar (nM) concentrations. In order to improve the specificity of tyrosine kinase inhibitors as competitive inhibitors of ATP, drugs with more complicated structures, involving multicyclic rings such as quinazoline and phenylaminopyrimidine, were developed. Quinazoline drugs, which have high specificity for the EGFR, were first discovered by AstraZeneca in 1992, leading to the release of gefitinib. In 1994, .W. Fry of Parke-Davis Pharmaceuticals reported tyrosine kinase inhibitor PD153035. In 1995, Oncogene Science discovered tyrosine kinase inhibitor CP-358774, which was developed as erlotinib. CGP 57148, a phenylaminopyrimidine inhibitor of Bcr-Abl, was reported by J. Zimmermann of Ciba Pharmaceuticals in 1995 and later developed as imatinib. In addition, tyrosine kinases such as vascular endothelial growth factor (VEGFR), RET proto-oncogene (RET), stem cell factor receptor (SCFR), PDGFR, Janus kinase 2 (JAK2), and Bruton's tyrosine kinase (BTK) were shown to play important roles in the progression of various types of tumors, leading to the development of kinase inhibitors that are now commonly used in the clinic.

The history and development processes for molecular targeted anticancer agents are discussed below in the order of their development, beginning with the earliest reported compounds.

9.1 Tretinoin (All-*Trans* Retinoic Acid, ATRA)

The first targeted anticancer agent was all-*trans* retinoic acid (ATRA), which was used in the treatment of acute promyelocytic leukemia (APL). APL is a rare form of leukemia, characterized by the acculumation of immature promyelocyte. In 1977, at the University of Chicago, oncocytologist J.D. Rowley discovered a common translocation of chromosomes 15 and 17 in cancer cells from APL patients, which she believed to be the cause of APL [1]. In 1990, three different research teams, including E. Solomon's group at the Imperial Cancer Research Fund in the United Kingdom and A. Dejean's group at France's Institut Pasteur, independently identified the genes in the area of the translocation identified in cancer cells from APL patients. As a result, they discovered that the translocation in APL cancer cells caused two genes, promyelocytic leukemia protein (*PML*) on chromosome 15 and retinoic acid receptor a (*RAR*A) on chromosome 17, to combine into a fusion gene encoding the tumor-specific fusion protein PML-RARα [2, 3].

A separate study was performed by T.R. Breitman et al. at the NCI to develop drugs to treat APL. Breitman had been interested by a 1971 report that Friend, at Mount Sinai Hospital, had induced cancer cell apoptosis by completely differentiating erythroleukemia cells using dimethyl sulfoxide (DMSO) [4]. In 1981, Breitman discovered that ATRA induced differentiation and killed HL60 human APL cells at a low concentration of 1 nM. The next year, Breitman observed that ATRA also specifically induced differentiation in cancer cells isolated from APL patients [5].

In 1988, leukemia researchers Z.Y. Wang et al. at Shanghai University first administered ATRA to 5-year old girl with refractory APL and observed a complete remission within 3 weeks of treatment. However, because relapse was frequently observed in patients treated with ATRA alone, conventional chemotherapy was performed in combination with ATRA treatment, showing a dramatic response, with no relapse within 5 years for 75 % of the patients [6]. Clinical trials conducted by R.P. Warrell at the Memorial Sloan-Kettering Cancer Center in the United States in 1991 demonstrated a similar therapeutic efficacy [7]. Based on these results, ATRA was finally approved by the FDA as a treatment for APL in 1995. ATRA was widely used and provided an opportunity to promote the development of targeted drugs. As research into the dramatic therapeutic effect of ATRA continued, H. de Thé et al. identified the anticancer mechanism of ATRA in 1999, discovering that ATRA binds to the RAR, a part of the PML-RARα protein, eliminating the transcription inhibition by the fusion protein and inducing transcription of differentiation-related genes (Fig. 9.3) [8].

9.2 Bcr-Abl Inhibitors

Imatinib was approved as a treatment for chronic myeloid leukemia (CML) in 2001. It is a highly specific inhibitor of the oncoprotein Bcr-Abl tyrosine kinase, which acts as an important oncogene during the progression of CML. Imatinib was the first protein kinase inhibitor to be approved as an anticancer agent, and it is known as the most pioneering and successful targeted anticancer drug. However, reports of imatinib-resistant mutant Bcr-Abl proteins in CML patients spurred the development of second generation Bcr-Abl inhibitors such as dasatinib, nilotinib, and bosutinib, which are currently introduced in the clinics (Fig. 9.4).

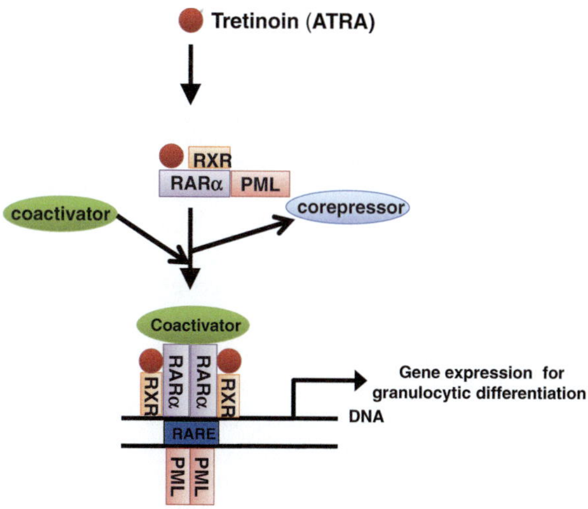

Fig. 9.3 Tretinoin therapeutic mechanism of action in acute promyelocytic leukemia. When all-*trans* retinoic acid (ATRA; tretinoin) binds to RARα in the PML-RARα fusion protein, the corepressors bound to it is separated and coactivators bind instead. PML-RARα complexes bound to coactivators have increased transcription activity and thus promote expression of genes related to cell differentiation, causing immature marrow cells to differentiate into mature marrow cells

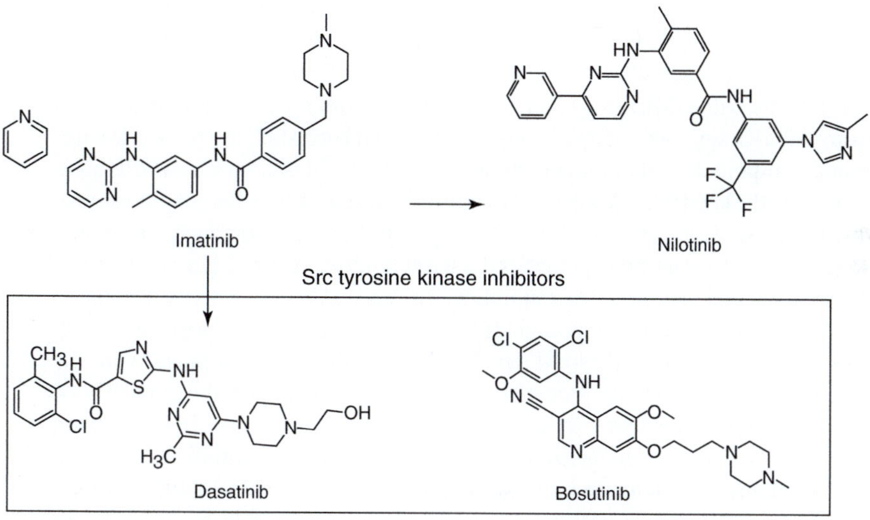

Fig. 9.4 The structure of Bcr-Abl inhibitors and the process of their development

9.2.1 First Generation Bcr-Abl Inhibitor: Imatinib

APL treatment using ATRA is not a perfect targeted anticancer therapy from a methodological perspective, because the discovery of the drug was not based on the discovery and understanding of oncogenes, but rather depended on experimental serendipity and inspiration. Accordingly, the first drug fitting the definition of a targeted anticancer agent was imatinib, which was used to treat CML in 1996.

In 1960, P.C. Nowell at the University of Pennsylvania was studying chromosomes in CML patients when he discovered a very small chromosome that was not observed in healthy individuals or patients with other forms of leukemia; he named this construct the "Philadelphia chromosome" [9]. Later, in the 1970s, as chromosome staining techniques improved, studies were conducted to investigate the origins of the Philadelphia chromosome. In 1973, before J.D. Rowley discovered the chromosomal translocation in APL in 1977, she discovered that the Philadelphia chromosome observed specifically in CML cells was the result of a chromosomal translocation in the part of chromosome 22 that binds to the long arm of chromosome 9 [10]. In 1982, A. de Klein et al. at Erasmus University in the Netherlands performed a further study of the translocation region in the Philadelphia chromosome and discovered that the Abl gene from chromosome 9 was fused with chromosome 22 [11]. In addition, in a collaborative study with N. Heisterkamp et al. at the NCI, who first determined the chromosomal location of c-Abl, de Klein et al. identified the Bcr gene on chromosome 22 as the gene bound to Abl and reported that the Philadelphia chromosomal translocation produced the oncogene Bcr-Abl in 1985 [12]. In 1980, D. Baltimore et al. at the MIT Whitehead Institute discovered that v-Abl protein showed tyrosine kinase activity related to its ability to induce cancer [13]. In 1986, Baltimore's group observed the tyrosine kinase activity of the oncoprotein Bcr-Abl and predicted that this function would be a cause of CML [14, 15].

Hemato-oncologist B. Druker at Oregon Health & Science University assumed that inhibition of the activity of the Bcr-Abl oncoprotein could be a treatment strategy for patients with CML. A. Matter and N. Lydon from the Swiss pharmaceutical company Ciba-Geigy (later merged with Novartis) had been studying protein kinase-inhibiting compounds and attempted to develop a Bcr-Abl inhibitor as a collaborative project. In the late 1980s, Matter and Lydon discovered 2-phenylaminopyrimidine, a protein kinase C (PKC) inhibitor, through large-scale compound screening. Subsequently, J. Zimmerman synthesized a large number of 2-phenylaminopyrimidine derivatives and measured their inhibitory effects on Bcr-Abl activity, leading to the discovery of a new lead compound [16]. After starting a collaborative study with B. Druker, Zimmerman synthesized derivatives from this lead compound with the goal of producing a specific Bcr-Abl inhibitor, leading to the development of CGP57148 (the previous name for imatinib) in 1992, in which a methyl group and benzamide were added to the benzene ring of 2-phenylaminopyrimidine before the addition of methylpiperazine to increase solubility (Fig. 9.5) [17]. In 1996, Druker performed preclinical trials with CGP57148 and observed a selective and potent cytotoxic effect on cultured CML cells, as well as a potent therapeutic efficacy in animal models of CML expressing Bcr-Abl [18].

Thereafter, beginning in 1998, Druker collaborated with C.L. Sawyers at Memorial Sloan-Kettering to conduct phase 1 clinical trials using imatinib as a monotherapy in CML patients. In 2001, Druker and Sawyrs reported the surprising result that leukemic cells had disappeared from the blood of 53 of 54 imatinib-treated CML patients receiving a dose ≥300 mg/day within a few weeks [19].

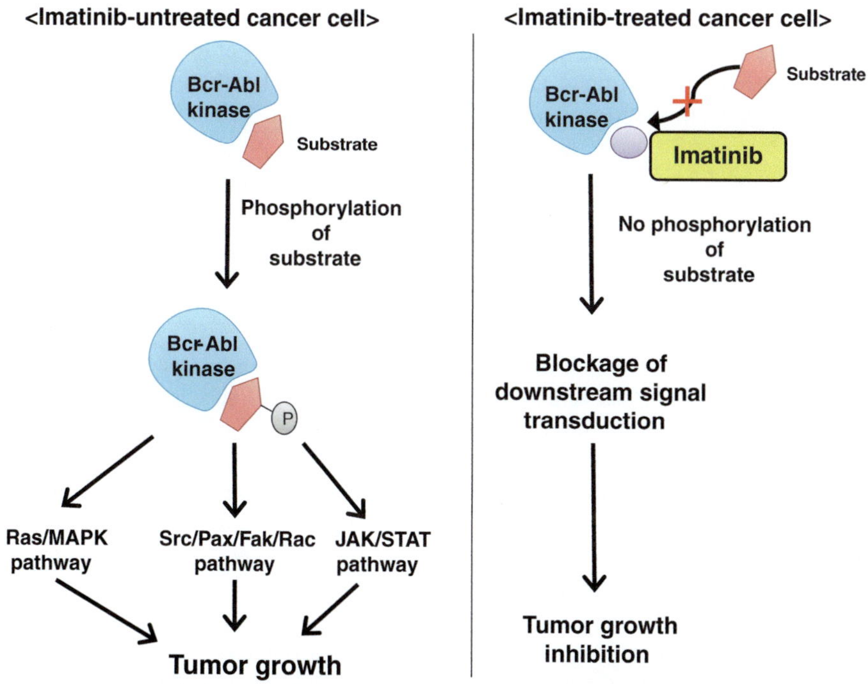

Fig. 9.5 Mechanism of action for imatinib. Imatinib binds to ATP binding pocket in Bcr-Abl and inhibits phosphorylation of its substrates, including GRB-2 and SHC. This action blocks important downstream signaling pathways for cancer cell proliferation and survival, including Ras/MAPK, Src/Pax/Fak/Rac, and JAK/STAT, preventing proliferation of cancer cells and inducing cell death. In this way, imatinib acts as an anticancer agent in chronic myeloid leukemia patients

In phase 2 and phase 3 clinical trials conducted in approximately 30 countries, 95 % of imatinib-treated CML patients showed a disappearance of cancer cells [20]. In 2001, after imatinib designated for priority review, , the drug was finally approved by the FDA as a treatment for CML. Imatinib is still widely used, but second generation Bcr-Abl inhibitors such as dasatinib, nilotinib, and bosutinib are used clinically in patients with imatinib resistance.

Studies of the molecular biology of cancer led directly to the development of imatinib, which acts with high specificity on a cancer-specific oncoprotein to treat a single type of cancer with minimal adverse events. As a result, imatinib serves as a model for the development of molecular targeted anticancer agents. In addition, the development of imatinib provided a demonstration of the effectiveness of molecular mechanism-based screening systems that were clearly distinct from previously existing systems for anticancer drug development.

Moreover, contrary to initial expectations, imatinib was found to have inhibitory activity against several cancer-related tyrosine kinases, as well as excellent therapeutic effects in patients with other types of cancer. The inhibitory activity of imatinib on PDGFR-α and PDGFR-β activities contributes to its therapeutic effects in patients with hypereosinophilic syndrome and medulloblastoma, while its inhibitory effect on c-KIT plays an important role in its therapeutic effect in patients with advanced gastrointestinal stromal tumors (GISTs) [21, 22]. Imatinib is currently used widely as a treatment for patients with CML and GISTs.

9.2.2 *Second Generation Bcr-Abl Inhibitors*

9.2.2.1 Dasatinib

After imatinib treatment, the majority of CML patients did not experienced relapse for a long period of time, but relapse was observed in a small subset of patients showing drug resistance. C.L. Sawyers, an oncologist at Memorial Sloan-Kettering Cancer Center, studied the molecular mechanisms of imatinib resistance, and in 2001 reported that the Bcr-Abl gene in resistant CML cells contained a mutation in the amino acid residue related to drug binding, which prevented the interaction of the drug with the oncoprotein [23]. These results stimulated the development of second generation Bcr-Abl inhibitors.

In the early 2000s, Sawyers performed studies aimed at developing second generation Bcr-Abl inhibitors together with the pharmaceutical company Bristol-Myers Squibb. J. Das et al. at Bristol-Myers Squibb synthesized derivatives of aminothiazole, which had been identified as an immunosuppressant. In 2004, a study of aminothiazole derivatives identified the thiazolyl-aminopyrimidine compound dasatinib, which had inhibitory activity on Bcr-Abl 300-fold stronger than that of imatinib (Fig. 9.6) [24, 25]. In 2004, Sawyers et al. reported that dasatinib inhibited Bcr-Abl activity in the 15 types of imatinib-resistant Bcr-Abl mutants that had been identified at the time, except for mutant T315I. Moreover, using cells expressing Bcr-Abl mutant proteins, they confirmed the therapeutic effect of dasatinib in an implantation tumor model [26]. In 2006, J.S. Tokarski et al. at Bristol-Myers Squibb performed structural analysis of human ABL kinase domain complexed with imatinib or dasatinib and discovered that the site of dasatinib action on Bcr-Abl was different from the site of imatinib action, demonstrating the molecular mechanism for inhibiting imatinib-resistant Bcr-Abl [27]. Based on these results, Sawyers conducted clinical trials of dasatinib in imatinib-resistant CML patients, and in 2006 reported successful therapeutic responses, with CML cells completely disappearing in 82 % of patients [28]. In 2006, dasatinib was approved as a treatment for imatinib-resistant CML. Dasatinib is still widely used.

9.2.2.2 Nilotinib

Novartis, the developer of imatinib, also conducted studies aimed at developing second generation Bcr-Abl inhibitors together with J.D. Griffin's group at the Dana-Farber Cancer Institute. In 2005, based on the structural analysis of the Abl-imatinib

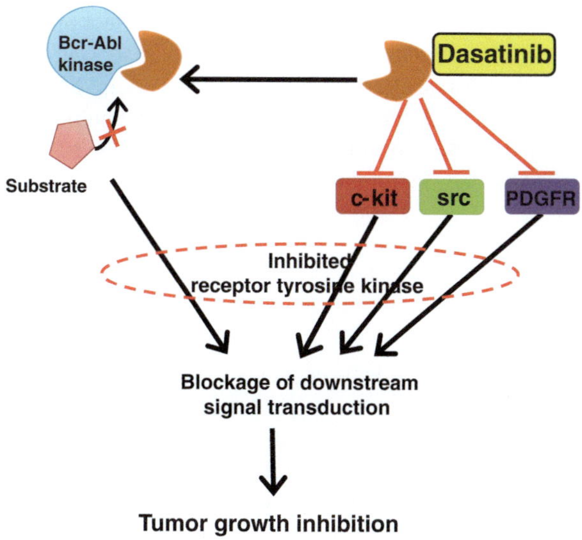

Fig. 9.6 Mechanism of action for dasatinib. Dasatinib binds Bcr-Abl to prevent phosphorylation of its substrates, including GRB-2 and SHC. Unlike imatinib, dasatinib has low conformational requirements for its Bcr-Abl binding site, which is attributable to its stronger efficacy; therefore, it is used in imatinib-resistant chronic myeloid leukemia patients. In addition, because dasatinib also inhibits other tyrosine kinases, including SCFR, Src, PDGFRs, and ephrin receptors, which is also related to the proliferation of cancer cells

complex by J. Kuriyan's group at Rockefeller University, J.D. Griffin's group and Novartis altered the N-methylpiperazine group on imatinib to a methylimidazole group and added a trifluoro-methyl group to the benzamide part of the molecule, producing the phenylamino-pyrimidine compound nilotinib [29, 30]. Nilotinib has approximately 20-fold stronger binding affinity than imatinib and higher specificity for Abl. Nilotinib inhibited the activity of all imatinib-resistant Bcr-Abl mutants except for the T315I mutant [30]. In 2006, Novartis cooperated with O.G. Ottman at the M.D. Anderson Cancer Center to perform clinical trials in CML patients with an imatinib-resistant Philadelphia chromosome, wherein nilotinib showed an outstanding therapeutic efficacy, eliminating resistant leukemic cells in 72 % of patients [31]. Based on these results, nilotinib was approved by the FDA as a treatment for imatinib-resistant CML in 2006.

9.2.2.3 Bosutinib

Bosutinib is a 4-anilino-3-quinolinecarbonitrile that was discovered in 2001 by D.H Boschelli et al. at the pharmaceutical company Wyeth Research (merged with Pfizer in 2009) during screening for Src tyrosine kinase inhibitors based on quinoline [32]. In 2003, J.M. Golas et al. at Wyeth Research investigated the inhibitory effect of bosutinib on Abl and found that it was stronger than the inhibitory effect of bosutinib against Src, which was 50 times stronger than the inhibitory effect of imatinib [33]. In 2006, in a collaborative study with M. Puttini et al., Golas showed that bosutinib inhibited several imatinib-resistant Bcr-Abl mutant proteins except for T315I mutant [34]. In a clinical trial on imatinib-resistant CML patients, bosutinib showed a clear effect in 82% of patients. In 2012, bosutinib was approved by the FDA as the third second generation Bcr-Abl inhibitor for the treatment of imatinib-resistant CML [35].

9.3 EGFR Inhibitors

The success of molecular targeted anticancer agents in the field of hemato-oncology promoted the development of molecular targeted drugs for the treatment of solid cancers. The first target protein to receive attention for molecular targeted therapy of solid cancers was the EGFR, because the EGF/EGFR signaling pathway plays a core role in the progression of various solid tumor cells. EGFR inhibitors include the monoclonal antibody drugs cetuximab and panitumumab, as well as first generation small molecular tyrosine kinase inhibitors gefitinib and erlotinib and second generation tyrosine kinase inhibitor afatinib (Fig. 9.7).

Research into the EGF/EGFR signaling pathway started with the study of S. Cohen at Washington University in 1960. Cohen had been studying nerve growth factor (NGF) in extract from the submaxillary gland of mice, when he observed a new, unexpected activity that could not be attributed to NGF: opening of the eyelids and early tooth eruption in newborn mice [36, 37]. Cohen continued research into this new activity at Vanderbilt University, and in 1963 he revealed that the phenomenon resulted from stimulation of epidermal growth within tissues [38]. In 1972, he isolated the EGF peptide from submaxillary gland extract.

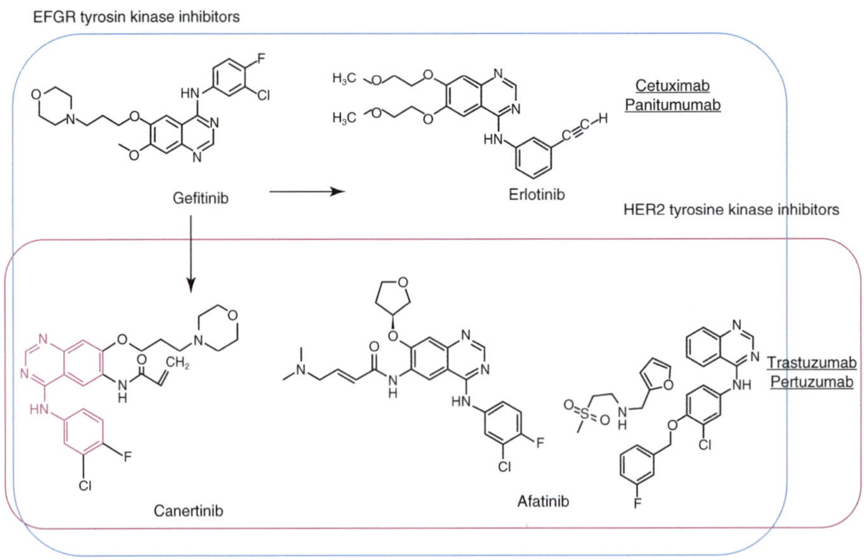

Fig. 9.7 The structure of EGFR and HER2 inhibitors and the process of their development

Thereafter, several researchers observed a strong effect of EGF on cell growth, while studies of human-derived EGF were conducted. In 1975, Cohen purified human EGF [39] and in 1982 he purified the EGFR, which transmits the growth signal after binding with EGF [40]. Cohen's group and T. Hunter's group separately discovered that tyrosine residues on the EGFR are phosphorylated when the receptor binds EGF, leading both groups to propose that this tyrosine phosphorylation was important for growth signal transduction, as well as the possibility that the EGFR might be a tyrosine kinase [41, 42]. In 1986, Cohen was awarded the Nobel Prize in Physiology or Medicine for his work discovering and understanding the function of the EGF/EGFR system.

In 1984, J. Downward et al. at the Imperial Cancer Research Fund performed purification of the EGFR and partially determined its amino acid sequence [43]. Shortly afterward, A. Ullrich and the research team of M.G. Rosenfeld at UCSD discovered the gene encoding the EGFR (Erb-B1) and resolved its entire sequence [44]. Interestingly, EGFR showed high homology with the oncoprotein v-Erb-B, discovered in avian erythroblastosis virus (AEV), which suggested that this protein's activity might be related to the development or progression of cancer.

Later, various studies reported that EGFR expression and activity were upregulated in a large number of solid cancers, including lung cancer, head and neck cancer, colorectal cancer, pancreatic cancer, breast cancer, and glioblastoma multiforme [45]. This series of studies clearly demonstrated the correlation of EGFR expression and activity with cancer, leading to numerous studies aimed at treating cancer by EGFR inhibition.

9.3.1 First Generation EGFR Inhibitors

9.3.1.1 Gefitinib

In 1992, A.J. Barker et al. at the pharmaceutical company Zeneca (now AstraZeneca) discovered the anilinoquinazoline class inhibitor AG1478, with high specificity for the EGFR, by screening a library of 250,000 compounds [46, 47]. AG1478 has a similar structure to ATP and inhibits the kinase activity of the EGFR by binding to the ATP binding pocket within its tyrosine kinase domain and competing with ATP. However, AG1478 had low solubility and was unstable; therefore, in 1997, these shortcomings were improved upon with the development of gefitinib [48]. The activity of gefitinib was confirmed in an implantation tumor model. In 2003, clinical trials of gefitinib were conducted in patients with non-small cell lung cancer (NSCLC), which was known to show increased EGFR activity. Gefitinib produced partial response in 10–15 % of NSCLC patients and was approved by the FDA for advanced NSCLC that does not respond to conventional chemotherapy [49]. However, in an additional large-scale clinical trial, gefitinib did not show a clinical benefit in terms of overall survival. In 2005, the FDA restricted the use of gefitinib to patients in which the drug had already shown an efficacy.

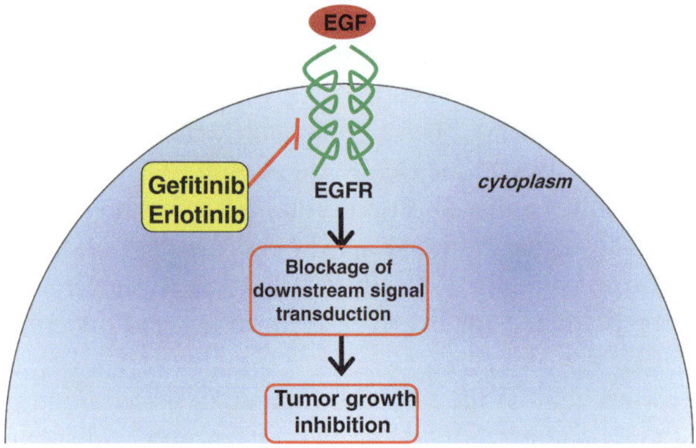

Fig. 9.8 Mechanism of action for gefitinib and erlotinib. Gefitinib and erlotinib compete with ATP for the ATP binding site on EGFR, and thereby inhibit the activity of EGFR. This action blocks the activation of downstream signaling required for survival and proliferation of cancer cells

Several studies were conducted in the 2000s with the goal of determining why gefitinib was not as effective as was expected by preclinical studies. In independent studies in 2004, T.J Lynch et al. of Harvard Medical School and J.G. Paez et al. revealed that the presence of EGFR mutations in lung cancer patients was strongly predictive of the efficacy of gefitinib [50, 51]. Specifically, in NSCLC patients in which gefitinib was particularly effective, mutations were frequently observed in the EGFR, such as the deletion of exon 19 (which suppressed apoptosis) or an L858R mutation, in which the leucine at position 858 in exon 21 was substituted with arginine. The mutated EGFR strongly activated the Akt-1 pathway, which is related to the EGFR-mediated cell survival, rather on cell proliferation; thus, when EGFR activity was inhibited by gefitinib in the cells with mutated EGFR, apoptosis was induced more effectively than in other cancer cells (Fig. 9.8). These EGFR mutations were particularly frequent in non-smoking Asian female patients with lung adenocarcinoma (non-smoking Asian female patients: 25 %, non-smoking US female patients: 10 %).

Based on thes results, a new comparative clinical trial using gefitinib as the first-line treatment was conducted in advanced NSCLC in East Asia. In comparison with conventional combination treatment with carboplatin plus paclitaxel, gefitinib treatment produced a significant improvement in progression-free survival for NSCLC patients with EGFR mutations [52]. In 2015, the FDA approved gefitinib as a first-line treatment for advanced NSCLC with EGFR mutations.

9.3.1.2 Erlotinib

Around the same time that gefitinib was developed, another anilinoquinazoline-class EGFR inhibitor, erlotinib, was developed by L.D. Arnold et al. at OSI Pharmaceuticals [53]. Similar to gefitinib, erlotinib also enters the ATP binding site within the EGFR kinase domain and competitively inhibits ATP binding (Fig. 9.8).

Erlotinib has a strong inhibitory effect on the EGFR, with an IC_{50} value of 20 nM for purified EGFR. In addition, erlotinib halts the cell cycle in G1 and induces apoptosis in human colon cancer cells [54].

Following preclinical studies of erlotinib, clinical trials were performed in collaboration with Genentech. When erlotinib was administered to patients with advanced NSCLC that did not respond to conventional chemotherapy, the median overall survival improved from 4.7 months (for the placebo group) to 6.7 months (for the treatment group) [55]. In 2004, the FDA approved erlotinib as a treatment for advanced NSCLC when conventional chemotherapy is ineffective.

Like gefitinib, erlotinib was highly effective in NSCLC patients with activating EGFR mutations; therefore, independent phase 3 clinical trials were conducted in NSCLC patients in Asia and Europe, which reported that erlotinib produced a therapeutic effect superior to that of standard chemotherapy in 2011 and 2012 [56, 57]. Accordingly, the FDA approved the use of erlotinib as a first-line treatment in NSCLC patients with an exon 19 deletion or L858R mutation in exon 21 of the EGFR.

In addition, a clinical trial of erlotinib was conducted in patients with locally advanced or metastatic pancreatic cancer, wherein erlotinib was administered with gemcitabine. Erlotinib treatment extended the median overall survival by 0.4 months in comparison with that of patients who were treated with gemcitabine alone [58]. Erlotinib has been in active use as a treatment for pancreatic cancer since its approval by the FDA in 2005.

9.3.2 Afatinib: Second Generation EGFR Inhibitor

Similar to imatinib, long-term use of gefitinib or erlotinib has been observed to induce resistance. In 2005, in independent studies by H. Varmus and W. Pao et al. at the Memorial Sloan-Kettering Cancer Center and by S. Kobayashi et al. at Harvard Medical School, the mechanisms of erlotinib resistance were investigated in patients who had an exon 19 deletion or an L858R mutation, but had relapsed after treatment with gefitinib or erlotinib. The researchers discovered that resistance was acquired when there was a secondary T790M mutation, in which the threonine at position 790 in the ATP binding site of the EGFR was replaced with methionine, reducing the inhibitory effect of erlotinib [59, 60]. The threonine at position 790 performs a similar role to the residue involved in the T315I mutation in Bcr-Abl, which is known to cause strong resistance to imatinib; mutation of T790 weakens binding of gefitinib and erlotinib. Approximately 50 % of patients who showed resistance after treatment with gefitinib or erlotinib were shown to have acquired a T790M mutation.

Beginning in 2005, second generation EGFR inhibitors were developed with the goal of overcoming drug resistance conferred by the T790M mutation. Second generation inhibitors are characterized by irreversible inhibition of the EGFR kinase domain, in contrast with the reversible inhibition produced by first generation drugs.

S. Kobayashi et al. discovered that the anilinoquinazoline-class irreversible inhibitor CL-387785, developed in 1999 by Wyeth Research, suppressed the activity of resistant $EGFR^{T790M}$ [61], while E.L. Kwak et al. at Harvard Medical School observed that the same effect was produced by another anilinoquinazoline class irreversible inhibitor, HKI-272, which was developed by Wyeth Research in 2004 [62]. Afatinib, an anilinoquinazoline-class compound developed by Boehringer Ingelheim in 2008, acts as an irreversible EGFR inhibitor because of its acrylamide group [63]. In a collaborative study by D. Li et al. at the Dana-Farber Cancer Institute, afatinib was found to covalently bind Cys773 of the EGFR and Cys805 of human epidermal growth factor receptor 2 (HER2), strongly inhibiting $EGFR^{L858R}$ and $EGFR^{T790M}$, which are resistant to first generation drugs. Afatinib was also shown to have a significant therapeutic effect when administered with rapamycin in an xenograft model with lung cancer cells possessing the L858R/T790M EGFR mutations, leading to the expectation that afatinib would be developed into an effective drug for patients with lung cancer.

Subsequently, an investigation was carried out using afatinib together with standard chemotherapy as a first-line treatment in patients with advanced NSCLC possessing a deletion of exon 19 or L858R mutation in exon 21 of the EGFR. In 2013, progression-free survival was found to be extended by 4.2 months when standard chemotherapy and afatinib were administered together, in comparison with that of patients exposed to standard chemotherapy alone [64]. Following these results, in 2013, the FDA approved afatinib as a first-line treatment in advanced NSCLC, for which it is presently in clinical use. Afatinib was also found to increase progression-free survival by 2.1 months in comparison with placebo in second-line treatment of advanced NSCLC patients who did not respond to gefitinib or erlotinib [65]. Moreover, because afatinib also displays HER2 inhibitory activity, a phase 2 clinical trial was conducted in patients with HER2-positive metastatic breast cancer, in which 19 of 41 patients showed improvement from afatinib treatment, suggesting a possible use for the drug as a treatment for patients with breast cancer [66].

9.3.3 Monoclonal Antibodies Against EGFR

9.3.3.1 Cetuximab

In addition to the aforementioned small molecule inhibitors, targeted anticancer treatments that act by suppressing EGFR activity have also been developed using antibodies. In 1983, J. Mendelsohn's group at UCSD developed a monoclonal mouse anti-EGFR antibody that inhibited EGFR activity by binding to the EGFR and interfering with the action of ligand EGF [67]. Subsequently, the monoclonal anti-EGFR antibody was shown to be capable of inhibiting tumor growth in a xenograft model [68]. Together with G. Sato's group (also at UCSD), Mendelsohn's group performed the development of cetuximab, a chimeric human-mouse antibody comprising parts the monoclonal mouse anti-EGFR antibody and human immunoglobulin G (IgG1), in 1995 (Fig. 9.9) [69].

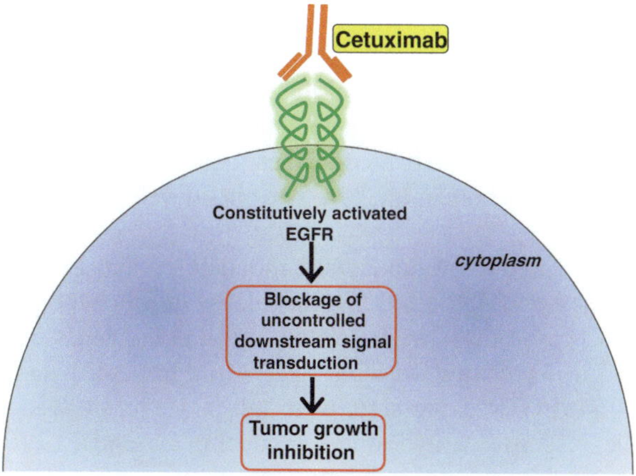

Fig. 9.9 Mechanism of action for cetuximab. Growth factor receptors induce proliferation signals when they are bound by growth factors, but these receptors undergo mutations in some cancer cells that enable them to activate the signaling pathway for proliferation without growth factors, meaning that cell proliferation cannot be controlled. Cetuximab is a monoclonal antibody for EGFR that prevents proliferation of cancer cells by inhibiting downstream pathways through binding to normal EGFR and mutated EGFR

In 1988, M. Sela and J. Schlessinger, immunologists at Israel's Weizmann Institute of Science, independently developed a monoclonal antibody for EGFR. After binding the radioisotope iodine-125 to their monoclonal anti-EGFR antibody, Sela and Schlessinger found that it inhibited the growth of human oral carcinoma cells implanted into immunodeficient mice. With the support of Bristol-Myers Squibb, clinical trials were conducted in patients with metastatic colorectal cancer to investigate the effects of cetuximab in combination with irinotecan chemotherapy. In 2004, an improved therapeutic effect of combination treatment with irinotecan and cetuximab was observed, with progression-free survival prolongation by 2.6 months in comparison with that produced by treatment with chemotherapy alone [70]. Based on these results, cetuximab was approved by the FDA in 2004 as a treatment for metastatic colorectal cancer, becoming the first molecular targeted monoclonal antibody targeting the EGFR. Because there was no benefit in colorectal cancer patients with K-ras mutation, FDA modified the indication for cetuximab for EGFR-expressing metastatic colorectal cancer patients with K-ras wildtype on 2012. Moreover, in 2006, cetuximab in combination with radiotherapy was confirmed to have a therapeutic efficacy against head and neck cancer. In 2011, cetuximab was also proved to have a therapeutic efficacy in combination with carboplatin/5-FU in patients with recurrent or metastatic head and neck cancer, after which it was approved by the FDA as a treatment for head and neck cancer. Cetuximab is currently used to treat patients with metastatic colorectal cancer with wild-type Ras, head and neck cancer, and metastatic NSCLC.

9.3.3.2 Panitumumab

Because cetuximab is a chimeric antibody of the mouse IgG1 isotype, it is accompanied by immunological adverse effects and cytotoxicity caused by activation of the complement pathway. In order to overcome these adverse events, panitumumab, an anti-EGFR antibody with a human IgG2 isotype, was developed by X.D. Yang at Abgenix in 1999 [71].

In 1997, in order to produce a humanized monoclonal anti-EGFR antibody, Abgenix established the XenoMouse, a transgenic mouse in which the genes encoding the IgG light and heavy chains were deleted, whereas the genes encoding the human IgG light and heavy chains were inserted [72]. After A431 human cancer cells, which show high EGFR expression, were injected into the XenoMouse to produce an immune response, a hybridoma producing an anti-EGFR antibody (panitumumab) was established. In xenograft experiments using A431, panitumumab showed a clear therapeutic effect, even when it was not combined with chemotherapeutic agents. In a clinical trial for panitumumab monotherapy in patients with metastatic colon cancer expressing EGFR, extended progression-free survival was observed (comparison group, 60 days; panitumumab administration group, 98 days) [73]. In 2006, panitumumab was approved as a treatment for EGFR-expressing colorectal cancer. In 2009, the indication was modified to include the information on KRAS mutation status.

9.4 HER2 Inhibitors

In 1982, R.A. Weinberg induced neurogliomas in rats, extracted DNA from the tumors, and fragmented it in order to identify causative oncogenes. Then, he injected the DNA fragments generated from tumor DNA into mouse cell lines, separated the cell colonies with enhanced proliferation, and transplanted them into young mice to induce cancer. Because the cancer cells from which the fragments originated were derived from rats, Weinberg anticipated the possibility that the mice would produce antibodies against the oncoprotein following DNA fragment injection, so he collected serum from the mice and performed an immune response test with the proteins extracted from the rat tumor cells, leading to the discovery of the oncoprotein HER2, also known as neu [74].

In 1985, A. Ullrich and Weinberg isolated and sequenced the gene encoding HER2 [75]. Analysis of the sequence of HER2 revealed that the protein possessed tyrosine kinase activity, similar to EGFR, and therefore, it was classified into the EGFR/Erb-b1/HER1 class and named Erb-b2/HER2. Subsequent studies revealed that HER2 does not bind directly with EGF; its endogenous ligand remains unknown. Moreover, HER2 is constitutively active and forms homodimers without ligand binding. HER2 also acts as a co-receptor that readily forms heterodimers with EGFR, HER3, or HER4 after they have been activated by ligand binding.

Using Ullrich's HER2 cDNA as a probe, oncologist D.J. Slamon at UCLA investigated HER2 expression in various types of cancer, revealing that HER2 is highly expressed in 25–30 % of breast cancer tissues because of gene amplification. Moreover, Slamon determined that high expression of HER2 is correlated with tumor progression and poor prognosis in breast cancer [76, 77]. Following the results described above, development of treatments targeting HER2 began.

9.4.1 Monoclonal Antibodies Against HER2

9.4.1.1 Trastuzumab

After encountering Slamon's results, Ullrich at Genentech collaborated with Slamon in an attempt to use monoclonal anti-HER2 antibodies in the treatment of breast cancer. In 1989, Ullrich first acquired mouse monoclonal anti-HER2 antibodies and confirmed that they suppressed the proliferation of HER2-overexpressing cells, as well as the growth of implanted tumor in mice [78]. After selecting the clone that showed the strongest growth-inhibiting effect among several monoclonal anti-HER2 antibodies, Genentech's P. Carter et al. used gene recombination techniques to develop the humanized antibody, trastuzumab (Herceptin) in 1992 [79].

Trastuzumab binds to the extracellular domain of the HER2 protein and has been shown to reduce its stability and suppress the heterodimer formation (Fig. 9.10). When HER2 activity is inhibited by trastuzumab, Akt activity is also suppressed, leading to higher levels of p27KIP1 and interfering with the cell cycle progression. Moreover, it has been reported that trastuzumab is also accompanied by an antibody-dependent cellullar cytotoxic (ADCC) effect. Slamon conducted clinical trials using trastuzumab in combination with standard chemotherapy in metastatic breast cancer patients with HER2 overexpression. The therapeutic effect of the combination

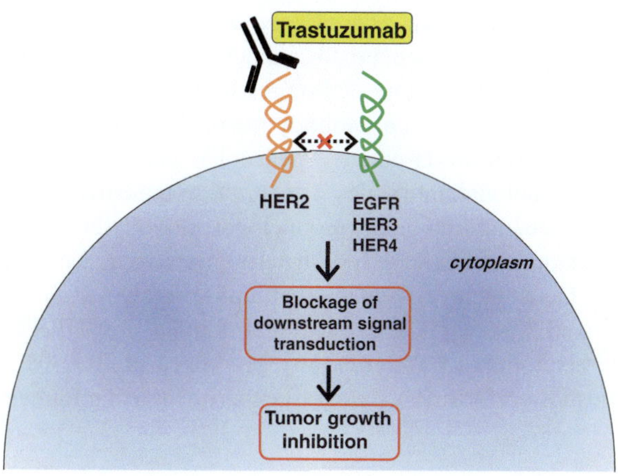

Fig. 9.10 Mechanism of action for trastuzumab. Trastuzumab is a monoclonal antibody that binds to the extracellular domain of HER2 and prevents HER2 from forming heterodimers with other receptor tyrosine kinases (*EGFR*, *HER3*, *HER4*). This action suppresses cancer cell proliferation by inhibiting downstream signaling pathways activated by HER2

of trastuzumab and standard chemotherapy was confirmed in 1998, with median progression-free survival extended by ~2.9 months and the median overall survival extended by 5 months [80]. Later in 1998, the FDA approved the use of trastuzumab as a treatment for patients with metastatic breast cancer with HER2 overexpression.

In 2010, Y.J. Bang et al. of Seoul National University Hospital, Korea implemented treatment of trastuzumab in combination with standard chemotherapy for patients with metastatic gastric or gastro-esophageal junction cancer with HER2 overexpression. For the combined patient group, median overall survival was extended by 2.7 months, from 11.1 to 13.8 months, whereas the tumor response rate improved from 35 to 47 % [81]. Based on these results, the FDA approved the use of trastuzumab as a treatment for patients who have gastric or gastro-esophageal junction cancer with HER2 overexpression in 2011. Currently, trastuzumab is a widely used and important treatment for patients with HER2-positive breast and gastric cancer.

9.4.1.2 Pertuzumab

Of the patients who showed therapeutic effects in clinical trials of trastuzumab, 15 % relapsed [82]. Therefore, studies were soon conducted to determine the mechanism of trastuzumab resistance, followed by efforts aimed at developing drugs able to overcome such resistance. An initial clue as to the causes of trastuzumab resistance, which provided possible methods of overcoming it, was reported by D.B. Agus et al. in 2002. Agus et al. reported that trastuzumab did not significantly suppress formation of HER2-HER3 heterodimers; instead, another type of monoclonal antibody, known as 2C4, strongly inhibited formation of HER2-HER3 heterodimers [83]. Protein structure analysis revealed that, of the extracellular domains (II and VI) that are associated with HER2 heterodimer formation, domain II plays a more important role in dimerization, whereas domain VI, where trastuzumab binds, was found to promote dimerization indirectly, through structural changes induced by ligand binding [84]. Accordingly, when HER2 or the HER3 ligand is overexpressed in patients, trastuzumab cannot entirely block the activation signal resulting from dimerization, leading to drug resistance.

In order to develop an antibody treatment capable of overcoming trastuzumab resistance based on its putative molecular mechanism, Genentech returned to the mouse monoclonal antibodies it acquired in the early stages of trastuzumab development, focusing first on the monoclonal antibody 2C4, which strongly suppressed the formation of HER2-HER3 heterodimers [85]. Next, in 2004, M.C. Franklin et al. at Genentech performed structural analysis and discovered that pertuzumab, humanized 2C4, binds to extracellular domain II of HER2, which plays a decisive role in heterodimer formation [86]. Moreover, in 2009, W. Scheuer et al. at Roche Diagnostics performed a xenograft experiment using human cancer cells and found that pertuzumab and trastuzumab had a synergistic inhibitory effect when administered in combination, because each drug had a distinct binding site on HER2 [87].

Later, a clinical trial was performed to compare the therapeutic efficacy of pertuzumab in combination with trastuzumab/docetaxel in patients with HER2-positive metastatic breast cancer. In this trial, the combination treatment of pertuzumab/trastuzumab/docetaxel delayed breast cancer progression by 6.3 months and extended median overall survival by 15.7 months in comparison with the those of patients treated with trastuzumab/docetaxel only [88]. Based on these results, the FDA approved a use of pertuzumab as a first-line treatment in patients with HER2-positive metastatic breast cancer in 2012.

9.4.2 HER2 Small Molecule Inhibitors

9.4.2.1 Lapatinib

In addition to targeted antibody treatments, there has also been active development of small molecule inhibitors that suppress HER2 activity. In 1999, GlaxoSmithKline's M.C. Carter et al. developed lapatinib, a 4′-benzyloxy derivative of quinazoline that inhibits EGFR and HER2 activity (Fig. 9.11) [89]. While the quinazoline in lapatinib inhibits the EGFR, it is thought that the newly added 4′-benzloxy group contributes to the inhibition of HER2, which explains why lapatinib has this inhibitory effect while gefitinib and erlotinib do not [90].

In 2001, D.W. Rusnak et al. at GlaxoSmithKline found that lapatinib had a strong inhibitory effect on EGFR and HER2 activity, with IC_{50} values of 10.2 and 9.8 nM, respectively, and showed that it was effective at inhibiting the growth of several cancer cell lines with high expression of EGFR and HER2, as well as suppressing AKT activation [91]. A clear anticancer effect of lapatinib was also reported in xenograft tumor experiments. In 2006, D.J Slamon et al. at UCLA performed in vitro and xenograft

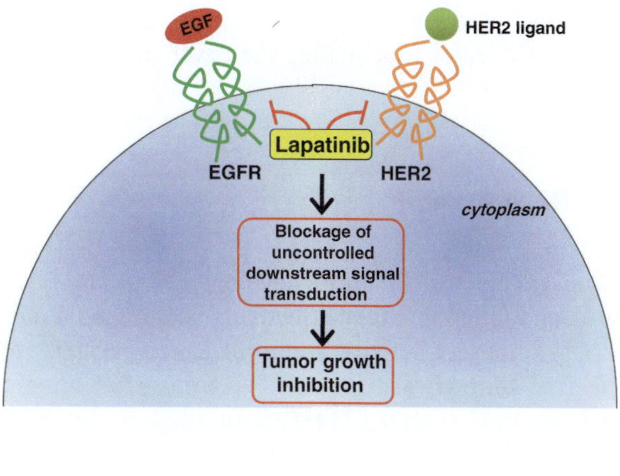

Fig. 9.11 Mechanism of action for lapatinib. Lapatinib is a small molecular agent that inhibits receptor tyrosine kinases EGFR and HER2. Lapatinib binds to the ATP binding site on the kinase domain of EGFR/HER2 and prevents cancer cell proliferation by inhibiting downstream signal transmission related to cell growth

experiments using breast cancer cell lines with overexpression of HER2 or trastuzumab resistance and observed a clear and durable anticancer effect of lapatinib [92].

Based on preclinical results obtained with lapatinib, a clinical trial was conducted using lapatinib in combination with capecitabine for HER2-positive metastatic breast cancer patients who had previously been treated with anthracycline, taxane, and trastuzumab. The results, released in 2006, showed that lapatinib/capecitabine treatment suppressed the progression of breast cancer approximately 50% as effectively as capecitabine alone [93]. Based on these results, the FDA approved the use of lapatinib as a treatment for metastatic breast cancer in 2007. In 2012, lapatinib in combination with the aromatase inhibitor letrozole was found to prolong the progression-free survival by 5.2 months in comparison with that of patients treated with letrozole alone (lapatinib/letrozole, 8.2 months; letrozole alone, 3.0 months) in postmenopausal hormone receptor (HR) positive and HER2 positive metastatic breast cancer. Lapatinib was also approved as a treatment for patients with HER2/HR-positive breast cancer and is widely used for this indication.

9.5 Angiogenesis Inhibitors

Since J. Folkman proposed that angiogenesis was a prerequisite for tumor growth and metastasis in 1971, angiogenesis has received attention as a major target for anticancer therapy [94]. However, until a biological understanding of angiogenesis was achieved at the molecular level, no actual anti-angiogenic cancer treatments were established. In 1989, the pivotal regulator of tumor angiogenesis, vascular endothelial growth factor (VEGF), was discovered by Genentech's N. Ferrara et al. and several other groups [95, 96]. In 1992, L.T. Wiliams's group at UCSF discovered the VEGF receptor VEGFR-1 [97]. VEGFR-2 was also discovered independently by B.I. Trerman at New York's Lederle Laboratories in 1992 and by A. Ullrich's group at the Max Planck Institute in 1993 [98, 99]. The identification of VEGF and its receptors allowed the investigation of detailed molecular mechanisms of angiogenesis, facilitating the development of several molecular targeted drugs.

9.5.1 Bevacizumab

In 1993, Genentech's N. Ferrara developed mouse monoclonal antibodies against VEGF-A and found that they effectively suppressed tumor angiogenesis and had a obvious anticancer activity in murine cancer models [100]. Ferrara developed a humanized antibody against VEGF-A for use in clinical trials, designated bevacizumab, in 1997 (Fig. 9.12) [101]. In 2004, a clinical trial was conducted on

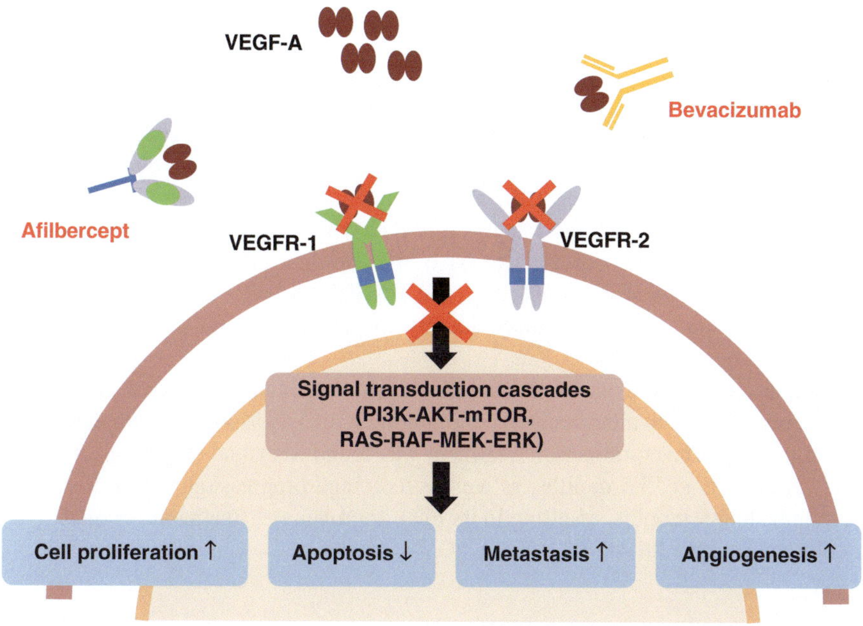

Fig. 9.12 Mechanism of action for bevacizumab and aflibercept. Bevacizumab is an anti-VEGF-A monoclonal antibody that prevents VEGF-A binding to VEGFR and is used as a treatment for patients with metastatic colorectal cancer, metastatic non-small cell lung cancer, progressive glioblastoma, and metastatic renal cell carcinoma. VEGF-A binds to VEGFR-1 and VEGFR-2 expressed on the surface of vascular epithelial cells. However, bevacizumab interferes with VEGF-A binding to VEGFR, which inhibits signaling pathways invoked by VEGFR-1 and VEGFR-2, thereby impairing angiogenesis, and survival of cancer cells. Aflibercept, which is also used as a treatment for patients with metastatic colorectal cancer, acts as a decoy receptor for VEGF-A. Aflibercept is composed of the extracellular domain of VEGFR and the Fc region of human IgG1; therefore, it intercepts VEGF-A and interferes with its action at VEGFRs on the surface of vascular endothelial cells

metastatic colorectal cancer patients using bevacizumab with standard chemotherapy (IFL, irinotecan/5-fluorouracil (5FU)/leucovorin) as a first-line treatment. The results showed a 5-month prolongation of overall survival and a 4-month prolongation of progression-free survival, resulting in approval of bevacizumab by the FDA [102]. In 2006, bevacizumab was approved as a second-line treatment in combination with standard chemotherapy (FOLFOX4, 5-FU/leucovorin/oxaliplatin) for patients with metastatic colorectal cancer. Bevacizumab has since been approved as a first-line treatment for metastatic NSCLC in combination with standard chemotherapy (carboplatin/paclitaxel) (2006), as a second-line monotherapy for advanced glioblastoma (2009), and as a first-line treatment for metastatic renal cell carcinoma in combination with interferon-α (2009).

9.5.2 *Aflibercept*

Aflibercept is a VEGFR fusion protein that was developed at Regeneron Pharmaceuticals in 2002 and binds with VEGF to inhibit angiogenesis via the VEGF/VEGFR pathway (Fig. 9.12) [103]. The Aflibercept fusion protein is synthesized from an artificial gene using DNA recombination techniques to fuse the extracellular domains of VEGFR-1 and VEGFR-2 with the Fc region of human IgG1. Aflibercept has been observed to have high binding affinity to VEGF165 (Kd = 1 pM), VEGF121 (Kd = 1–10 pM), and PIGF-2 (Kd = 45 pM). Moreover, aflibercept showed a strong anticancer activity in xenograft tumor model using human breast cancer cell lines.

In 2012, a clinical trial was conducted, wherein metastatic colorectal cancer patients were treated with aflibercept in combination with 5-FU/folinic acid/irinotecan chemotherapy. The combination treatment was found to extend the overall survival by 1.4 months to 13.5 months, as well as to extend progression-free survival by 2.2 months to 6.9 months, resulting in its FDA approval as a treatment for metastatic colorectal cancer [104].

9.5.3 *Small Molecule VEGFR Inhibitors: Multi-targeted Kinase Inhibitors*

In addition to protein drugs such as the anti-VEGF monoclonal antibody bevacizumab and the decoy receptor aflibercept, small molecule VEGFR inhibitors have also been developed, including sorafenib and sunitinib. More small molecule VEGFR inhibitors pazopanib, regorafenib, axitinib, and vandetanib were later developed and are currently used in clinics (Fig. 9.13). These inhibitors are multi-targeted kinase inhibitors; therefore, although they suppress angiogenesis by inhibiting VEGFR-1/2, they also exert their anticancer effect through inhibition of other tyrosine kinases related to tumorigenesis, including PDGFRB, colony stimulating factor 1 receptor (CSF1R), SCFR, Fms-like tyrosine kinase 3 (FLT-3), and RET.

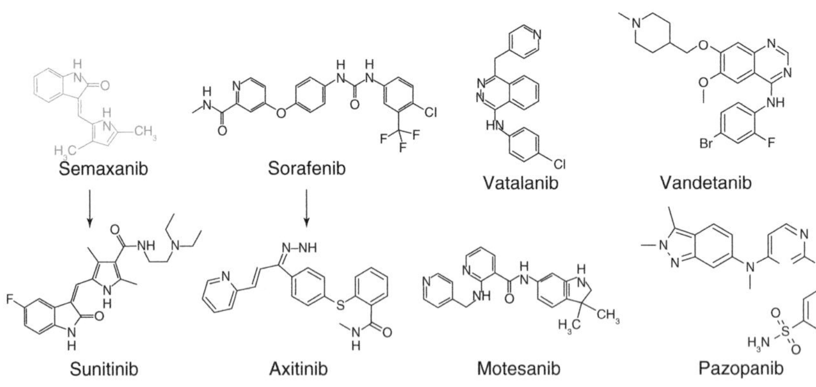

Fig. 9.13 Structures of VEGFR inhibitors and the process of their development

9.5.3.1 Sunitinib

The development of small molecule drugs inhibiting VEGFR activity started in the mid-1990s. Because angiogenesis and VEGF/VEGFR signaling were known to be closely related to the growth and metastasis of various cancers, A. Ullrich, who discovered VEGFR-2, established the company Sugen with J. Schlessinger in 1994, with the aim of developing drugs that treat cancer patients by suppressing tumor angiogenesis. In 1997, while screening for fibroblast growth factor receptor (FGFR) inhibitors, Schlessinger identified a novel class of tyrosine kinase inhibitor as lead compounds called indolineones [105]. Next, Schlessinger synthesized indolinone derivatives, leading to the discovery of SU5416 and SU6668, which inhibit VEGFR-2, in 1998 [106, 107]. However, SU5416 and SU6668 failed in clinical trials owing to inappropriate pharmacokinetic properties, resulting in additional studies to overcome these limitations, which in 2003 led to the development of SU11248 (sunitinib). In comparison with SU5416 and SU6668, sunitinib has a 20-fold stronger inhibitory effect on VEGFR-2 and improved solubility and bioavailability [108]. Like sorafenib, sunitinib was revealed to inhibit various protein tyrosine kinases related to tumor growth and angiogenesis, specifically angiogenesis-related growth factor receptors (VEGFR-1/2/3, PDGFR-β, CSF1R), and oncogenic growth factor receptors (SCFR, FLT-3, RET) [109]. This inhibitory activity of sunitinib was verified in vascular endothelial cells and implantation tumor models. Based on these preclinical evidences, clinical trials were conducted for sunitinib in renal cell carcinoma and pancreatic neuroendocrine tumors, which are highly angiogenic, as well as in gastrointestinal stromal tumors (GIST) involving c-KIT mutations and acute lymphocytic leukemia involving FLT-3 mutations.

Renal cell carcinoma (RCC) is a representative cancer with VEGF overexpression and robust angiogenesis. VEGFR overexpression in RCC is usually the result of a loss-of-function mutation in the von Hippel-Lindau (VHL) gene, which normally induces degradation of hypoxia-inducible factor-1α (HIF-1α) protein, a VEGF transcription regulator. Because of this loss-of-function, HIF-1α accumulates and transcription of VEGF mRNA takes place continuously, leading to oversecretion of VEGF.

When sunitinib was used in a clinical trial for metastatic RCC patients, it was found to increase progression-free survival from 5 months to 11 months compared to standard treatment with IFN-α [110], resulting in approval of sunitinib as a first-line treatment for patients with metastatic RCC by the FDA in 2006. In a clinical trial for patients with GIST that showed resistance to imatinib treatment, sunitinib showed an excellent effect and was approved by the FDA in 2006 [111]. In well-differentiated pancreatic neuroendocrine tumor patients, sunitinib was found to extend progression-free survival from 5.4 months to 10.2 months and was approved by the FDA in 2011 [112]. Sunitinib is currently being used for above indications.

9.5.3.2 Sorafenib

Sorafenib is a VEGFR-2 inhibitor developed by the pharmaceutical companies Bayer and Onyx. In 1995, Bayer and Onyx established a rapid drug screening method to search for Raf inhibitors that blocked the Ras-Raf-MEK-ERK pathway,

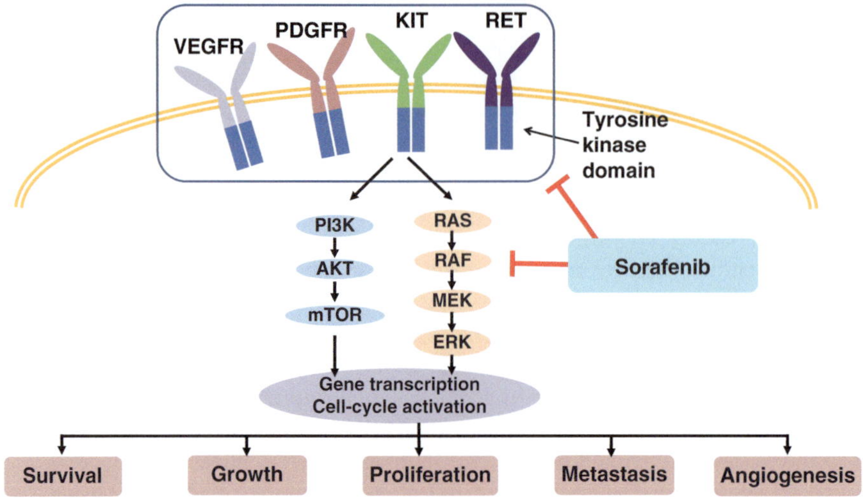

Fig. 9.14 Mechanism of action for sorafenib. Sorafenib inhibits the activity of VEGFR-1 at the cell surface and RAF within the cytoplasm in order to regulate the RAF-MEK-ERK signaling pathway. Sorafenib is used as a treatment for patients with renal cell carcinoma and hepatocellular carcinoma in which VEGF is overexpressed. Sorafenib also inhibits VEGFR-2/3, platelet-derived growth factor receptor-β (PDGFR-β), fibroblast growth factor receptor 1 (FGFR1), SCFR, FLT-3, and RET, which are associated with the development of cancer. Thereby, sorafenib inhibits growth, spreading, metastasis of cancer cells, as well as angiogenesis

through which they tested 200,000 natural substances and synthetic compounds. As a result, Bayer and Onyx identified the hit compound 3-thienyl urea, with an IC_{50} of 17 mM for Raf. Several rounds of 3-thienyl urea derivative synthesis and screening led to the production of the lead compound N-3-thienyl N′-aryl in 2001, with an IC_{50} of 0.5 mM for Raf [113]. Bayer's T.B. Lowinger and S. Wilhelm et al. increased the activity of N-3-thienyl N′-aryl and improved its biosuitability, ultimately leading to the development of sorafenib, with an IC_{50} of 6 nM for Raf, in 2001 [114, 115].

In 2004, S. Wilhelm et al. investigated the kinases targeted by sorafenib and found that, in addition to Raf-1, the drug strongly inhibited various other oncogenic tyrosine kinases. Specifically, sorafenib inhibited normal B-Raf, oncogenic B-Raf^{V600E}, pro-angiogenenic growth factor receptors (VEGFR-1/2/3, PDGFR-β, FGFR1), and oncogenic growth factor receptors (SCFR, FLT-3, RET) (Fig. 9.14) [116]. In addition, S. Wilhelm et al. performed xenograft experiments using cancer cells with various mutations, including B-Raf^{V600E}, and found an inhibitory activity of sorafenib in various types of cancer. Sorafenib was expected to have an anticancer effect because it affected angiogenesis by suppressing VEGFR-1/2 and PDGFRβ, in addition to B-Raf [117].

Based on preclinical results obtained with sorafenib, clinical trials were conducted in patients with metastatic RCC, which is highly angiogenic. In 2005, when sorafenib was administered as a treatment for patients with metastatic RCC, it increased progression-free survival from 2.8 months (that of the placebo group) to 5.5 months [118]. Following these promising results, sorafenib was approved by the FDA for metastatic RCC patients in 2005. Clinical trials were also conducted in patients with metastatic hepatocellular carcinoma (HCC), which are also highly angiogenic. The overall survival and progression-free survival were increased by approximately 3 months in HCC patients with liver cirrhosis [119], leading to the approval of sorafenib by the FDA as a treatment for HCC patients in 2007.

Sorafenib has also been tested in patients with locally advanced or metastatic thyroid cancer that was refractory to radioactive iodine treatment, where it was found to improve progression-free survival from 5.8 months to 10.8 months, resulting in approval of the drug by the FDA in 2013. Sorafenib is currently widely used to treat patients with metastatic RCC, HCC, and thyroid cancer.

9.5.3.3 Regorafenib

Regorafenib is a multi-targeted kinase inhibitor developed by Bayer in 2005 that is also called fluoro-sorafenib, because it is a fluorine-substituted analogue of the diphenyl urea compound sorafenib [120]. In 2011, Bayer's S. Wilhelm et al. reported that regorafenib inhibited VEGFR-2 at lower concentrations than sorafenib and inhibited more types of tyrosine kinases [121]. Specifically, regorafenib is known to inhibit the receptor tyrosine kinases VEGFR-1,2,3, SCFR, PDGFR-α/β, FGFR1,2, angiopoietin-1 receptor (TIE2), discoidin domain-containing receptor 2 (DDR2), putative potassium ion transporter isoform 2A (TRK2A), ephrin type-A receptor 2 (EPH2A), protein tyrosine kinase 5 (PTK5), Abl, and RET, as well as RAF-1, BRAF, $BRAF^{V600E}$ and stress-activated protein kinase 2 (SAPK2), (Fig. 9.15). The effects of regorafenib were investigated closely in various xenograft models, wherein the drug was found to suppress tumor blood perfusion into malignant glioma, to suppress angiogenesis caused by colon carcinoma, and to delay tumor growth of implanted breast cancer or RCC models.

Based on preclinical findings obtained with regorafenib, phase 1 clinical trials were performed, in which regorafenib produced a profound efficacy in metastatic colon cancer patients who are refractory to conventional treatment. Therefore, phase 3 clinical trials were performed in patients with metastatic colorectal cancer who had not responded to fluoropyrimidine/oxaliplatin/irinotecan combination chemotherapy, anti-VEGF therapy, or anti-EGFR therapy, wherein a 1.4-month extension of overall survival and 0.3-month extension of progression-free survival occurred as a result of regorafenib treatment [122]. In 2012, regorafenib was approved by the FDA as a treatment for patients with colorectal cancer. In 2013, clinical trials were conducted in patients with GIST that were unresponsive to imatinib and sunitinib, in which progression-free survival was improved by 3.9 months in comparison with that of the placebo group (4.8 vs 0.9 months) [123], resulting in approval of regorafenib by the FDA as a drug to treat GIST in 2013.

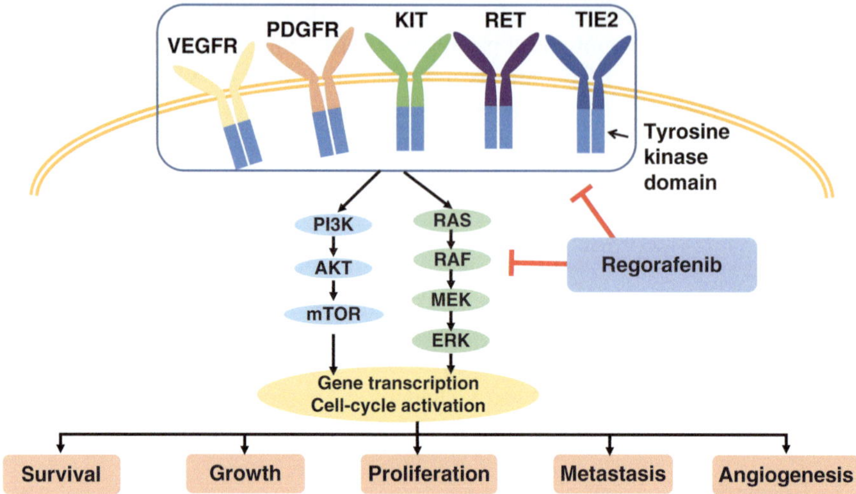

Fig. 9.15 Mechanism of action for regorafenib. Regorafenib is a small molecular multi-targeted kinase inhibitor that suppresses various signaling mechanisms that contribute to the promotion of angiogenesis and proliferation of cancer cells. Regorafenib is used as a treatment for patients with metastatic colorectal cancer. Regorafenib targets to VEGFR-1,3, RAD, and TIE-2, as well as the mutant tumor-forming kinases SCFR, RET, and BRAF. Regorafenib interferes with kinase autophosphorylation, preventing downstream signaling through several pathways (PI3K-Akt-mTOR, Ras-RAF-MEK-MAPK, etc.). Regorafenib inhibits VEGFR-2 at a lower concentration than sorafenib, and it is known to inhibit more types of tyrosine kinases

9.5.3.4 Pazopanib

Pazopanib is a dianilino-pyrimidine class multi-targeted tyrosine kinase inhibitor developed by GlaxoSmithKline in 2007. P.A. Harris et al. identified a dianilino-pyrimidine derivative with an IC_{50} of 400 nM for inhibition of VEGFR-2 during a drug screening, which served as a lead molecule and led in 2008 to the development pazopanib, with an IC_{50} of 30 nM for VEGFR-2 and excellent solubility [124].

In 2007, R. Kumar et al. at GlaxoSmithKline found that pazopanib inhibits receptor tyrosine kinases associated with angiogenesis and cancer growth, such as VEGFR-1,2,3, PDGFR-α/β, and SCFR. In addition, they observed VEGF-dependent growth suppression in vascular endothelial cells exposed to pazopanib, as well as an anticancer effect of pazopanib in xenograft tumor models using several types of human-derived cancer cells [125].

Subsequently, a clinical trial was conducted using pazopanib in metastatic RCC patients with various treatment histories. Pazopanib prolonged progression-free survival by 5 months, from 4.2 to 9.2 months, compared to control [126]. In 2009, pazopanib was approved as a treatment for metastatic RCC patients. In 2012, pazopanib was used in a clinical trial for patients with soft tissue sarcoma that progressed after first-line treatment, wherein progression-free survival increased from 1.6 months to 4.6 months [127]. Based on these results, the FDA approved pazopanib as a treatment for patients with advanced soft tissue sarcoma in 2012. Pazopanib is currently widely used in patients with metastatic RCC or soft tissue sarcoma.

9.5.3.5 Axitinib

Axitinib is an indazole derivative developed by Pfizer's R.S Kania in 2003 as a multi-targeted receptor tyrosine kinase inhibitor [128]. In 2008, D.D. Hu-Lowe et al. at Pfizer found that axitinib inhibited receptor tyrosine kinases associated with angiogenesis and cancer growth, including VEGFR-1,2,3, PDGFR-α/β, and SCFR. In addition, axitinib inhibited VEGFR more potently than sorafenib, sunitinib, or pazopanib [129]. A definite anticancer effect of axitinib was confirmed in xenograft tumor models of lung, colon, and breast cancer, as well as in a clinical trial comparing axitinib with sorafenib in RCC patients with various treatment histories. In 2011, the axitinib-treated group was reported to prolong progression-free survival by 2 months compared to sorafenib group [130]. Based on these results, axitinib was approved for patients with metastatic RCC in 2012.

9.5.3.6 Vandetanib

Vandetanib, an anilinoquinazoline-class drug, was developed by AstraZeneca's L.F. Hennequin et al. as a VEGFR-2 inhibitor during the process of developing the EGFR inhibitor gefitinib. Vandetanib showed an IC_{50} of 40 nM for VEGFR-2 [131]. Later, in 2002, S.R. Wedge et al. at AstraZeneca discovered that vandetanib inhibited receptor tyrosine kinases such as VEGFR-3 and EGFR [132], VEGF-dependent growth in vascular endothelial cells, and angiogenesis in xenograft tumor model implanted with human lung cancer cells. Administration of vandetanib at high concentrations directly inhibited the growth of various cancer cell lines and had an anticancer effect in xenograft tumor models.

In 1990, M. Grieco and M. Santoro et al. from Italy's Napoli University discovered that metastatic medullary thyroid cancer (MTC), a rare form of cancer, developed as a result of mutations in RET, a tyrosine kinase that acts as the receptor for the glial-derived neurotrophic factor (GDNF) family [133]. Following this discovery, they confirmed that 40–50 % of MTC cases involved an activating RET mutation. While investigating inhibition of mutated RET as a way of treating cancer, the researchers found that vandetanib inhibited RET kinase with an IC_{50} of 100 nM and suppressed the growth of MTC cells possessing a RET mutation (Fig. 9.16) [134]. In a clinical trial conducted in metastatic MTC patients using vandetanib as a monotherapy, vandetanib extended progression-free survival by 6.2 months (22.6 vs 16.4 moths) in comparison with that of the placebo group [135]. Vandetanib was approved by the FDA as a treatment for patients with MTC in 2011.

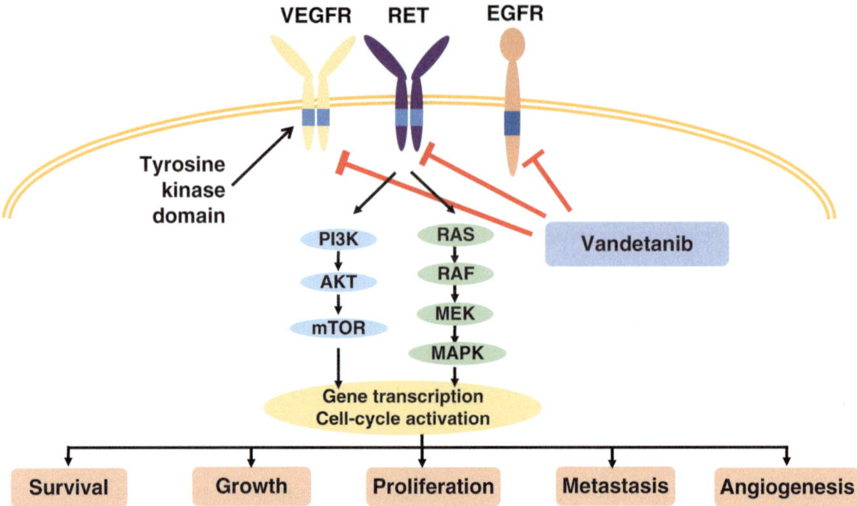

Fig. 9.16 Mechanism of action for vandetanib. Vandetanib acts as an inhibitor of VEGFR-2, EGFR, and RET, which are involved in the development of thyroid medullary carcinoma. By inhibiting these kinases, vandetanib interferes with the PI3K-Akt-mTOR and Ras-RAF-MEK-MAPK signaling pathways. As a result, vandetanib suppresses survival, growth, spreading, metastasis of cancer cells, and angiogenesis. In particular, vandetanib strongly inhibits RET kinase in thyroid medullary carcinoma caused by RET mutations

9.5.3.7 Cabozantinib

Cabozantinib is a quinolone-class multi-targeted tyrosine kinase inhibitor that was developed by Exelixis in 2009 [136]. In 2011, F.M. Yakes et al. at Exelixis investigated the inhibitory effects of cabozantinib and found that it had a very strong inhibitory effect against MET proto-oncogene receptor tyrosine kinase (c-MET) and VEGFR-2, with IC_{50} values of 1.3 and 0.035 nM, respectively. Cabozantinib also showed strong inhibitory effects against SCFR, RET, AXL, TIE2, and FLT3, with IC_{50} values in the range of 4.6–11.3 nM [137].

Based on these results, Exelixis performed intensive studies on the applicability of cabozantinib in metastatic MTC cancers, which showed a high frequency of RET mutations. In a clinical trial in metastatic MTC patients, Exelixis found that cabozantinib lengthened progression-free survival by 7.2 months [138]. In 2012, the FDA approved cabozantinib as a treatment for patients with MTC.

9.6 Other Kinase Inhibitors

9.6.1 Ruxolitinib: JAK-1,2 Inhibitor

Janus tyrosine kinase (JAK) is an intracellular tyrosine kinase that is activated when cytokines, which modulate cell growth and the immune response, bind with cytokine receptors in the cell membrane. Activated JAK phosphorylates transcription

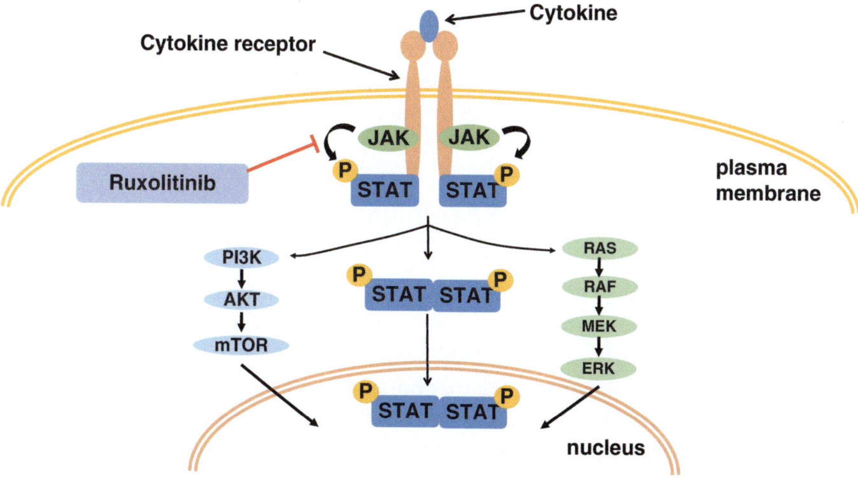

Fig. 9.17 Mechanism of action for ruxolitinib. JAK is an intracellular tyrosine kinase that is activated when cytokines bind to their receptors and phosphorylates the transcription factor STAT to induce nuclear translocation. Once STAT enters the nucleus, it binds to DNA and activates transcription of genes that regulate cell movement, differentiation, and proliferation. $JAK2^{V617F}$ mutations, which are frequently observed in myeloproliferative neoplasms, activate the PI3K-Akt-mTOR and Ras-RAF-MEK-ERK signaling pathways to aid survival and spreading of cancer cells. During this process, ruxolitinib inhibits JAK2 specifically, suppressing the growth of myeloproliferative cancer cells

factors of the signal transducer and activator of transcription (STAT) family, causing them to move into the nucleus and promote expression of genes related to cell proliferation and the immune response.

In 2005, University Hospital Basel's R. Kralovics et al. investigated the DNA sequence of the domain in chromosome 9p where loss of heterozygosity (LOH) has been reported in myeloproliferative neoplasm (MPN) patients. They discovered that almost all 9p LOH patients showed a mutation to a phenylalanine codon in place of the valine codon at position 617 in JAK2, while the same mutation was found in only approximately 30 % of MPN patients without LOH [139]. $JAK2^{V617F}$ was observed in 35–50 % of patients with primary myelofibrosis, 32–57 % of patients with polycythemia, and more than 95 % of patients with essential thrombocythemia (all of which are forms of MPN); moreover, these mutants were revealed to have important functions in regulating tumor cell growth [140, 141]. Accordingly, there was active research into the development of inhibitors capable of suppressing the activity of $JAK2^{V617F}$.

Ruxolitinib is a cyclopentylpropionitrile-class JAK inhibitor that was developed in 2009 by Incyte Pharmaceuticals' Q. Lin et al. by adding cyclopentylacrylaldehyde to pyrazole [142]. In 2010, in a collaborative study between Incyte and A. Quintás-Cardama et al. at the M.D. Anderson Cancer Center, ruxolitinib was found to strongly inhibit JAK1 and JAK2, with IC_{50} values of 3.3 nM and 2.8 nM, respectively. In addition, ruxolitinib specifically inhibited the proliferation of $JAK2^{V617F}$-positive cancer cells (Fig. 9.17) [143].

Based on preclinical results obtained with ruxolitinib, phase 3 clinical trials were conducted on patients with various types of myelofibrosis, in which 29–42 % of patients showed decreased spleen size and 46 % of patients were alleviated in symptoms [144, 145]. Ruxolitinib was approved by the FDA in 2011.

9.6.2 Crizotinib: ALK and ROS1 Inhibitor

Crizotinib is an aminopyridine compound developed by Pfizer in 2006 that acts as a c-Met (also known as hepatocyte growth factor receptor, HGFR) inhibitor. Pfizer first discovered the high inhibitory PHA-665752 using indolin-2-one as a precursor structure, but it was found to be unsuitable for clinical use. Later, researchers J.J. Cui et al. synthesized 2-aminopyridine derivatives based on the crystal structure analysis of PHA-665752/c-Met complex. After identifying a lead compound, J.J. Cui et al. developed crizotinib for oral administration through a process of optimization [146]. In 2007, Pfizer's H.Y. Zou et al. investigated the inhibitory effects of crizotinib and found that it strongly inhibited c-Met (IC_{50} of 5 nM) and anaplastic lymphoma kinase (ALK) (IC_{50} of 24 nM) (Fig. 9.18) [147].

Understanding of ALK mutations and their association with cancer began with a study in 1994 by S.W. Morris at St. Jude Children's Research Hospital, in which the t(2;5) chromosome translocation observed in large cell lymphoma and the genetic

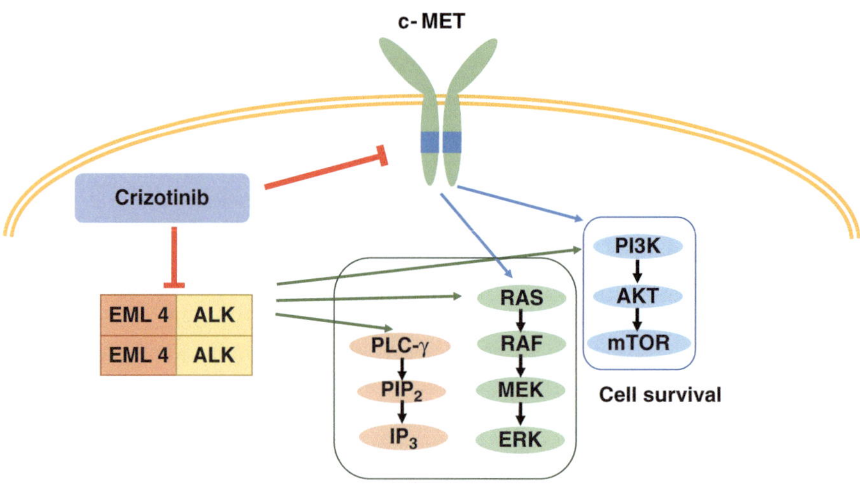

Fig. 9.18 Mechanism of action for crizotinib. Crizotinib inhibits c-Met (also known as hepatocyte growth factor receptor, HGFR), upon which the consequent suppression of Ras-RAF-MEK-ERK and PI3K-Akt-mTOR pathways limits growth and proliferation of cancer cells. In non-small cell lung cancer, a chromosomal translocation causes two genes to fuse and form the EML4-ALK oncogene, which activates the PLCγ-PIP_2-IP_3 and Ras-RAF-MEK-ERK signaling pathways. Crizotinib suppresses proliferation of cancer cells by inhibiting EML4-ALK

mutations caused by this translocation were investigated [148]. As a result of the t(2;5) chromosome translocation, two genes, NPM and ALK, were fused to form the oncogene NPM-ALK, which had kinase activity that was essential to cancer cell proliferation. In 2007, H. Mano et al. at the Japan Science and Technology Agency were investigating genetic mutations in lung cancer when they discovered that approximately 7 % of NSCLC patients possess an EML4-ALK oncogene formed by chromosomal translocation [149]. As this fusion oncogene was found to be related to the tumorigenesis of lung cancer, ALK emerged as an important molecular target for targeted therapy. Moreover, in 2008, ALK was reported to be mutated in 15 % of neuroblastomas, a rare form of cancer [150].

Phase 2 clinical trials for crizotinib were conducted twice in metastatic NSCLC patients. Because a dramatic response was observed in crizotinib-treated patients with ALK mutations [151], crizotinib was granted accelerated approval by FDA in patients with ALK-mutant metastatic NSCLC in 2011. In 2013, in a phase 3 clinical trial comparing crizotinib to standard chemotherapy, an increased response rate and 4.4-month prolongation of progression-free survival (7.4 vs 3.0 months) were observed in the crizotinib-treated patients [152]; therefore, the drug was officially approved as a treatment for metastatic NSCLC. Crizotinib is currently used in metastatic lung cancer patients with ALK mutations.

9.6.3 B-Raf Kinase Inhibitors

9.6.3.1 Vemurafenib

Vemurafenib is an azaindole class B-Raf kinase inhibitor developed by Plexxikon in 2010. In 1983, G.E. Mark and U.R. Rapp at the NCI first discovered the oncogene v-Raf in murine sarcoma virus (MSV) 3611, which causes sarcoma in mice [153]. Later, Mark and Rapp discovered the proto-oncogenes RAF1 (CRAF), ARAF, and BRAF in the human genome. Raf was subsequently revealed to be the protein kinase that mediates signal transduction in the Ras-Raf-MEK-ERK pathway, which plays a central role in promoting cell proliferation in many cancers.

In 2002, R. Wooster et al. at the Wellcome Trust Sanger Institute revealed that a specific point mutation of B-RAF ($BRAF^{V600E}$) occurs in approximately 50 % of malignant melanoma patients [154]. Plexxikon's J. Tsai et al. developed the mutated B-Raf^{V600E} inhibitor PLX4720 (IC_{50} 13 nM) in 2008 based on protein structure analysis [155]. PLX4720 showed inhibitory activity against wild type B-Raf with an IC_{50} of 160 nM, as well as strong anticancer effects in melanoma cells and animal models expressing B-Raf^{V600E}. Plexxikon's G. Bollag et al. developed PLX4032 (vemurafenib) in 2010 through lead optimization of PLX4720 [156]. Vemurafenib inhibits B-Raf^{V600E} with an IC_{50} of 31 nM and inhibits c-Raf with an IC_{50} of 48 nM, while it inhibits wild type B-Raf with an IC_{50} of 100 nM (Fig. 9.19). In 2010, a phase 1 clinical trial was conducted using vemurafenib in metastatic melanoma patients possessing the B-Raf^{V600E} mutation, in which a drug response rate of 81 %

was observed [157]. In a phase 3 clinical trial in 2011 in B-Raf^{V600E}-positive melanoma patients, vemurafenib prolonged overall survival by 1.7 months (6.2 vs 4.5) and progression-free survival by 3.7 months (5.3 vs 1.6) [158]. Therefore, vemurafenib was approved by FDA as a treatment for melanoma patients.

9.6.3.2 Dabrafenib

In 2009, S. Laquerre et al. at GlaxoSmithKline developed dabrafenib, an aminopyrimidine-class drug that inhibits wild type B-Raf, B-Raf^{V600E}, and c-Raf more strongly than vemurafenib, and confirmed its anticancer effect in an animal cancer model using human melanoma cells expressing B-Raf^{V600E} (Fig. 9.19) [159]. Subsequently, a clinical trial was conducted using dabrafenib in B-Raf^{V600E}-positive melanoma patients, wherein it extended the survival duration by 2.4 months in comparison with that of dacarbazine chemotherapy [160]. In 2013, dabrafenib was approved by the FDA as a treatment for B-Raf^{V600E}-positive melanoma.

9.6.4 Trametinib: MEK Inhibitor

KRas, NRas, and HRas show a high frequency of mutations in many cancers and are known to promote cell proliferation by activating the p42/p44 mitogen-activated protein kinase (MAPK) pathway. MEK1/2 is a protein kinase that mediates signal

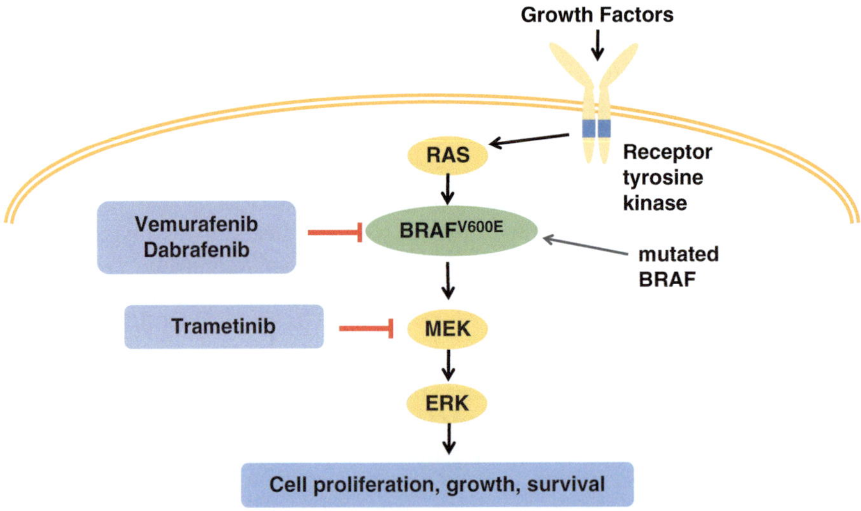

Fig. 9.19 Mechanism of action for vemurafenib, dabrafenib, and trametinib. B-RAF is known to undergo a point mutation (*B-RAF*^{V600E}) in half of malignant melanoma patients. Vemurafenib and dabrafenib inhibit the function of this mutant B-RAF^{V600E}, whereas trametinib inhibits the action of MEK, interfering with the Ras-RAF-MEK-ERK signaling pathway, and thus suppressing survival, growth, and proliferation of cancer cells

transduction leading to cell proliferation downstream of RAF in this pathway (Fig. 9.19). There have been several attempts to treat cancer by inhibiting MEK1/2 to block MAPK signaling, but the development of MEK1/2 inhibitors as anticancer agents has frequently been halted because of severe toxicity in normal tissue, because MAPK signaling is very active in normal cells.

In 2007, T. Yamaguchi et al. at Japan Tobacco's pharmaceutical development laboratories discovered the pyrido-pyrimidine derivative JTP-70902 as an inducer of gene expression for p15INK4b, a protein that inhibits CyclinD-CDK4/6 interaction. An investigation of the mechanism of JTP-70902 showed that the drug inhibited MEK1/2 activity [161]. Subsequently, JTP-70902 underwent a process of lead optimization, leading to the development of JTP-74057 (trametinib). In 2011, A.G. Gilmartin et al. at GlaxoSmithKline discovered that trametinib was a selective inhibitor of MEK1/2, acting as an allosteric inhibitor rather than a competitive ATP inhibitor [162]. Because of these properties, Gilmartin et al. investigated the efficacy of trametinib in $BRAF^{V600E}$-positive cancer cells and animal models using these cells, revealing significant anticancer effects with few adverse effects (Fig. 9.19). Subsequently, a clinical trial was performed using trametinib in $B\text{-}Raf^{V600E}$-expressing melanoma patients, in which the drug showed a 14 % increased response rate and 2.2-month longer progression-free survival in comparison with patients treated with conventional chemotherapy [163]. In 2014, trametinib was registered as an FDA-approved drug.

9.6.5 *Ibrutinib*

In 1993, S. Tsukada at UCLA discovered that X-linked agammaglobulinemia, wherein B-lymphocytes and plasma cells are not produced, results from a loss-of-function mutation in Bruton's tyrosine kinase (BTK) [164]. Subsequently, BTK was revealed to act as a mediating factor that is essential to signal transduction via the B-cell antigen receptor (BCR), which is required for development and maintenance of B-lymphocytes. BTK signaling thus promotes survival, proliferation, and antibody production in B-cells by activating phospholipase-Cγ and inducing nuclear translocation of NF-kB. Moreover, BTK was observed to be frequently activated in B-cell lymphocytic leukemia. Based on these findings, BTK inhibitors were developed for the treatment of these cancers.

In 2007, based on structural analysis of BTK, S. Pan et al. at Celera Genomics developed ibrutinib, which irreversibly inhibits BTK by reacting with its cysteine-481 residue close to the ATP binding site (Fig. 9.20) [165]. In 2010, L.A. Honigberg et al. at Pharamcyclics, which had merged with Celera Genomics, found that ibrutinib strongly inhibited BTK (IC_{50} 0.5 nM) and showed an anticancer effect in animal models of B-cell non-Hodgkin lymphoma [166]. In 2013, L.A. Honigberg et al. conducted phase 2 clinical trials using ibrutinib in patients with mantle cell lymphoma, a type of tumor formed from B-cells, and reported a drug response rate of 68 % [167]. The drug also showed a high response rate of 71 % against chronic lymphocytic leukemia [168], and was temporarily approved by the FDA in 2013 and 2014.

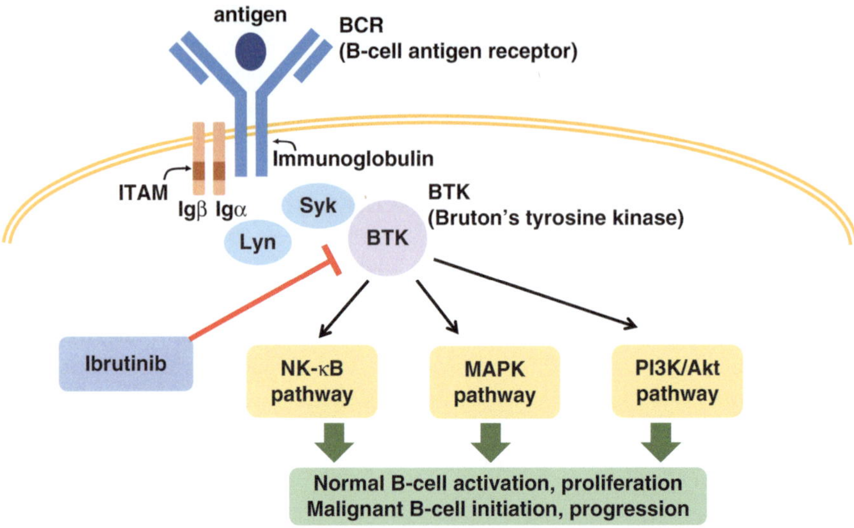

Fig. 9.20 Mechanism of action for ibrutinib. When an antigen binds to the B-cell receptor (*BCR*), the kinases Lyn and Syk bind to the ITAM motif and tyrosine residue in them are phosphorylated. Phosphorylated Lyn and Syk then phosphorylate BTK, activating downstream signaling transmission via NFκB, MAPK, and PI3K/AKT pathways, which causes activation and proliferation of normal B-cells as well as B-lymphoma cells. In this process, ibrutinib produces an anticancer effect by inhibiting BTK activity

9.7 mTOR Inhibitors

In 1975, S.N. Sehgal, a microbiologist at Ayerst Research Laboratories in Canada, discovered rapamycin, a macrolide antibiotic with antifungal activity, in the culture medium of *Streptomyces hygroscopicus* that had been collected from Easter Island (local name: Rapa Nui) [169]. In 1977, Ayerst researchers R.R. Martel et al. discovered that rapamycin alleviated symptoms in rat models of encephalomyelitis and rheumatoid arthritis, revealing its potential as an immunosuppressant [170]. In 1987, T. Kino et al. from Japan's Fujisawa Pharmaceutical Co. discovered FK-506, a compound similar to rapamycin, in the culture medium of another *Streptomyces* species and found that this substance inhibited T-cell proliferation induced by antigen stimulation [171].

In 1990, F.J. Dumont at Merck Sharp and Dohrne Research Laboratories investigated the effects of rapamycin and FK-506 on T-cells, focusing on their structural similarities. They found that FK-506 inhibits ionomycin-induced T-cell proliferation, whereas rapamycin inhibits T-cell proliferation induced by interleukin-2 (IL-2) or IL-4 [172]. As its ability to inhibit T-cell proliferation became known, rapamycin was developed as an immunosuppressant. In 1999, rapamycin was approved as an immunosuppressant to reduce rejection responses in tissue transplant.

In addition, in 1984, Ayerst's Sehgal et al. investigated the anticancer effects of rapamycin in various implanted tumor models and found that a high concentration of rapamycin produced excellent anticancer effects with minimal adverse effects

[173]. Next, they showed that rapamycin suppressed the growth of cancer cells derived from various tissues and the proliferation of vascular endothelial cells. Moreover, they revealed that rapamycin suppressed angiogenesis in xenograft tumor models using tumor cell lines with high angiogenic activity.

Studies of the molecular mechanisms through which rapamycin inhibits cell proliferation revealed that rapamycin binds with FK506-binding protein 12 (FKBP12) to inhibit mammalian target of rapamycin(mTOR) signaling, which is important for cell survival and growth. S.L. Schreiber's group at Harvard University discovered that rapamycin binds strongly to FKBP12 in 1990 [174]. In 1994, Schreiber's group discovered that the rapamycin-FKBP12 complex interacts with the mTOR complex [175]. Following this discovery, it was revealed that mTOR is activated by the phosphatidylinositol 3-kinase (PI3K)/AKT pathway, known to be an important pathway promoting cell growth and survival, upon which mTOR increases the mRNA translation efficiency of ribosomes in order to provide the proteins required for growth by inducing phosphorylation of downstream molecules S6 kinase-1 (S6K1) and eukaryotic initiation factor 4E-binding protein-1 (4EBP1). Moreover, mTOR plays an important role in cancer energetics by promoting glucose metabolism.

The report that the rapamycin-FKBP12 complex inhibits mTOR activity led to the development of rapamycin as an anticancer agent. However, rapamycin possesses inappropriate pharmacokinetic properties for an anticancer agent; therefore, numerous rapamycin derivatives were developed (Fig. 9.21).

9.7.1 Temsirolimus

Temsirolimus is a C-42 hydroxyester of rapamycin that was developed in 2001 as an mTOR inhibitor by Wyeth Pharmaceuticals, which merged with Ayerst [176]. In preclinical trials, temsirolimus clearly suppressed angiogenesis and showed a significant anticancer effect in xenograft tumor models using RCC cells, which accompany robust angiogenesis [177]. Based on these results, a clinical trial was conducted using temsirolimus in advanced RCC. The temsirolimus treatment group showed a 3.6-month prolongation of overall survival and a 2.4-month prolongation of progression-free survival in comparison with the group treated with interferon [178], leading to approval of this drug by the FDA as a treatment for advanced RCC in 2007. Temsirolimus still remains in treatment for patients with RCC (Fig. 9.22).

9.7.2 Everolimus

The second mTOR inhibitor approved as an anticancer agent was everolimus, a hydroxyethyl derivative of rapamycin developed by Novartis in 1997 [179]. Clinical trials were conducted in patients with cancers with high levels of angiogenesis, such as RCC, pancreatic neuroendocrine tumor (PNET), subependymal giant cell astrocytoma (SEGA), and advanced breast cancer. When everolimus was used in a

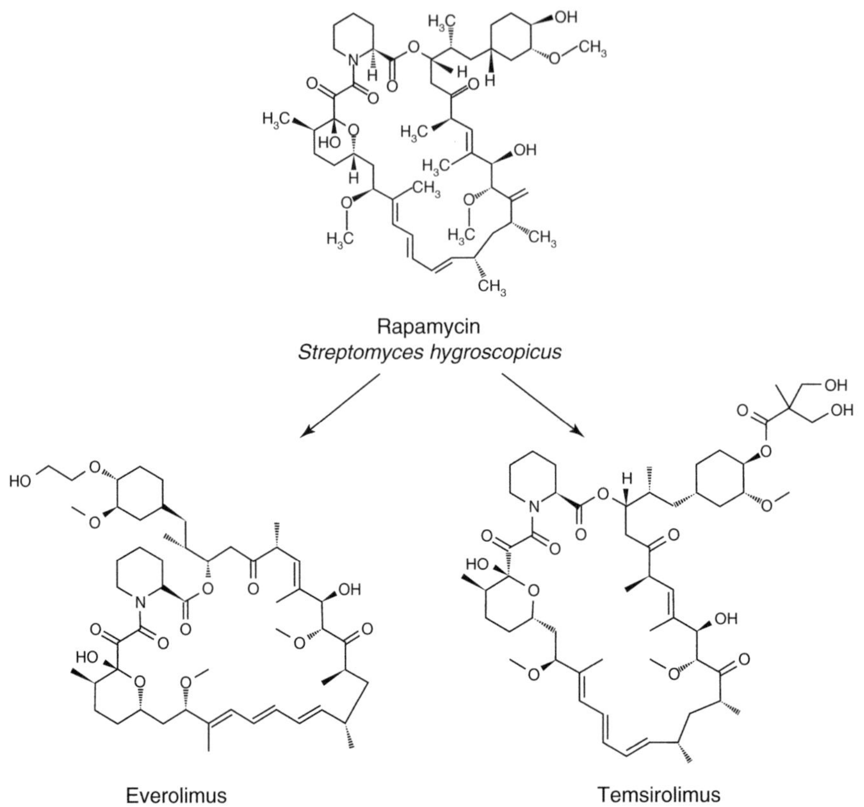

Fig. 9.21 The structures of mTOR inhibitors and the process of their development

clinical trial for patients with metastatic RCC that did not respond to sunitinib and sorafenib, progression-free survival was prolonged by 3 months (4.9 vs 1.9) [180]. Everolimus was approved as an anticancer agent in 2009. Clinical trials of everolimus were conducted in patients with SEGA in 2010 [181], progressive PNET in 2011 [182], and advanced hormone receptor-positive HER2-negative breast cancer in 2012 [183]. Everolimus was successful in each clinical trial and is currently used as an anticancer agent in patients with several types of cancer.

9.8 Other Targeted Anticancer Antibody Drugs

9.8.1 Rituximab

Rituximab was the first targeted anticancer antibody drug to be developed. Developed in 1994 by IDEC Pharmaceuticals, rituximab is a chimeric antibody combining the human IgG1k constant domain and mouse variable domain [184], which recognizes the B lymphocyte-specific cell surface antigen CD20 (Fig. 9.23).

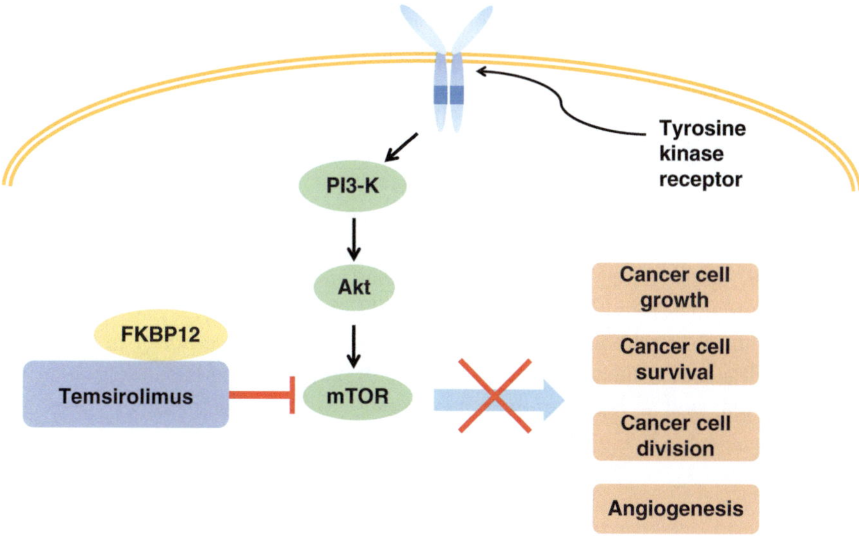

Fig. 9.22 Mechanism of action for temsirolimus. Temsirolimus is used as an inhibitor of mTOR kinase, decreasing translation of cyclin D mRNA, which is important for progression of the cell cycle, and thus suppressing cancer cell proliferation. In addition, temsirolimus inhibits translation of HIF-1α mRNA, reducing synthesis of VEGF and thereby inhibiting angiogenesis

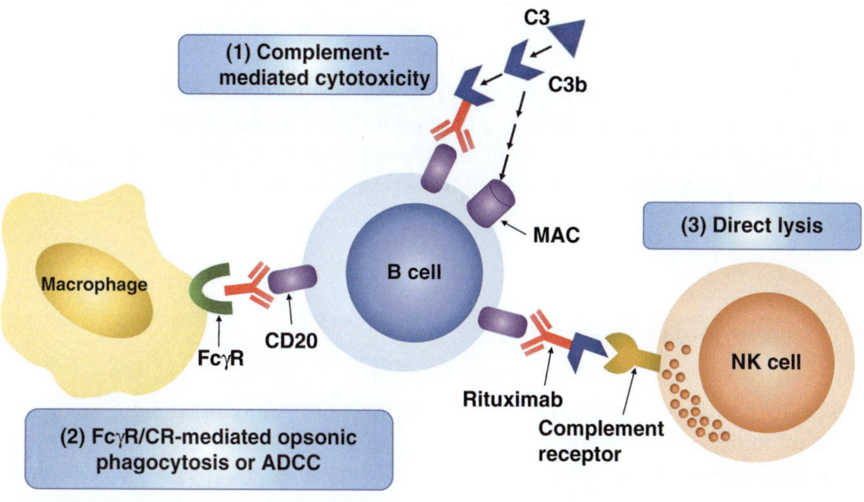

Fig. 9.23 Mechanism of action for rituximab. Rituximab is used in the treatment for non-Hodgkin lymphoma. It is a chimeric monoclonal antibody combining the human IgG1k constant domain with the mouse variable domain. Rituximab binds to the B-cell-specific membrane protein CD20, which activates the complement cascade and forms a membrane attack complex, thereby causing complement-dependent cytotoxicity (CDC) (*1*). In addition, when the complement pathway is activated, C3b/iC3b fragments accumulate on B- lymphoma cells. When accumulated C3b/iC3b fragments and the Fc domain of rituximab are recognized by complement receptors and Fcγ receptors on macrophages, phagocytosis and antibody-dependent cell-mediated cytotoxicity (ADCC) is induced (*2*). Moreover, when rituximab binds CD20, ADCC is induced via natural killer (NK) cells (*3*). These three pathways cause the death of malignant B-cells by rituximab treatment

CD20 is expressed on the surface of B cells from initial pre-B cell stage to mature B-cells., but it is not expressed by fully differentiated plasma cells. When rituximab binds to CD20 on B-cells, it induces complement-mediated lysis or kills the B-cell through a process of antibody-dependent cell-mediated cytotoxicity (ADCC), following recognition of the complex by natural killer (NK) cells.

A clinical trial was conducted in which rituximab was used as monotherapy in patients with B-cell non-Hodgkin lymphoma showing resistance to chemotherapy, in which an objective response rate was observed in 46% of patients [185]. Rituximab was approved as a molecular targeted treatment for recurrent or refractory B-cell non-Hodgkin lymphoma in 1997. Subsequently, rituximab in combination with chemotherapy showed an excellent therapeutic efficacy in various other B-cell cancers, such as diffuse large B-cell lymphoma and acute/chronic B-cell lymphoma, and it is currently being widely used in treatment of these cancers.

9.8.2 *Ibritumomab Tiuxetan*

Ibritumomab tiuxetan is a monoclonal antibody radioimmunotherapy treatment developed in 1996 by IDEC Pharmaceuticals [186]. Ibritumomab is the anti-CD20 mouse monoclonal antibody (IgG1) used in the production of rituximab. Ibritumomab tiuxetan is manufactured by linking ibritumomab to tiuxetan, which coordinated with yttrium-90 or indium-111 [187].

Ibritumomab tiuxetan was used in a clinical trial for patients with rituximab-resistant or recurrent B-cell non-Hodgkin lymphoma and showed a response rate of 80%, which was an increase of 24% in comparison with that of rituximab treatment[188]. Ibritumomab tiuxetan was approved as a treatment for B-cell non-Hodgkin lymphoma in 2002.

9.8.3 *Tositumomab Iodine-131*

Tositumomab iodine-131 is an radioimmunotherapy drug developed by Corixa (now GlaxoSmithKline) in 1992, in which iodine-131 is joined to the anti-CD20 mouse monoclonal antibody (IgG2a) directly by a covalent bond [189].

A clinical trial was conducted for follicular lymphoma patients who had experienced relapse after chemotherapy or had shown resistance to rituximab, in which tositumomab iodine-131 showed a response rate of 63% [190]. Tositumomab iodine-131 was approved as a treatment for patients with follicular non-Hodgkin lymphoma in 2003.

9.8.4 Alemtuzumab

Alemtuzumab is a humanized anti-CD52 antibody developed by Genzyme. Alemtuzumab was derived from a rat antibody developed by H. Waldmann in 1983 at the University of Cambridge [191], which was developed into an IgG1k humanized antibody in 1992 by G. Winter, who invented the technique of antibody humanization [192, 193]. Because CD52 was known to be a cell surface protein expressed in mature lymphocytes, early studies focused on CLL treatment using alemtuzumab. In a phase 2 clinical trial of alemtuzumab in CLL patients who were refractory to fludarabine, an objective response rate of 33 % was observed [194], leading to the granting of accelerated approval by the FDA in 2001. Phase 3 clinical trials comparing alemtuzumab with chlorambucil treatment were conducted in CLL patients who were non-responsive to fludarabine, in which alemtuzumab showed a 38 % increase in response rate and an 8.6-month prolongation of progression-free survival (23.3 vs 14.7 months) [195], leading to its regular approval by the FDA as a treatment for CLL in 2007. However, alemtuzumab was later found to have severe toxicity against blood and immune cells because of the expression of CD52 in mononuclear cells and various other healthy blood cells, in addition to mature lymphocytes.

9.8.5 Ofatumumab

Ofatumumab is a third generation molecular targeted antibody consisting of a fully humanized anti-CD20 monoclonal antibody, which was developed in 2004 through collaboration between Genmab and GlaxoSmithKline [196]. Ofatumumab was developed via full humanization of rituximab in order to reduce the adverse immune reactions that result from the properties of chimeric antibodies. Moreover, the Fc region was manufactured for efficient ADCC, whereas the variable domain was improved to enhance the ability of the drug to kill cancer cells. A clinical trial of ofatumumab was conducted for patients with CLL that was resistant to fludarabine/alemtuzumab, in which a response rate was 42 % of patients [197], leading to the approval of ofatumumab by the FDA as a treatment for CLL in 2009.

9.8.6 Brentuximab Vedotin

Brentuximab vedotin is an antibody-drug conjugate (ADC) developed in 2003 by Seattle Genetics (Fig. 9.24). ADCs were developed to increase the efficacy of cytotoxic drugs by binding them to antibodies that do not show a sufficient anticancer

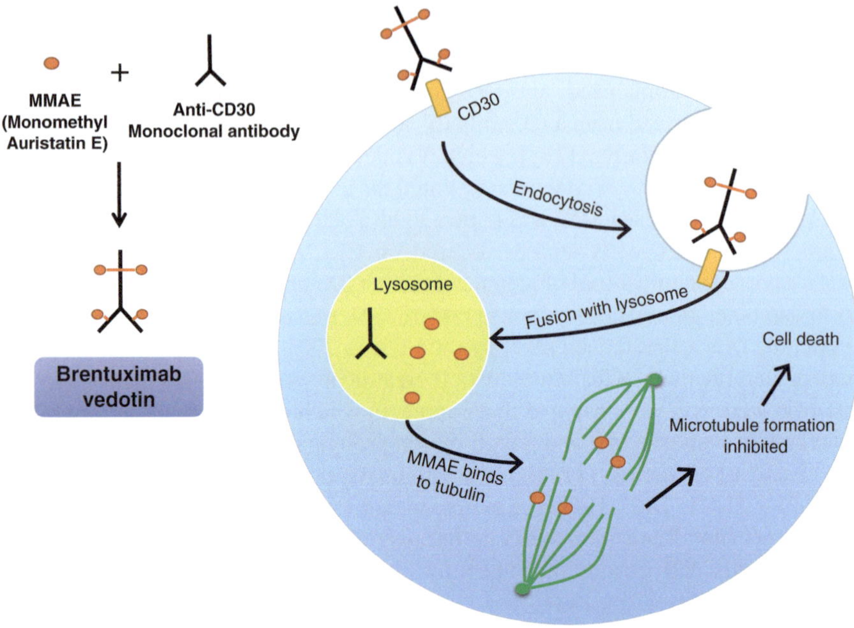

Fig. 9.24 Mechanism of action for brentuximab vedotin. Brentuximab vedotin is an antibody-drug conjugate (ADC) targeting CD30, which is overexpressed in B lymphoma cells. Brentuximab vedotin includes monomethyl auristatin E (MMAE), which is a mitosis inhibiting agent. When this brentuximab vedotin binds to CD30 on the surface of B lymphoma cells, it is endocytosed and transported in an intracellular lysosome, after which MMAE is dissociated by hydrolysis and released into the cytoplasm. MMAE binds to tubulin and interferes with microtubule formation, inducing cell cycle arrest and apoptosis

efficacy by themselves. Brentuximab is a human/mouse chimeric monoclonal antibody against CD30, a TNF receptor-class membrane protein. Because CD30 is highly expressed in Hodgkin's lymphoma and anaplastic large cell lymphoma (ALCL), it was selected as a target for antibody treatment, leading to the development of the mouse monoclonal anti-CD30 antibody brentuximab in 2002 [198]. In order to enhance the efficacy of brentuximab, monomethyl auristatin E (MMAE), which interferes with tubulin function, was conjugated to the antibody in 2003, producing brentuximab vedotin. The outstanding anticancer effect of brentuximab vedotin was confirmed in xenograft models of Hodgkin's lymphoma and ALCL in severe combined immunodeficiency (SCID) mice [199]. Brentuximab vedotin underwent phase 2 clinical trials in Hodgkin's lymphoma and ALCL patients, wherein it showed excellent response rates of 73 % and 86 %, respectively[200, 201]. In 2011, brentuximab vedotin was approved as a treatment for recurrent Hodgkin's lymphoma and ALCL.

9.8.7 *Obinutuzumab*

Obinutuzumab is a humanized anti-CD20 monoclonal antibody developed by E. Mössner et al. at Switzerland's Glycart Biotechnology in 2010 [202]. Obinutuzumab has the same CD20 binding site as rituximab, but it showed higher stability than that of rituximab. Moreover, improvement in the glycosylation site in the Fc region enhanced the ability of the drug to bind to the surface of NK cells and macrophages, increasing ADCC. In preclinical tests, obinutuzumab produced a strong anticancer effect in xenograft models of non-Hodgkin and follicular lymphoma and was more effective than rituximab [203]. In a clinical trial for CLL patients in which obinutuzumab was used in combination with chemotherapy, progression-free survival was extended by 10.6 months in comparison with that of the rituximab/chemotherapy group [204], leading to FDA approval in 2013.

9.9 Epigenetic Anticancer Drugs

Because of biomolecular research, it has been recognized that cancer develops as the result of genetic changes in DNA, such as mutations or deletions in genes that regulate growth and proliferation. However, in 1979, R. Holliday at the United Kingdom's Medical Research Council first proposed the hypothesis that cancer could develop as the result of changes in DNA methylation [205]. In 1983, A. Feinberg and B. Vogelstein at Johns Hopkins University discovered differences in the extent of DNA methylation of cancer cells and normal cells [206], suggesting the possibility that cancer might develop due to epigenetic changes, without changes in the DNA sequence. Later, these epigenetic changes were revealed to occur as the result of four mechanisms: DNA methylation, genomic imprinting, histone modification, and microRNA (miRNA) control. Subsequently, many efforts were aimed at producing drugs capable of regulating cancer-related epigenetic changes, which led to the development of DNA methylation inhibitors and histone deacetylase (HDAC) inhibitors currently used as anticancer agents.

9.9.1 *DNA Methylation Inhibitors: Azanucleosides*

9.9.1.1 Azacitidine (5-Azacytidine)

In 1963, Čihák et al. in Czechoslovakia synthesized various types of azapyrimidine and investigated their efficacy in transplanted tumor models, with the aim of developing drugs that produced anticancer effects by inhibiting nucleic acid synthesis. The efforts of Čihák et al. resulted in their discovery of 5-azacytidine, which had an outstanding anticancer effect [207]. By exploring the mechanism of action of 5-azacytidine, he found that phosphorylated 5-azacytidine is incoporated into various types of RNA and DNA. When phosphorylated 5-azacytidine is inserted into rRNA, it produces cytotoxicity by inhibiting ribosomal protein translation. However, in 1980, biochemist P.A. Jones at the University of Southern California reported that 5-azacytidine regulates cell differentiation by inhibiting DNA methylation [208]. In 1983, D.V. Santi et al. at UCSF identified the mechanism by which 5-azacytidine inhibits DNA methyltransferase [209]. Later, when DNA methylation was determined to play an important role in developmental processes and to contribute to the development and progression of cancer, 5-azacytidine emerged again as an important candidate anticancer drug, leading to clinical trials for the drug in patients with a wide range of cancers. In the most successful clinical trial conducted with 5-azacytidine, a 15 % increase in drug response rate was observed in 5-azacytidine-treated patients with myelodysplastic syndrome (MDS) in comparison with that of the placebo group [210], leading to approval of the drug by the FDA as a treatment for patients with MDS in 2004. 5-Azacytidine remains the mainstay of treatment for patients with MDS.

9.9.1.2 Decitabine (5-aza-2′-Deoxycytidine)

At about the same time that A. Čihák group developed 5-azacytidine, they also developed its 2′-deoxyribose form, decitabine [211]. Whereas 5-azacytidine inserts itself into RNA and DNA, decitabine is selectively incorporated into DNA. Moreover, decitabine inhibits DNA methylation more potently than 5-azacytidine (Fig. 9.25).

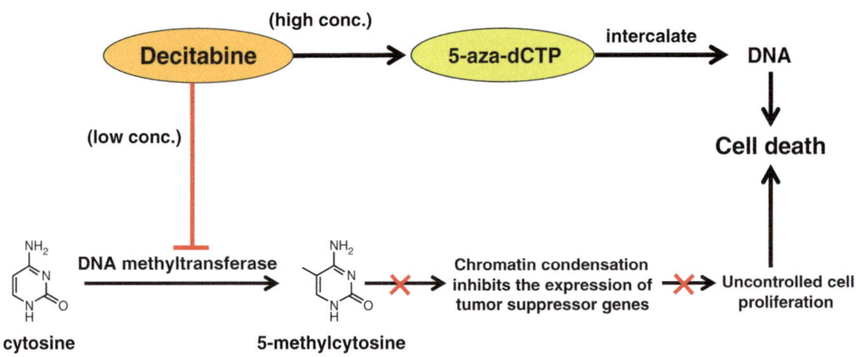

Fig. 9.25 Mechanism of action for decitabine and 5-azacytidine. At low concentrations, decitabine inhibits DNA methyltransferase, interfering with DNA methylation, while at high concentration, it exerts cytotoxicity by inserting itself into DNA during the process of replication. Under exposure to low-dose decitabine, hypomethylation of cytosine bases in the DNA allow expression of tumor-suppressing genes, preventing proliferation of cancer cells. The action of high-dose decitabine is similar to that of 5-azacytidine; however, unlike 5-azacytidine, which inserts itself into DNA and RNA, decitabine is only inserted into DNA. When the two drugs are incorporated in DNA synthesis, they inhibit DNA replication and produce DNA damage, resulting in cell death

Clinical trials in patients with MDS were conducted at about the same time for 5-azacytidine and decitabine, with the latter showing a 25 % higher response rate [212]. In 2006, decitabine was approved by the FDA as a treatment for MDS patients. Decitabine remains the mainstay of treatment for patients with MDS.

In MDS patients, 5-azacytidine and decitabine interfered with the commonly observed DNA methylation of the P15/INK4B gene, which promoted expression of P15/INK4B protein, delaying the cell cycle and suppressing the transfomation of MDS to leukemia [213].

9.9.2 Histone Deacetylase (HDAC) Inhibitors

Because genetic information is stored in a long, linear structure of DNA, it can easily undergo damage, such as breakage upon diverse physical stimuli. Through tight binding DNA with proteins like histones, eukaryotic organisms maintain their DNA in a highly folded chromatin structure for protection and further surround the chromatin with a nuclear membrane. Because histones form much of the compacted structure of chromatin, E. Stedman at the United Kingdom's Edinburgh University proposed in 1950 that histones might play an inhibitory role in gene expression, suggesting that gene expression could only take place after histones had separated [214]. In 1964, V.G. Allfrey and A.E. Mirsky at the Rockefeller Research Institute first discovered methylation and acetylation of histones, reporting that histone hyperacetylation was associated with chromatin regions that showed high rates of expression [215]. They also proposed that gene expression could arise simply from modifications caused by acetylation, without removal of the histones from the chromatin. From that point on, research was conducted on histone acetyltransferases (HATs), the enzymes responsible for histone acetylation. In 1996, D. Allis's group at Cold Spring Harbor identified the first HAT gene and demonstrated the important role of its encoded protein in gene expression [216]. Also during 1996, S. Schreiber's group at Harvard University discovered the first gene encoding a histone deacetylase (HDAC) enzyme, the product of which inhibits gene transcription via histone deacetylation [217].

However, research into HDAC inhibitors began before the discovery of HDACs. In 1957, virologist C. Friend discovered the Friend Leukemia Virus (FLV), which causes leukemia in mice. After investigating leukemia cells developed by FLV infection, Friend proposed the hypothesis that leukemia arises due to the interruption of normal differentiation of blood cells. In 1971, Friend made another important discovery by chance, when she performed an experiment in which she established Friend erythroleukemia cells by isolating FLV-induced leukemic cells from mice and reinfected the cells with FLV. In order to increase infection efficiency, she treated the cells with dimethyl sulfoxide (DMSO) before infection, but she observed that these cells, which had been in an undifferentiated state without hemoglobin expression, began to differentiate after DMSO treatment and had become fully differentiated erythrocytes that expressed high levels of hemoglobin, ceased cell division, and lost the characteristics of leukemic cells after 4 days [218]. Based on these observations, Friend proposed differentiation therapy as a method of treating leukemia by inducing differentiation of immature leukemic cells. This study stimulated a large amount of research on inducing differentiation in cancer, eventually leading to the development of HDAC inhibitors.

Because DMSO was used to induce differentiation of leukemic cells at a high concentration (greater than 100 mM) by C. Friend, several groups searched for more potent substances. In 1975, P. Leder at the National Institutes of Health (NIH) discovered that butyrate induced differentiation of Friend erythroleukemia cells into erythrocytes at a low concentration of 1 mM [219]. In 1977, M.G. Riggs et al. at MIT discovered that butyrate increased histone acetylation [220]. In 1978, J.R. Davie et al. at the University of British Columbia investigated this phenomenon more closely and found that the increase in histone acetylation caused by butyrate resulted from suppression of histone deacetylation, rather than enhancement of histone acetylation, leading them to propose the existence of HDACs and the possibility that butyrate could be an HDAC inhibitor [221].

Nevertheless, butyrate lacked the specificity to be used as a medicinal drug. The discovery of HDACs with high specificity did not occur until the 1990s. In 1987, M. Yoshida et al. at Tokyo University discovered that the antibiotic trichostatin A (TSA) induced differentiation of Friend erythroleukemia cells into erythrocytes at a very low concentration of 15 nM [222]. Trichostatin A is a hydroxamic acid class antibiotic that was discovered in 1976 as an antifungal extracted from *Streptomyces platensis* by N. Tsuji et al. at Shionogi Pharmaceuticals in Japan [223]. In 1990, M. Yoshida et al. discovered that TSA acts as an HDAC inhibitor like butyrate, although with a significant effect at a much lower concentration, and they proposed HDAC inhibition as the mechanism of action by which TSA inhibits growth and promotes differentiation in cancer cells [224]. This study was the first evidence of attempts to develop an HDAC inhibitor as an anticancer agent.

Thereafter, there were a number of studies on the association between histone-modification enzyme activity and cancer. In particular, HDAC inhibitors were highly studied as anticancer agents when several researchers showed that HDAC activity was related to the development of cancer through leukemia fusion oncogenes, such as PML-RARα and AML-ETO, which bind HDAC. Moreover, in 2001, K.W. Kim et al. in Seoul National University, Korea reported that HDAC activity promoted HIF-1α-induced cancer angiogenesis by suppressing expression of VHL [225]. K.W. Kim et al. also discovered that TSA suppressed angiogenesis by inhibiting HDAC activity and proposed angiogenesis suppression using HDAC inhibitors as a strategy for cancer treatment.

In 1993, T. Beppu's group discovered that the cyclotetrapeptide antibiotic trapoxin A, first isolated from *Helicoma ambiens* in 1990 by H. Itazaki et al. at Shionogi Pharmaceuticals, was a strong HDAC inhibitor acting at nM-level concentrations and predicted that cyclic peptide antibiotics could represent a new type of HDAC inhibitor [226]. Subsequently, several research groups discovered various cyclic peptide HDAC inhibitors.

9.9.2.1 Romidepsin

In 1998, M. Yoshida's group identified romidepsin (FR 901228), a new cyclic peptide drug [227]. Romidepsin is a bicyclic depsipeptide that was discovered as an anticancer antibiotic in *Chromobacterium violaceum* by H. Ueda et al. Fujisawa Pharmaceuticals. Romidepsin showed strong HDAC inhibition with efficacy similar to that of TSA. Trapoxin A and TSA were found to be unsuitable for use in patients owing to instability and toxicity, but romidepsin overcame these problems. Therefore, in 1997, clinical trials on romidepsin began with the support of the NCI. Phase 2 clinical trials were conducted in patients with various cancers, leading to the observation of a clear drug response rate of 34 % in cutaneous T-cell lymphomas (CTCLs) and peripheral T-cell lymphomas (PTCLs) [228]. Romidepsin was approved by the FDA as a treatment for patients with CTCL in 2009.

The anticancer mechanisms of romidepsin were found to be suppression of cell growth due to increased expression of p21 via HDAC inhibition, promotion of apoptosis through HSP90 acetylation, increased expression of apoptosis-promoting genes such as Fas and Fas ligand, and suppression of angiogenesis through increased expression of VHL.

9.9.2.2 Vorinostat (SAHA)

Vorinostat was the first FDA-approved HDAC inhibitor and was developed as the result of 30 years of research by P. Marks at the Sloan Kettering Cancer Center and R. Breslow at Columbia University (Fig. 9.26). In the mid-1970s, P. Marks was studying hemoglobin gene expression when he encountered C. Friend's study of the differentiation-inducing effects of DMSO in leukemia cells, after which he began collaborative research with R. Breslow to investigate the molecular mechanisms underlying this phenomenon, with the goal of developing an effective inducer of differentiation.

In 1975, Marks and Breslow showed that low-molecular-weight polar compounds similar to DMSO also had similar differentiation-inducing effects [229]. In 1976, Marks and Breslow developed hexamethylene bisacetamide (HMBA), which is effective at a concentration approximately 20-fold lower than that of DMSO (5 mM) [230]. HMBA was used in a clinical trial for myelodysplastic syndrome and acute myeloid leukemia in 1992, but its therapeutic effect was weak and the drug required improvement. In 1996, the methyl groups at either end of HMBA were swapped for hydroxyl groups; the resulting hydroxamic acid substance, suberoyl bis-hydroxamic acid (SBHA), contained six methylenes and was found to have a therapeutic effect 100 times stronger than that of HMBA [231]. Using SBHA as a template, several derivatives were synthesized. SBHA-derivative vorinostat (suberoyl anilide hydroxamic acid, SAHA) showed a therapeutic effect 6 times stronger than that of SBHA.

In 1998, V. Richon from P. Marks' laboratory noticed on the similarity in structure between SAHA and the known HDAC inhibitor TSA, revealing that the two

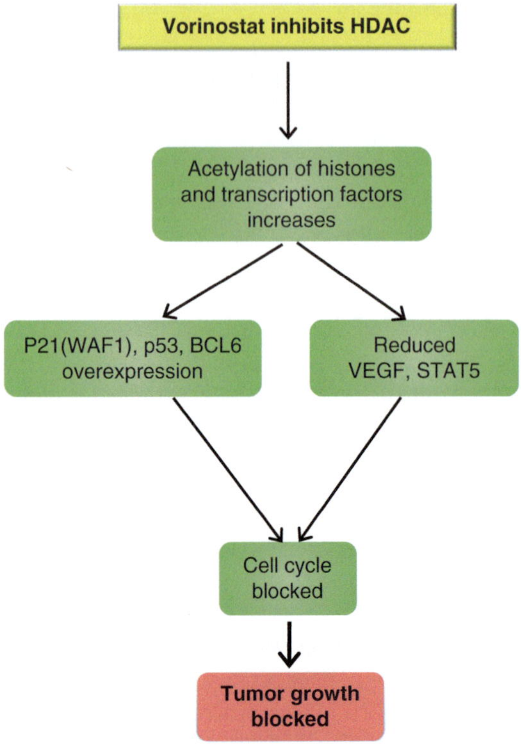

Fig. 9.26 Mechanism of action for vorinostat. Vorinostat inhibits HDACs, which are overexpressed in cancer cells, thus inducing histone acetylation and allowing transcription factors access to DNA. p21 (WAF1) protein induced as the result of histone acetylation inhibits cyclin-dependent kinase (CDK) activity, leading to cell cycle arrest and suppressing cancer cell proliferation

substances were both HDAC inhibitors with similar levels of activity [232]. Following this finding, it became clear that SAHA, in comparison with other HDAC inhibitors, had the advantage of low toxicity while maintaining its inhibitory strength. Beginning in 2001, clinical trials were conducted for SAHA in patients with various types of cancer. In 2006, in phase 2 clinical trials of SAHA in patients with CTCL, a drug response rate of 29.5–33 % was observed [233]. Therefore, SAHA was approved by the FDA as a treatment for CTCL in 2006.

9.10 Proteasome Inhibitors

9.10.1 Bortezomib

Bortezomib is a proteasome inhibitor that was developed by Myogenics (merged with Millennium Pharmaceuticals) in 1995. The ubiquitin-proteasome system is responsible for degradation of 80 % of intracellular proteins. Proteasome-mediated protein degradation modulates important signaling pathways that regulate cell proliferation and differentiation. After studying the physiological functions of proteasomes in 1992, A. Goldberg at Harvard Medical School conducted research into

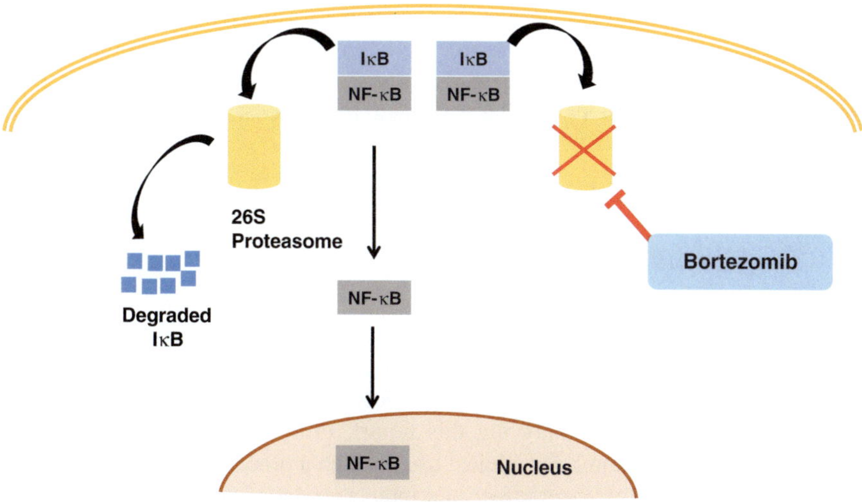

Fig. 9.27 Mechanism of action for bortezomib. Bortezomib was the first proteasome inhibitor. Bortezomib is currently used to treat patients with multiple myeloma and mantle cell lymphoma. When bortezomib inhibits the proteasome, which usually acts to degrade intracellular proteins, impaired protein degradation causes an imbalance of proteins. Proteasome inhibitors are used as anticancer agents because they induce the death of cancer cells by exploiting this phenomenon. In multiple myeloma cells, IkB is degraded by the proteasome, after which NFκB moves into the nucleus, where it induces expression of genes related to the development of cancer. However, when bortezomib inhibits the proteasome, NFκB is prevented from entering the nucleus, leading to an anticancer effect

inhibition of proteasomes to alleviate cachexia. In 1994, Goldberg developed various types of proteasome inhibitors that suppressed proteasome activity by binding to chemotrypsin-like protease, one of the proteolytic enzymes that make up the proteasome. Of the inhibitors produced by Goldberg, the peptide aldehyde derivative MG-132 became a candidate compound for development into a clinical drug [234]. Subsequently, in 1995, J. Adams from Myogenics developed the dipeptide boronate MG-132 derivative MG-341 (bortezomib) as an improvement on MG-132 that was suitable as a clinical drug [235].

In 1999, J. Adams et al. confirmed that bortezomib increased sensitivity to chemotherapy or radiotherapy in various types of cultured cancer cells and a mouse model of lung cancer [236]. In 2001, in a collaborative study with K.C. Anderson's group at the Dana Farber Cancer Institute, bortezomib demonstrated 1,000-fold stronger toxicity in myeloma cells in comparison with its toxicity in normal plasma cells, because NFκB, which is necessary for survival and growth and is constitutively active in myeloma cells, was inhibited by bortezomib (Fig. 9.27) [237]. In addition, bortezomib was observed to inhibit proliferation of vascular endothelial cells, which have an important function in the tumor microenvroment for myeloma cells.

During phase 2 clinical trials of bortezomib in refractory multiple myeloma patients, K.C. Anderson et al. observed a complete or partial response in 35 % of patients [238]. Bortezomib was approved as a treatment for refractive myeloma in 2003. In 2006, in clinical trials for mantle cell lymphoma, bortezomib-treated patients showed 31 % response rate with median duration of 15.4 months, leading to approval of the drug by the FDA as a treatment for patients with mantle cell lymphoma.

9.10.2 Carfilzomib

Carfilzomib was the second proteasome inhibitor to be approved as an anticancer agent. In 1999, C. Crews at Yale University discovered that epoxomicin produced by Actinomyces irreversibly inhibited the proteolytic activity of chemotrypsin within the proteasome [239]. Following this report, Proteolix Inc., founded by C. Crews, developed carfilzomib for clinical use through a process of drug optimization and confirmed its anticancer effect in a mouse model of multiple myeloma [240]. Next, under the guidance of Onyx Pharmaceuticals, clinical trials of carfilzomib were conducted in patients with relapsed or refractive multiple myeloma and a history of bortexomib or thalidomide/lenalidomide treatment, in which an objective response was observed in 22.9 % of patients [241]. In 2012, carfilzomib was approved by the FDA as an anticancer agent for patients with multiple myeloma.

9.11 Vismodegib: Hedgehog Pathway Blocker

In the 1950s, the birth of lambs with immature brains and cyclopia was often witnessed at a particular sheep pasture in Idaho in the United States [242]. In 1957, the Department of Agriculture began an investigation into the cause. After a 11-year investigation, L. James et al. revealed that cyclopamine (11-deoxojervine) contained in African corn lilies had caused deformities by affecting fetal development [243]. However, it was not until almost 30 years later that the mechanisms by which cyclopamine caused these deformities were revealed.

Sonic hedgehog (Shh) is an extracellularly secreted protein that is endocytosed after binding the receptor Patched (PTCH1). When Shh binds to PTCH1, the membrane protein Smoothened (SMO) dissociates from PTCH1 and increases the stability of GLI transcription factors in the cytoplasm, causing them to translocate into the nucleus and induce expression of downstream genes.

In 1996, P.A. Beachy's group at Johns Hopkins University generated genetically defective mice in order to study the functions of Shh in the development of the central nervous system in more detail. The mice lacking Shh showed cyclopia and under-developed brains [244].

In 1996, M.P Scott's group at Stanford University and H. Hahn et al. at Queensland University in Australia observed a high frequency of PTCH1 mutations in patients with nevoid basal cell carcinoma syndrome and discovered that the hedgehog pathway was activated by these mutations [245]. Moreover, in 1998, in a collaborative study between E.H. Epstein Jr's group at UCSF and F.J. de Sauvage's group at Genentech, activating mutations of SMO were discovered in basal cell carcinomas (BCCs) [246]. Subsequently, as the result of a full investigation of mutations in the hedgehog pathway in BCCs, mutations were found in the tumors of a majority of patients with BCC, with 90 % of the mutations in PTCH1 and the remaining 10 % in SMO.

In 1998, P.A. Beachy's group had been investigating candidate drugs that could modulate the hedgehog pathway when they became interested in cyclopamine-induced deformities, such as brain immaturity and cyclopia, in Shh-deficient mice, leading them to investigate the relationship between cyclopamine and the hedgehog pathway. They discovered that cyclopamine binds to SMO to suppress hedgehog signaling [247]. In 2000, Beachy's group observed that cyclopamine suppressed activation of the hedgehog pathway caused by the PTCH1 and SMO mutantions discovered in BCC tumors and suggested the possibility that cyclopamine could represent a new type of anticancer agent [248].

However, cyclopamine is unsuited for use as a chemotherapeutic because it is chemically unstable, and it has low solubility. Therefore, several researchers have attempted to develop additional hedgehog inhibitors. In 2009, Genentech's K.D. Robarge et al. developed vismodegib, which competes with cyclopamine to bind to mutant SMO protein, and observed an anticancer effect in a medulloblastoma xenograft animal model (Fig. 9.28) [249]. Later, clinical trials of cyclopa-

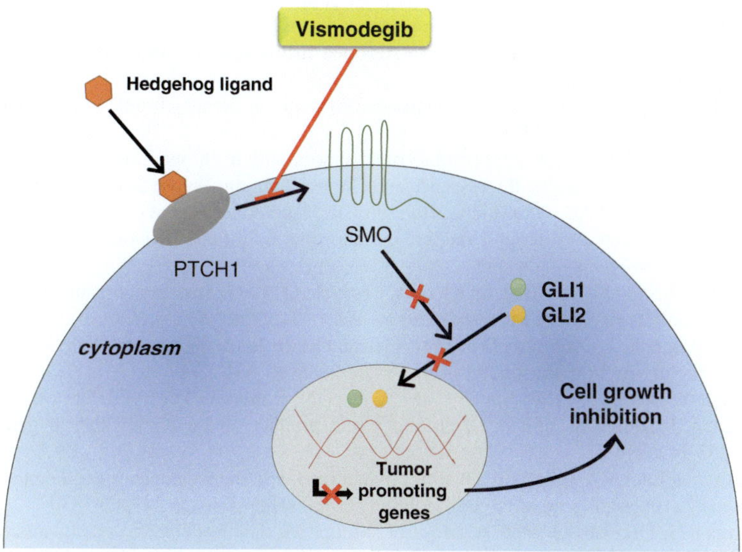

Fig. 9.28 Mechanism of action for vismodegib. In basal cell carcinoma, activating mutations arise in proteins required for the hedgehog signaling pathway. Vismodegib acts on Smoothened (*SMO*), a membrane protein, to inhibit nuclear translocation of downstream transcription factors GLI1 and GLI2, thereby preventing expression of proto-oncogenes related to the hedgehog pathway

mine were conducted in patients with metastatic BCC, in which vismodegib showed a response rate of 43 % with median response duration of 7.6 months [250]. Cyclopamine was subsequently approved by the FDA as a treatment for metastatic BCC.

References

1. Rowley JD, Golomb HM, Dougherty C (1977) 15/17 translocation, a consistent chromosomal change in acute promyelocytic leukaemia. Lancet 309:549–550
2. Borrow J, Goddard AD, Sheer D, Solomon E (1990) Molecular analysis of acute promyelocytic leukemia breakpoint cluster region on chromosome 17. Science 249:1577–1580
3. de Thé H, Chomienne C, Lanotte M, Degos L, Dejean A (1990) The t(15;17) translocation of acute promyelocytic leukaemia fuses the retinoic acid receptor alpha gene to a novel transcribed locus. Nature 347:558–561
4. Friend C, Scher W, Holland JG, Sato T (1971) Hemoglobin synthesis in murine virusinduced leukemic cells in vitro: stimulation of erythroid differentiation by dimethyl sulfoxide. Proc Natl Acad Sci U S A 68:378–382
5. Breitman TR, Collins SJ, Keene BR (1981) Terminal differentiation of human promyelocytic leukemic cells in primary culture in response to retinoic acid. Blood 57:1000–1004
6. Huang ME, Ye YC, Chen SR, Chai JR, Lu JX, Zhoa L, Gu LJ, Wang ZY (1988) Use of all-trans retinoic acid in the treatment of acute promyelocytic leukemia. Blood 72:567–572
7. Warrell RP Jr, Frankel SR, Miller WH Jr, Scheinberg DA, Itri LM et al (1991) Differentiation therapy of acute promyelocytic leukemia with tretinoin (all-trans-retinoic acid). N Engl J Med 324:1385–1393
8. Zhu J, Gianni M, Kopf E, Honoré N, Chelbi-Alix M, Koken M, Quignon F, Rochette-Egly C, de Thé H (1999) Retinoic acid induces proteasome-dependent degradation of retinoic acid receptor alpha (RARalpha) and oncogenic RARalpha fusion proteins. Proc Natl Acad Sci 96:14807–14812
9. Nowell PC, Hungerford DA (1960) A minute chromosome in human chronic granulocytic leukemia. Science 132:1497–1501
10. Rowley JD (1973) A new consistent chromosomal abnormality in chronic myelogenous leukaemia identified by quinacrine fluorescence and Giemsa staining. Nature 243:290–293
11. de Klein A, van Kessel AG, Grosveld G, Bartram CR, Hagemeijer A et al (1982) A cellular oncogene is translocated to the philadelphia chromosome in chronic myelocitic leukemia. Nature 300:765–767
12. Heisterkamp N, Stam K, Groffen J, de Klein A, Grosveld G (1985) Structural organization of the Bcr gene and its role in the Ph' translocation. Nature 315:758–761
13. Witte ON, Dasgupta A, Baltimore D (1980) Abelson murine leukemia virus protein is phosphorylated in vitro to form phosphotyrosine. Nature 283:826–831
14. Ben-Neriah Y, Daley GQ, Mes-Masson AM, Witte ON, Baltimore D (1986) The chronic myelogenous leukemia-specific P210 protein is the product of the bcr/abl hybrid gene. Science 233:212–214
15. Daley GQ, Van Etten RA, Baltimore D (1990) Induction of chronic myelogenous leukemia in mice by the P210bcr/abl gene of the Philadelphia chromosome. Science 247:824–830
16. Zimmermann J, Caravatti G, Mett H, Meyer T, Miiller M, Fabbro D (1996) Phenylaminopyrimidine (PAP) derivatives: a new class of potent and selective inhibitors of protein kinase C (PKC). Arch Pharm 329:371–376
17. Buchdunger E, Zimmermann J, Mett H, Meyer T, Miiller M, Druker BJ, Lydon NB (1996) Inhibition of the Abl protein-tyrosine kinase in vitro and in vivo by a 2-phenylaminopyrimidine derivative. Cancer Res 56:100–104

18. Druker BJ, Tamura S, Buchdunger E, Ohno S, Segal GM, Fanning S, Zimmermann J, Lydon NB (1996) Effects of a selective inhibitor of the ABL tyrosine kinase on the growth of BCR-ABL positive cells. Nat Med 2:561–566
19. Druker BJ, Talpaz M, Resta D et al (2001) Efficacy and safety of a specific inhibitor of the Bcr-Abl tyrosine kinase in chronic myeloid leukemia. N Engl J Med 344:1031–1037
20. Kantarjian H, Sawyer C, Hochhaus A, Guilhot F, Schiffer C et al (2002) Hematologic and cytogenetic responses to imatinib mesylate in chronic myelogenous leukemia. N Engl J Med 346:645–652
21. Gleich GJ, Leiferman KM, Pardanani A et al (2002) Treatment of hypereosinophilic syndrome with imatinib mesilate. Lancet 359:1577–1578
22. Demetri GD, von Mehren M, Blanke CD et al (2002) Efficacy and safety of imatinib mesylate in advanced gastrointestinal stromal tumors. N Engl J Med 347:472–480
23. Gorre ME, Mohammed M, Ellwood K, Hsu N, Paquette R, Rao PN, Sawyers CL (2001) Clinical resistance to STI-571 cancer therapy caused by Bcr-Abl gene mutation or amplification. Science 293:876–880
24. Wityak J, Das J, Moquin RV, Shen Z, Lin J, Chen P, Doweyko AM et al (2003) Discovery and initial SAR of 2-amino-5-carboxamidothiazoles as inhibitors of the Src-family kinsae p56lck. Bioorg Med Chem Lett 13:4007–4010
25. Lombardo LJ, Lee FY, Chen P, Norris D, Barrish JC, Behnia K, Castaneda S et al (2004) Discovery of N-(2-chloro-6-methylphenyl)-2-(6-(4-(2-hydroxyethyl)piperazin-1-yl)-2-methylpyrimidin-4-ylamino)thiazole-5-carboxamide (BMS-354825), a dual Src/Abl kinase inhibitor with potent anti-tumor activity in preclinical assays. J Med Chem 47:6658–6661
26. Shah NP, Tran C, Lee FY, Chen P, Norris D, Sawyers CL (2004) Overriding imatinib resistance with a novel ABL kinase inhibitor. Science 305:399–401
27. Tokarski JS, Newitt JA, Chang CY, Cheng JD, Wittekind M, Kiefer SE et al (2006) The structure of dasatinib (BMS-354825) bound to activated ABL kinase domain elucidates its inhibitory activity against imatinib-resistant ABL mutants. Cancer Res 66:5790–5797
28. Talpaz M, Shah NP, Kantarjian H, Donato N, Nicoll J, Paquette R et al (2006) Dasatinib in imatinib-resistant Philadelphia chromosome-positive leukemias. N Engl J Med 354:2531–3541
29. Schindler T, Bornmann W, Pellicena P, Miller TW, Clarkson B, Kuriyan J (2000) Structural mechanism of STI-571 inhibition of abelson tyrosine kinase. Science 289:1938–1942
30. Weisberg E, Manley PW, Breitenstein W et al (2005) Characterization of AMN107, a selective inhibitor of native and mutant Bcr-Abl. Cancer Cell 7:129–141
31. Kantarjian H, Giles F, Wunderle L, Bhalla K, O'Brien S, Wassmann B et al (2006) Nilotinib in imatinib-resistant CML and Philadelphia chromosome-positive ALL. N Engl J Med 354:2542–2551
32. Boschelli DH, Ye F, Wang YD, Dutia M, Johnson SL, Wu B, Miller K et al (2001) Optimization of 4-phenylamino-3-quinolinecarbonitriles as potent inhibitors of Src kinase activity. J Med Chem 44:3965–3977
33. Golas JM, Arndt K, Etienne D et al (2003) SKI-606, a 4-anilino-3-quinolinecarbonitrile dual inhibitor of Src and Abl kinases, is a potent antiproliferative agent against chronic myelogenous leukemia cells in culture and causes regression of K562 xenografts in nude mice. Cancer Res 3:375–381
34. Puttini M, Coluccia AM, Boschelli F et al (2006) In vitro and in vivo activity of SKI-606, a novel Src-Abl inhibitor, against imatinib resistant Bcr-Abl+neoplastic cells. Cancer Res 66:11314–11322
35. Cortes JE, Kantarjian HM, Brümmendorf TH, Kim DW, Turkina AG et al (2011) Safety and efficacy of bosutinib (SKI-606) in chronic phase Philadelphia chromosome-positive chronic myeloid leukemia patients with resistance or intolerance to imatinib. Blood 118:4567–4576
36. Cohen S (1960) Purification of a nerve-growth promoting protein from the mouse salivary gland and its neuro-cytotoxic antiserum. Proc Natl Acad Sci 46:302–311
37. Cohen S (1962) Isolation of a mouse submaxillary gland protein accelerating incisor eruption and eyelid opening in the new-born animal. J Biol Chem 237:1555–1562

38. Cohen S, Elliot GA (1963) The stimulations of epidermal keratinization by a protein isolated from the submaxillary gland of the mouse. J Invest Dermatol 40:1–5
39. Starkey RH, Cohen S, Orth DN (1975) Epidermal growth factor: identification of a new hormone in human urine. Science 89:800–802
40. Cohen S, Ushiro H, Stoscheck CM, Chinkers M (1982) A native 170,000 epidermal growth factor receptor-kinase complex from shed plasma membrane vesicles. J Biol Chem 257: 1523–1531
41. Ushiro H, Cohen S (1980) Identification of phosphotyrosine as a product of epidermal growth factor-activated protein kinase in A-431 cell membranes. J Biol Chem 255:8363–8365
42. Hunter T, Cooper JA (1981) Epidermal growth factor induces rapid tyrosine phosphorylation of proteins in A431 human tumor cells. Cell 24:741–752
43. Downward J, Yarden Y, Mayes E, Scrace G, Totty N, Stockwell P, Ullrich A, Schlessinger J, Waterfield MD (1984) Close similarity of epidermal growth factor receptor and v-erb-B oncogene protein sequences. Nature 307:521–527
44. Ullrich A, Coussens L, Hayflick JS, Dull TJ, Gray A, Tam AW, Lee J et al (1984) Human epidermal growth factor receptor cDNA sequence and aberrant expression of the amplified gene in A431 epidermoid carcinoma cells. Nature 309:418–425
45. Hong WK, Ullrich A (2000) The role of EGFR in solid tumors and implications for therapy. Oncol Biother 1:1–29
46. Barker AJ, Davies DH (1992) Therapeutic preparations containing quinazoline derivatives. European Patent, EP-520722-A
47. Wakeling AE, Barker AJ, Davies DH et al (1996) Specific inhibition of epidermal growth factor receptor tyrosine kinase by 4-anilinoquinazolines. Breast Cancer Res Treat 38:67–73
48. Woodburn JR, Barker AJ, Gibson KH et al (1997) ZD1839, an epidermal growth factor tyrosine kinase inhibitor selected for clinical development. Proc Am Assoc Cancer Res 38:633–634
49. Kris MG, Natale RB, Herbst RS et al (2003) Efficacy of gefitinib, an inhibitor of the epidermal growth factor receptor tyrosine kinase, in symptomatic patients with nonsmall cell lung cancer: a randomized trial. JAMA 290:2149–2158
50. Lynch TJ, Bell DW, Sordella R et al (2004) Activating mutations in the epidermal growth factor receptor underlying responsiveness of nonsmall-cell lung cancer to gefitinib. N Engl J Med 350:2129–2139
51. Paez JG, Janne PA, Lee JC et al (2004) EGFR mutations in lung cancer: correlation with clinical response to gefitinib therapy. Science 304:1497–1500
52. Mok TS, Wu Y-L, Thongprasert S et al (2009) Gefitinib or carboplatin—paclitaxel in pulmonary adenocarcinoma. N Engl J Med 361:947–957
53. Arnold LD, Schnur RC (1996) Novel anti-proliferative quinazoline derivatives useful for treating tumours, inflammatory disorders etc. World Patent Application W09630347
54. Moyer JD, Barbacci EG, Iwata KK, Arnold L, Boman B, Cunningham A et al (1997) Induction of apoptosis and cell cycle arrest by CP-358,774, an inhibitor of epidermal growth factor receptor tyrosine kinase. Cancer Res 57:4838–4848
55. Shepherd FA, Rodrigues Pereira J, Ciuleanu T et al (2005) Erlotinib in previously treated non-small-cell lung cancer. N Engl J Med 353:123–132
56. Zhou C, Wu Y-L, Chen G et al (2011) Erlotinib versus chemotherapy as first line treatment for patients with advanced EGFR mutation-positive non-small-cell lung cancer (OPTIMAL, CTONG- 0802): a multicentre, open-label, randomised, phase 3 study. Lancet Oncol 12: 735–742
57. Rosell R, Carcereny E, Gervais R et al (2012) Erlotinib versus standard chemotherapy as first-line treatment for European patients with advanced EGFR mutationpositive non-small-cell lung cancer (EURTAC): a multicentre, open-label, randomised phase 3 trial. Lancet Oncol 13:239–246
58. Moore MJ, Goldstein D, Hamm J et al (2007) Erlotinib plus gemcitabine compared with gemcitabine alone in patients with advanced pancreatic cancer: a phase III trial of the National Cancer Institute of Canada Clinical Trials Group. J Clin Oncol 25:1960–1966

59. Pao W, Wang TY, Riely GJ, Miller VA, Pan Q, Ladanyi M et al (2005) Acquired resistance of lung adenocarcinomas to gefitinib or erlotinib is associated with a second mutation in the EGFR kinase domain. PLoS Med 2:e73
60. Kobayashi S, Boggon TJ, Dayaram T et al (2005) EGFR mutation and resistance of nonsmall-cell lung cancer to gefitinib. N Engl J Med 352:786–792
61. Kobayashi S, Ji H, Yuza Y, Meyerson M, Wong KK, Tenen DG, Halmos B (2005) An alternative inhibitor overcomes resistance caused by a mutation of the epidermal growth factor receptor. Cancer Res 65:7096–7101
62. Kwak EL, Sordella R, Bell DW, Godin-Heymann N, Okimoto RA, Brannigan BW et al (2005) Irreversible inhibitors of the EGF receptor may circumvent acquired resistance to gefitinib. Proc Natl Acad Sci 102:7665–7670
63. Li D, Ambrogio L, Shimamura T, Kubo S, Takahashi M, Chirieac LR et al (2008) BIBW2992, an irreversible EGFR/HER2 inhibitor highly effective in preclinical lung cancer models. Oncogene 27:4702–4711
64. Passaro A, Gori B, de Marinis F (2013) Afatinib as first-line treatment for patients with advanced non-small-cell lung cancer harboring EGFR mutations: focus on LUX-Lung 3 and LUX-Lung 6 phase III trials. J Thorac Dis 5:383–384
65. Miller VA, Hirsh V, Cadranel J et al (2012) Afatinib versus placebo for patients with advanced, metastatic non-small-cell lung cancer after failure of erlotinib, gefitinib, or both, and one or two lines of chemotherapy (LUX-Lung 1): a phase 2b/3 randomised trial. Lancet Oncol 13:528–538
66. Lin NU, Winer EP, Wheatley D, Carey LA, Houston S, Mendelson D et al (2012) A phase II study of afatinib (BIBW 2992), an irreversible ErbB family blocker, in patients with HER2-positive metastatic breast cancer progressing after trastuzumab. Breast Cancer Res Treat 133:1057–1065
67. Kawamoto T, Sato JD, Le A, Polikoff J, Sato GH, Mendelsohn J (1983) Growth stimulation of A431 cells by epidermal growth factor: identification of high-affinity receptors for epidermal growth factor by an anti-receptor monoclonal antibody. Proc Natl Acad Sci 80:1337–1341
68. Masui H, Kawamoto T, Sato JD, Wolf B, Sato G, Mendelsohn J (1984) Growth inhibition of human tumor cells in athymic mice by anti-EGF receptor monoclonal antibodies. Cancer Res 44:1002–1007
69. Goldstein NI, Prewett M, Zuklys K, Rockwell P, Mendelsohn J (1995) Biological efficacy of a chimeric antibody to the epidermal growth factor receptor in a human tumor xenograft model. Clin Cancer Res 1:1311–1318
70. Cunningham D, Humblet Y, Siena S, Khayat D, Bleiberg H, Santoro A et al (2004) Cetuximab monotherapy and cetuximab plus irinotecan in irinotecan-refractory metastatic colorectal cancer. N Engl J Med 351:337–345
71. Yang XD, Jia XC, Corvalan JR, Wang P, Davis CG, Jakobovits A (1999) Eradication of established tumors by a fully human monoclonal antibody to the epidermal growth factor receptor without concomitant chemotherapy. Cancer Res 59:1236–1243
72. Mendez MJ, Green LL, Corvalan JR, Jia XC, Maynard-Currie CE, Yang XD et al (1997) Functional transplant of megabase human immunoglobulin loci recapitulates human antibody response in mice. Nat Genet 115:146–156
73. Van Cutsem E, Peeters M, Siena S, Humblet Y, Hendlisz A, Neyns B et al (2007) Open-label phase III trial of panitumumab plus best supportive care compared with best supportive care alone in patients with chemotherapy-refractory metastatic colorectal cancer. J Clin Oncol 25:1658–1664
74. Padhy LC, Shih C, Cowing D, Finkelstein R, Weinberg RA (1982) Identification of a phosphoprotein specifically induced by the transforming DNA of rat neuroblastomas. Cell 28:865–871
75. Coussens L, Yang-Feng TL, Liao YC, Chen E, Gray A, McGrath J et al (1985) Tyrosine kinase receptor with extensive homology to EGF receptor shares chromosomal location with neu oncogene. Science 230:1132–1139

76. Slamon DJ, Clark GM, Wong SG, Levin WJ, Ullrich A, McGuire WL (1987) Human breast cancer: correlation of relapse and survival with amplification of the HER-2/neu oncogene. Science 235:177–182
77. Slamon DJ, Godolphin W, Jones LA, Holt JA, Wong SG, Keith DE, Levin WJ et al (1989) Studies of the HER-2/neu proto-oncogene in human breast and ovarian cancer. Science 244:707–712
78. Hudziak RM, Lewis GD, Winget M, Fendly BM, Shepard HM, Ullrich A (1989) p185HER2 monoclonal antibody has antiproliferative effects in vitro and sensitizes human breast tumor cells to tumor necrosis factor. Mol Cell Biol 9:1165–1172
79. Carter P, Presta L, Gorman CM, Ridgway JB, Henner D, Wong WL et al (1992) Humanization of an anti-p185HER2 antibody for human cancer therapy. Proc Natl Acad Sci 89:4285–4289
80. Slamon D, Leyland-Jones B, Shak S, Paton V, Bajamonde A, Fleming T, Eiermann W, Baselga J, Norton L et al (1998) Proc Annu Meet Am Soc Clin Oncol 17:98a; Slamon DJ, Leyland-Jones B, Shak S et al (2001) Use of chemotherapy plus a monoclonal antibody against HER2 for metastatic breast cancer that overexpresses HER2. N Engl J Med 344:783–792
81. Bang YJ, Van Cutsem E, Feyereislova A, Chung HC, Shen L, Sawaki A et al (2010) Trastuzumab in combination with chemotherapy versus chemotherapy alone for treatment of HER2-positive advanced gastric or gastroesophageal junction cancer (ToGA): a phase 3, openlabel, randomised controlled trial. Lancet 376:687–697
82. Cobleigh MA, Vogel CL, Tripathy D, Robert NJ, Scholl S, Fehrenbacher L et al (1999) Multinational study of the efficacy and safety of humanized anti-HER2 monoclonal antibody in women who have HER2-overexpressing metastatic breast cancer that has progressed after chemotherapy for metastatic disease. J Clin Oncol 17:2639–2648
83. Agus DB, Akita RW, Fox WD et al (2002) Targeting ligand-activated ErbB2 signaling inhibits breast and prostate tumor growth. Cancer Cell 2:127–137
84. Cho HS, Mason K, Ramyar KX, Stanley AM, Gabelli SB, Denney DW Jr, Leahy DJ (2003) Structure of the extracellularregion of HER2 alone and in complex with the Herceptin Fab. Nature 421:756–760
85. Fendly BM, Winget M, Hudziak RM et al (1990) Characterization of murine monoclonal antibodies reactive to either the human epidermal growth factor receptor or HER2/neu gene product. Cancer Res 50:1550–1558
86. Franklin MC, Carey KD, Vajdos FF, Leahy DJ, de Vos AM, Sliwkowski MX (2004) Insights into ErbB signaling from the structure of the ErbB2-pertuzumab complex. Cancer Cell 5:317–328
87. Scheuer W, Friess T, Burtscher H et al (2009) Strongly enhanced antitumor activity of trastuzumab and pertuzumab combination treatment on HER2-positive human xenograft tumor models. Cancer Res 69:9330–9336
88. Baselga J, Cortes J, Kim SB et al (2012) Pertuzumab plus trastuzumab plus docetaxel for metastatic breast cancer. N Engl J Med 366:109–119
89. Carter MC, Cockerill GS, Guntrip SB, Lackey KE, Smith KJ (1999) Bicyclic heteroaromatic compounds [quinazolinamines and analogs] useful as protein tyrosine kinase inhibitors. PCT Int Appl WO9935146
90. Cockerill S, Stubberfield C, Stables J, Carter M, Guntrip S, Smith K, McKeown S, Shaw R, Topley P, Thomsen L (2001) Indazolylamino quinazolines and pyridopyrimidines as inhibitors of the EGFr and C-erbB-2. Bioorg Med Chem Lett 11:1401–1405
91. Rusnak DW, Lackey K, Affleck K, Wood ER, Alligood KJ, Rhodes N et al (2001) The effects of the novel, reversible epidermal growth factor receptor/ErbB-2 tyrosine kinase inhibitor, GW2016, on the growth of human normal and tumor-derived cell lines *in vitro* and *in vivo*. Mol Cancer Ther 1:85–94
92. Konecny GE, Pegram MD, Venkatesan N, Finn R, Yang G, Rahmeh M et al (2006) Activity of the dual kinase inhibitor lapatinib (GW572016) against HER-2-overexpressing and trastuzumab-treated breast cancer cells. Cancer Res 66:1630–1639

93. Geyer CE, Forster J, Lindquist D, Chan S, Romieu CG, Pienkowski T et al (2006) Lapatinib plus capecitabine for HER2-positive advanced breast cancer. N Engl J Med 355:2733–2743
94. Folkman J (1971) Tumor angiogenesis: therapeutic implications. N Engl J Med 285: 1182–1186
95. Ferrara N, Henzel WJ (1989) Pituitary follicular cells secrete a novel heparin-binding growth factor specific for vascular endothelial cells. Biochem Biophys Res Commun 161:851–858
96. Gospodarowicz D, Abraham JA, Schilling J (1989) Isolation and characterization of a vascular endothelial mitogen produced by pituitary-derived folliculo stellate cells. Proc Natl Acad Sci 86:7311–7315
97. de Vries C, Escobedo JA, Ueno H, Houck K, Ferrara N, Williams LT (1992) The fms-like tyrosine kinase, a receptor for vascular endothelial growth factor. Science 255:989–991
98. Terman BI, Dougher-Vermazen M, Carrion ME, Dimitrov D, Armellino DC et al (1992) Identification of the KDR tyrosine kinase as a receptor for vascular endothelial cell growth factor. Biochem Biophys Res Commun 187:1579–1586
99. Millauer B, Wizigmann-Voos S, Schnürch H, Martinez R, Møller NP, Risau W, Ullrich A (1993) High affinity VEGF binding and developmental expression suggest Flk-1 as a major regulator of vasculogenesis and angiogenesis. Cell 72:835–846
100. Kim KJ, Li B, Winer J, Armanini M, Gillett N, Phillips HS, Ferrara N (1993) Inhibition of vascular endothelial growth factor-induced angiogenesis suppresses tumour growth *in vivo*. Nature 362:841–844
101. Presta LG, Chen H, O'Connor SJ, Chisholm V, Meng YG, Krummen L, Ferrara N (1997) Humanization of an anti-vascular endothelial growth factor monoclonal antibody for the therapy of solid tumors and other disorders. Cancer Res 57:4593–4599
102. Hurwitz H, Fehrenbacher L, Novotny W, Cartwright T, Hainsworth J, Heim W, Kabbinavar F (2004) Bevacizumab plus irinotecan, fluorouracil, and leucovorin for metastatic colorectal cancer. N Engl J Med 350:2335–2342
103. Holash J, Davis S, Papadopoulos N, Croll SD, Ho L, Russell M, Rudge JS et al (2002) VEGF-Trap: a VEGF blocker with potent antitumor effects. Proc Natl Acad Sci U S A 99: 11393–11398
104. Van Cutsem E, Tabernero J, Lakomy R, Prenen H, Prausová J, Macarulla T, Allegra C (2012) Addition of aflibercept to fluorouracil, leucovorin, and irinotecan improves survival in a phase III randomized trial in patients with metastatic colorectal cancer previously treated with an oxaliplatin-based regimen. J Clin Oncol 30:3499–3506
105. Mohammadi M, McMahon G, Sun L, Tang C, Hirth P, Yeh BK, Hubbard SR, Schlessinger J (1997) Structures of the tyrosine kinase domain of fibroblast growth factor receptor in complex with inhibitors. Science 276:955–960
106. Millaurer B, Shawver LK, Plate KH, Risau W, Ullrich A (1994) Glioblastoma growth inhibited in vivo by a dominant-negative Flk-1 mutant. Nature 367:576–579
107. Sun L, Tran N, Tang F, App H, Hirth P, McMahon G, Tang C (1998) Synthesis and biological evaluations of 3-substituted indolin-2-ones: a novel class of tyrosine kinase inhibitors that exhibit selectivity toward particular receptor tyrosine kinases. J Med Chem 41: 2588–2603
108. Sun L, Liang C, Shirazian S, Zhou Y, Miller T, Cui J, Fukuda JY et al (2003) Discovery of 5-[5-fluoro-2-oxo-1,2-dihydroindol-(3Z)-ylidenemethyl]-2,4-dimethyl-1H-pyrrole-3--carboxylic acid (2-diethylaminoethyl)amide, a novel tyrosine kinase inhibitor targeting vascular endothelial and platelet-derived growth factor receptor tyrosine kinase. J Med Chem 46:1116–1119
109. Mendel DB, Laird AD, Xin X, Louie SG, Christensen JG, Li G, Schreck RE et al (2003) In vivo anti – tumor activity of SU11248, a novel tyrosine kinase inhibitor targeting vascular endothelial growth factor and platelet – derived growth factor receptors: determination of a pharmacokinetic/pharmacodynamic relationship. Clin Cancer Res 9:327–337
110. Motzer RJ, Hutson TE, Tomczak P, Michaelson MD, Bukowski RM et al (2007) Sunitinib versus interferon alfa in metastatic renal-cell carcinoma. N Engl J Med 356:15–24

111. Demetri GD, van Oosterom AT, Garrett CR et al (2006) Efficacy and safety of sunitinib in patients with advanced gastorointestinal stromal tumour after failure of imatinib: a randomised controlled trial. Lancet 368:329–338
112. Raymond E, Dahan L, Raoul JL, Bang YJ, Borbath I, Lombard-Bohas C et al (2011) Sunitinib malate for the treatment of pancreatic neuroendocrine tumors. N Engl J Med 364:501–513
113. Smith RA, Barbosa J, Blum CL, Bobko MA, Caringal YV, Dally R et al (2001) Discovery of heterocyclic ureas as a new class of raf kinase inhibitors: identification of a second generation lead by a combinatorial chemistry approach. Bioorg Med Chem Lett 11:2775–2778
114. Wilhelm S et al (2001) BAY 43–9006, a novel Raf-1 kinase inhibitor (RKI) blocks the Raf/MEK/ERK pathway in tumor cells. Proc Am Assoc Cancer Res 42:923
115. Lowinger TB, Riedl B, Dumas J, Smith RA (2002) Design and discovery of small molecules targeting raf-1 kinase. Curr Pharm Des 8:2269–2278
116. Wilhelm SM, Carter C, Tang L, Wilkie D, McNabola A, Rong H, Trail PA et al (2004) BAY 43-9006 exhibits broad spectrum oral antitumor activity and targets the RAF/MEK/ERK pathway and receptor tyrosine kinases involved in tumor progression and angiogenesis. Cancer Res 64:7099–7109
117. Chang YS, Henderson A, Xue D, Chen C, McNabola A, Wilkie D et al (2005) BAY 43-9006 (Sorafenib) inhibits ectopic and orthotopic growth of a murine model of renal adenocarcinoma (Renca) predominantly through inhibition of tumor angiogenesis. Proc Am Assoc Cancer Res 46:5831
118. Escudier B, Eisen T, Stadler WM, Szczylik C, Oudard S, Siebels M, Bukowski RM et al (2007) Sorafenib in advanced clear-cell renal-cell carcinoma. N Engl J Med 356:125–134
119. Llovet JM, Ricci S, Mazzaferro V, Hilgard P, Gane E, Blanc JF, Bruix J et al (2008) Sorafenib in advanced hepatocellular carcinoma. N Engl J Med 359:378–390
120. Bayer Pharmaceutical Corporation (2005) Fluoro substituted omega- carboxylaryl diphenyl urea for the treatment and prevention of diseases and conditions. US Patent, US2004023500
121. Wilhelm SM, Dumas J, Adnane L et al (2011) Regorafenib (BAY 73-4506): a new oral multikinase inhibitor of angiogenic, stromal and oncogenic receptor tyrosine kinases with potent preclinical antitumor activity. Int J Cancer 129:245–255
122. Grothey A, Van Cutsem E, Sobrero A, Siena S, Falcone A, Ychou M et al (2013) Regorafenib monotherapy for previously treated metastatic colorectal cancer (CORRECT): an international, multicentre, randomised, placebo-controlled, phase 3 trial. Lancet 381:303–312
123. Demetri GD, Reichardt P, Kang YK, Blay JY, Rutkowski P, Gelderblom H et al (2013) Efficacy and safety of regorafenib for advanced gastrointestinal stromal tumours after failure of imatinib and sunitinib (GRID): an international, multicentre, randomised, placebo-controlled, phase 3 trial. Lancet 381:295–302
124. Harris PA, Boloor A, Cheung M, Kumar R, Crosby RM, Davis-Ward RG et al (2008) Discovery of 5-[[4-[(2,3-dimethyl-2H-indazol-6-yl)methylamino]-2-pyrimidinyl]amino]-2-methylbenzenesulfonamide (pazopanib), a novel and potent vascular endothelial growth factor receptor inhibitor. J Med Chem 51:4632–4640. Boloor A et al (2006) Pyrimidineamines as angiogenesis modulators. U.S. Patent, 7105530
125. Kumar R, Knick VB, Rudolph SK, Johnson JH, Crosby RM, Crouthamel MC et al (2007) Pharmacokinetic-pharmacodynamic correlation from mouse to human with pazopanib, a multikinase angiogenesis inhibitor with potent antitumor and antiangiogenic activity. Mol Cancer Ther 6:2012–2021
126. Sternberg CN, Davis ID, Mardiak J, Szczylik C, Lee E, Wagstaff J et al (2010) Pazopanib in locally advanced or metastatic renal cell carcinoma: results of a randomized phase III trial. J Clin Oncol 28:1061–1068
127. van der Graaf WT, Blay JY, Chawla SP, Kim DW, Bui-Nguyen B et al (2012) Pazopanib for metastatic soft-tissue sarcoma(PALETTE): a randomised, double-blind, placebo-controlled phase 3 trial. Lancet 379:1879–1886
128. Kania RS (2003) Indazole compounds and pharmaceutical compositions for inhibiting protein kinases, and methods for their use. US Patent, US 6534524

129. Hu-Lowe DD, Zou HY, Grazzini ML et al (2008) Nonclinical antiangiogenesis and antitumor activities of axitinib (AG-013736), an oral, potent, and selective inhibitor of vascular endothelial growth factor receptor tyrosine kinases 1, 2, 3. Clin Cancer Res 14:7272–7283
130. Rini BI, Escudier B, Tomczak P, Kaprin A, Szczylik C, Hutson TE, Michaelson MD et al (2011) Comparative effectiveness of axitinib versus sorafenib in advanced renal cell carcinoma (AXIS): a randomised phase 3 trial. Lancet 378:1931–1939
131. Hennequin LF, Stokes ES, Thomas AP, Johnstone C, Plé PA, Ogilvie DJ et al (2002) Novel 4-anilinoquinazolines with C-7 basic side chains: design and structure activity relationship of a series of potent, orally active, VEGF receptor tyrosine kinase inhibitors. J Med Chem 45:1300–1312
132. Wedge SR, Ogilvie DJ, Dukes M et al (2002) ZD6474 inhibits vascular endothelial growth factor signaling, angiogenesis, and tumor growth following oral administration. Cancer Res 62:4645–4655
133. Grieco M, Santoro M, Berlingieri MT, Melillo RM, Donghi R, Bongarzone I, Pierotti MA et al (1990) PTC is a novel rearranged form of the ret proto-oncogene and is frequently detected *in vivo* in human thyroid papillary carcinomas. Cell 60:557–563
134. Carlomagno F, Vitagliano D, Guida T, Ciardiello F, Tortora G, Vecchio G et al (2002) ZD6474, an orally available inhibitor of KDR tyrosine kinase activity, efficiently blocks oncogenic RET kinases. Cancer Res 62:7284–7290
135. Wells SA Jr, Robinson BG, Gagel RF, Dralle H, Fagin JA, Santoro M et al (2012) Vandetanib in patients with locally advanced or metastatic medullary thyroid cancer: a randomized, double-blind phase III trial. J Clin Oncol 30:134–141
136. Bannen LC, Chan DS, Forsyth TP, Khoury RG, Leahy JW, Mac MB et al (2009) inventors; Exelixis, Inc., assignee. c-Met modulators and methods of use. U.S. patent US7579473
137. Yakes FM, Chen J, Tan J, Yamaguchi K, Shi Y, Yu P, Qian F, Chu F et al (2011) Cabozantinib (XL184), a novel MET and VEGFR2 inhibitor, simultaneously suppresses metastasis, angiogenesis, and tumor growth. Mol Cancer Ther 10:2298–2308
138. Kurzrock R, Sherman SI, Ball DW, Forastiere AA, Cohen RB, Mehra R, Pfister DG et al (2011) Activity of XL184 (Cabozantinib), an oral tyrosine kinase inhibitor, in patients with medullary thyroid cancer. J Clin Oncol 29:2660–2666
139. Kralovics R, Passamonti F, Buser AS et al (2005) A gain-of-function mutation of JAK2 in myeloproliferative disorders. N Engl J Med 352:1779–1790
140. Baxter EJ, Scott LM, Campbell PJ et al (2005) Acquired mutation of the tyrosine kinase JAK2 in human myeloproliferative disorders. Lancet 365:1054–1061
141. James C, Ugo V, Le Couedic JP et al (2005) A unique clonal JAK2 mutation leading to constitutive signalling causes polycythaemia vera. Nature 434:1144–1148
142. Lin Q, Meloni D, Pan Y, Xia M, Rodgers J, Shepard S, Li M, Galya L et al (2009) Enantioselective synthesis of Janus kinase inhibitor INCB018424 via an organocatalytic aza-Michael reaction. Org Lett 11:1999–2002
143. Quintás-Cardama A, Vaddi K, Liu P, Manshouri T, Li J, Scherle PA et al (2010) Preclinical characterization of the selective JAK1/2 inhibitor INCB018424: therapeutic implications for the treatment of myeloproliferative neoplasms. Blood 115:3109–3117
144. Harrison C, Kiladjian JJ, Al-Ali HK, Gisslinger H, Waltzman R et al (2012) JAK Inhibition with ruxolitinib versus best available therapy for myelofibrosis. N Engl J Med 366:787–798
145. Verstovsek S, Mesa RA, Gotlib J, Levy RS, Gupta V, DiPersio JF et al (2012) A double-blind, placebo-controlled trial of ruxolitinib for myelofibrosis. N Engl J Med 366:799–807
146. Cui JJ et al (2006) Pyrazole-substituted aminoheteroaryl compounds as protein kinase inhibitors. U. S. Patent Application 20060128724; Cui JJ, Tran-Dubé M, Shen H, Nambu M, Kung PP, Pairish M, Jia L et al (2011) Structure based drug design of crizotinib (PF-02341066), a potent and selective dual inhibitor of mesenchymal-epithelial transition Factor (c-MET) kinase and anaplastic lymphoma kinase (ALK). J Med Chem 54:6342–6363
147. Zou HY, Li Q, Lee JH, Arango ME, McDonnell SR, Yamazaki S et al (2007) An orally available small-molecule inhibitor of c-Met, PF-02341066, exhibits cytoreductive antitumor efficacy through antiproliferative and antiangiogenic mechanisms. Cancer Res 67:4408–4417

148. Morris SW, Kirstein MN, Valentine MB, Dittmer KG, Shapiro DN et al (1994) Fusion of a kinase gene, ALK, to a nucleolar protein gene, NPM, in non-Hodgkin's lymphoma. Science 263:1281–1284
149. Soda M, Choi YL, Enomoto M, Takada S, Yamashita Y, Ishikawa S et al (2007) Identification of the transforming EML4-ALK fusion gene in non-small-cell lung cancer. Nature 448: 561–566
150. Chen Y, Takita J, Choi YL, Kato M, Ohira M, Sanada M, Wang L, Soda M et al (2008) Oncogenic mutations of ALK kinase in neuroblastoma. Nature 455:971–974
151. Kim DW, Ahn MJ, Shi Y, De Pas TM, Yang CY et al (2012) Results of a global phase II study with crizotinib in advanced ALK-positive non-small cell lung cancer. J Clin Oncol 30:suppl 7533
152. Shaw AT, Kim DW, Nakagawa K, Seto T, Crinó L, Ahn MJ, De Pas T et al (2013) Crizotinib versus chemotherapy in advanced ALK-positive lung cancer. N Engl J Med 368:2385–2394
153. Rapp UR, Goldsborough MD, Mark GE, Bonner TI, Groffen J, Reynolds FH Jr, Stephenson JR (1983) Structure and biological activity of v-raf, a unique oncogene transduced by a retrovirus. Proc Natl Acad Sci 80:4218–4222
154. Davies H, Bignell GR, Cox C, Stephens P, Edkins S, Clegg S et al (2002) Mutations of the BRAF gene in human cancer. Nature 417:949–954
155. Tsai J, Lee JT, Wang W, Zhang J, Cho H, Mamo S, Bremer R, Gillette S et al (2008) Discovery of a selective inhibitor of oncogenic B-Raf kinase with potent antimelanoma activity. Proc Natl Acad Sci 105:3041–3046
156. Bollag G, Hirth P, Tsai J, Zhang J, Ibrahim PN, Cho H, Spevak W et al (2010) Clinical efficacy of a RAF inhibitor needs broad target blockade in BRAF-mutant melanoma. Nature 467:596–599
157. Flaherty KT, Puzanov I, Kim KB, Ribas A, McArthur GA, Sosman JA et al (2010) Inhibition of mutated, activated BRAF in metastatic melanoma. N Engl J Med 363:809–819
158. Chapman PB, Hauschild A, Robert C, Haanen JB, Ascierto P, Larkin J et al (2011) Improved survival with vemurafenib in melanoma with BRAF V600E mutation. N Engl J Med 364:2507–2516
159. Laquerre S, Arnone M, Moss K, Yang J, Fisher K, Kane-Carson LS et al (2009) A selective Raf kinase inhibitor induces cell death and tumor regression of human cancer cell lines encoding B-Raf^{V600E} mutation. Mol Cancer Ther 8 suppl:B88
160. Hauschild A, Grob JJ, Demidov LV, Jouary T, Gutzmer R, Millward M et al (2012) Dabrafenib in BRAF-mutated metastatic melanoma: a multicentre, open-label, phase 3 randomised controlled trial. Lancet 380:358–365
161. Yamaguchi T, Yoshida T, Kurachi R, Kakegawa J, Hori Y, Nanayama T et al (2007) Identification of JTP-70902, a p15INK4b-inductive compound, as a novel MEK1/2 inhibitor. Cancer Sci 98:1809–1816
162. Gilmartin AG, Bleam MR, Groy A, Moss KG, Minthorn EA et al (2011) GSK1120212 (JTP-74057) is an inhibitor of MEK activity and activation with favorable pharmacokinetic properties for sustained *in vivo* pathway inhibition. Clin Cancer Res 17(5):989–1000
163. Flaherty KT, Robert C, Hersey P, Nathan P, Garbe C, Milhem M et al (2012) Improved survival with MEK inhibition in BRAF-mutated melanoma. N Engl J Med 367:107–114
164. Rawlings DJ, Saffran DC, Tsukada S, Largaespada DA, Grimaldi JC et al (1993) Mutation of unique region of Bruton's tyrosine kinase in immunodeficient XID mice. Science 261: 358–361
165. Pan Z, Scheerens H, Li SJ, Schultz BE, Sprengeler PA, Burrill LC et al (2007) Discovery of selective irreversible inhibitors for Bruton's tyrosine kinase. Chem Med Chem 2:58–61
166. Honigberg LA, Smith AM, Sirisawad M, Verner E, Loury D, Chang B et al (2010) The Bruton tyrosine kinase inhibitor PCI-32765 blocks B-cell activation and is efficacious in models of autoimmune disease and B-cell malignancy. Proc Natl Acad Sci 107:13075–13080
167. Wang ML, Rule S, Martin P, Goy A, Auer R, Kahl BS, Jurczak W et al (2013) Targeting BTK with ibrutinib in relapsed or refractory mantle-cell lymphoma. N Engl J Med 369:507–516

168. Byrd JC, Furman RR, Coutre SE, Flinn IW, Burger JA, Blum KA et al (2013) Targeting BTK with ibrutinib in relapsed chronic lymphocytic leukemia. N Engl J Med 369:32–42
169. Vézina C, Kudelski A, Sehgal SN (1975) Rapamycin (AY-22,989), a new antifungal antibiotic. I Taxonomy of the producing streptomycete and isolation of the active principle. J Antibiot 28:721–726
170. Martel RR, Klicius J, Galet S (1977) Inhibition of the immune response by rapamycin a new antifungal antibiotic. Can J Physiol Pharmacol 55:48–51
171. Kino T, Hatanaka H, Hashimoto M, Nishiyama M, Goto T, Okuhara M et al (1987) FK-506. a novel immunosuppressant isolated from a Streptomycetes. I. Fermentation, isolation, and physicochemical and biological characteristics. J Antibiot 60:1249–1255
172. Dumont FJ, Melino MR, Staruch MJ, Koprak SL, Fisher PA, Signal NH (1990) The immunosupressive macrolides FK506 and rapamycin act as reciprocal antagonist in murine T cells. J Immunol 144:1418–1424
173. Eng CP, Sehgal SN, Vézina C (1984) Activity of rapamycin (AY-22,989) against transplanted tumors. J Antibiot 37:1231–1237
174. Bierer BE, Somers PK, Wandless TJ, Burakoff SJ, Schreiber SL (1990) Probing immunosuppressant action with a nonnatural immunophilin ligand. Science 250:556–559
175. Brown EJ, Albers MW, Shin TB, Ichikawa K, Keith CT, Lane WS, Schreiber SL (1994) A mammalian protein targeted by G1-arresting rapamycin-receptor complex. Nature 369:756–768
176. Skotnicki JS, Leone CL, Smith AL (2001) Design, synthesis, and biological evaluation of C-42 hydroxyesters of rapamycin: the identification of CCI-779. Clin Cancer Res 7: S3749–S3750
177. Thomas GV, Tran C, Mellinghoff IK, Welsbie DS, Chan E, Fueger B, Czernin J, Sawyers CL (2006) Hypoxia-inducible factor determines sensitivity to inhibitors of mTOR in kidney cancer. Nat Med 12:122–127
178. Hudes G, Carducci M, Tomczak P, Dutcher J, Figlin R, Kapoor A (2007) Temsirolimus, interferon alfa, or both for advanced renal-cell carcinoma. N Engl J Med 356:2271–2281
179. Schuurman HJ, Cottens S, Fuchs S, Joergensen J, Meerloo T, Sedrani R et al (1997) SDZ RAD, a new rapamycin derivative: synergism with cyclosporine. Transplantation 64:32–35
180. Motzer RJ, Escudier B, Oudard S, Hutson TE, Porta C, Bracarda S et al (2008) Efficacy of everolimus in advanced renal cell carcinoma: a double-blind, randomised, placebo-controlled phase III trial. Lancet 372:449–456
181. Darcy AK, Marguerite MC, Katherine H, Karen A, Cynthia T, Prajakta M et al (2010) Everolimus for subependymal giant-cell astrocytomas in tuberous sclerosis. N Engl J Med 363:1801–1811
182. James CY, Manisha HS, Tetsuhide I, Catherine LB, Edward MW, Eric VC et al (2011) Everolimus for advanced pancreatic neuroendocrine tumors. N Engl J Med 364:514–523
183. José B, Mario C, Martine P, Howard AB, Hope SR, Tarek S et al (2012) Everolimus in postmenopausal hormone-receptor-positive advanced breast cancer. N Engl J Med 366:520–529
184. Reff ME, Carner K, Chambers KS, Chinn PC, Leonard JE, Rabb R et al (1994) Depletion of B cells *in vivo* by a chimeric mouse human monoclonal antibody to CD20. Blood 83: 435–445
185. David GM, Antonio JG, Christine AW, David B, Russell JS, James AN et al (1997) IDEC-C2B8 (Rituximab) Anti-CD20 monoclonal antibody therapy in patients with relapsed low-grade non-Hodgkin's lymphoma. Blood 90:2188–2195
186. Knox SJ, Goris ML, Trisler K et al (1996) Yttrium-90-labeled anti-CD20 monoclonal antibody therapy of recurrent B-cell lymphoma. Clin Cancer Res 2:457–470
187. Roselli M, Schlom J, Gansow OA et al (1991) Comparative biodistribution studies of DTPA-derivative bifunctional chelates for radiometal labeled monoclonal antibodies. Int J Radiat Appl Instrum B Nucl Med Biol 18:389–394
188. Witzig TE, Gordon LI, Cabanillas MS et al (2002) Randomized controlled trial of yttrium-90-labeled ibritumomab tiuxetan radioimmunotherapy versus rituximab immunotherapy for

patients with relapsed or refractory, low grade, follicular, or transformed B-cell non-Hodgkin's lymphoma. J Clin Oncol 20:2453–2463
189. Kaminski MS, Fig LM, Zasadny KR et al (1992) Imaging, dosimetry, and radioimmunotherapy with iodine 131-labeled anti-CD37 antibody in B-cell lymphoma. J Clin Oncol 10:1696–1711
190. Kaminski MS, Zelenetz AD, Press OW et al (2001) Pivotal study of Bexxar (iodine I 131 tositumomab) for chemotherapy-refractory low-grade or transformed low-grade B-cell non-Hodgkin's lymphomas. J Clin Oncol 19:3918–3928
191. Hale G, Bright S, Chumbley G, Hoang T, Metcalf D, Munro AJ, Waldmann H (1983) Removal of T cells from bone marrow for transplantation: a monoclonal antilymphocyte antibody that fixes human complement. Blood 62:873–882
192. Riechmann L, Clark M, Waldmann H, Winter G (1988) Reshaping human antibodies for therapy. Nature 332:323–327
193. Crowe JS, Hall VS, Smith MA, Cooper HJ, Tite JP (1992) Humanized monoclonal antibody CAMPATH-1H: myeloma cell expression of genomic constructs, nucleotide sequence of cDNA constructs and comparison of effector mechanisms of myeloma and Chinese hamster ovary cell-derived material. Clin Exp Immunol 87:105–110
194. Keating MJ, Flinn I, Jain V et al (2002) Therapeutic role of alemtuzumab (Campath-1H) in patients who have failed fludarabine: results of a large international study. Blood 99:3554–3561
195. Hillmen P, Skotnicki AB, Robak T, Jaksic B, Dmoszynska A, Wu J, Sirard C, Mayer J (2007) Alemtuzumab compared with chlorambucil as first-line therapy for chronic lymphocytic leukemia. J Clin Oncol 25:5616–5623
196. Teeling JL, French RR, Cragg MS, van den Brakel J, Pluyter M, Huang H et al (2004) Characterization of new human CD20 monoclonal antibodies with potent cytolytic activity against non-Hodgkin lymphomas. Blood 104:1793–1800
197. Wierda WG, Kipps TJ, Mayer J, Stilgenbauer S, Williams CD et al (2010) Ofatumumab as single-agent CD20 immunotherapy in fludarabine refractory chronic lymphocytic leukemia. J Clin Oncol 28:1749–1755
198. Wahl AF et al (2002) The anti-CD30 monoclonal antibody SGN-30 promotes growth arrest and DNA fragmentation *in vitro* and affects antitumor activity in models of Hodgkin's disease. Cancer Res 62:3736–3742
199. Francisco JA, Cerveny CG, Meyer DL, Mixan BJ, Klussman K et al (2003) cAC10-vcMMAE, an anti-CD30-monomethyl auristatin E conjugate with potent and selective antitumor activity. Blood 102:1458–1465
200. Younes A, Gopal AK, Smith SE, Ansell SM, Rosenblatt JD, Savage KJ et al (2012) Results of a pivotal phase II study of brentuximab vedotin for patients with relapsed or refractory Hodgkin's lymphoma. J Clin Oncol 30:2183–2189
201. Pro B, Advani R, Brice P, Bartlett NL, Rosenblatt JD, Illidge T et al (2012) Brentuximab vedotin (SGN-35) in patients with relapsed or refractory systemic anaplastic large-cell lymphoma: results of a phase II study. J Clin Oncol 30:2190–2196
202. Mössner E, Brunker P, Moser S et al (2010) Increasing the efficacy of CD20 antibody therapy through the engineering of a new type II anti-CD20 antibody with enhanced direct and immune effector cell-mediated B-cell cytotoxicity. Blood 115:4393–4402
203. Dalle S, Reslan L, Besseyre de Horts T et al (2011) Preclinical studies on the mechanism of action and the anti-lymphoma activity of the novel anti-CD20 antibody GA101. Mol Cancer Ther 10:178–185
204. Goede V, Fischer K, Busch R, Engelke A, Eichhorst B et al (2014) Obinutuzumab plus chlorambucil in patients with CLL and coexisting conditions. N Engl J Med 370:1101–1110
205. Holliday R (1979) A new theory of carcinogenesis. Br J Cancer 40:513–522
206. Feinberg AP, Vogelstein B (1983) Hypomethylation distinguishes genes of some human cancers from their normal counterparts. Nature 301:89–92
207. Čihák A, Škoda J, Šorm F (1963) Inhibition of biosynthesis of the nucleic acid pyrimidine bases by N-formylbiuret, a degradation product of 5-azauracil. Biochim Biophys Acta 72: 125–127

208. Jones PA, Taylor SM (1980) Cellular differentiation, cytidine analogs and DNA methylation. Cell 20:85–93
209. Santi DV, Garrett CE, Barr PJ (1983) On the mechanism of inhibition of DNA-cytosine methyltransferases by cytosine analogs. Cell 33:9–10
210. Silverman LR, Demakos EP, Peterson BL et al (2002) Randomized controlled trial of azacitidine in patients with the myelodysplastic syndrome: a study of the cancer and leukemia group B. J Clin Oncol 20:2429–2440
211. Veselý J, Cihák A (1980) Kinetics of 5-aza-2′-deoxycytidine phosphorylation in mouse spleen and L1210 leukemic cell extracts. Neoplasma 27:121–127
212. Kantarjian H, Issa JP, Rosenfeld CS, Bennett JM, Albitar M, DiPersio J et al (2006) Decitabine improves patient outcomes in myelodysplastic syndromes: results of a Phase III randomized study. Cancer 106:1794–1803
213. Daskalakis M, Nguyen TT, Nguyen C, Guldberg P, Köhler G, Wijermans P, Jones PA, Lübbert M (2002) Demethylation of a hypermethylated P15/INK4B gene in patients with myelodysplastic syndrome by 5-aza-2′-deoxycytidine (decitabine) treatment. Blood 100: 2957–2964
214. Stedman E (1950) Cell specificity of histones. Nature 166:780–781
215. Allfrey VG, Faulkner R, Mirsky AE (1964) Acetylation & methylation of histones and their possible role in the regulation of RNA synthesis. Proc Natl Acad Sci 51:786–794
216. Brownell JE, Zhou J, Ranalli T, Kobayashi R, Edmondson DG, Roth SY, Allis CD (1996) Tetrahymena histone acetyltransferase A: a homolog to yeast Gcn5p linking histone acetylation to gene activation. Cell 84:843–851
217. Taunton J, Hassig CA, Schreiber SL (1996) A mammalian histone deacetylase related to the yeast transcriptional regulator Rpd3p. Science 272:408–411
218. Friend C, Scher W, Holland JG, Sato T (1971) Hemoglobin synthesis in murine virus-induced leukemic cells *in vitro:* stimulation of erythroid differentiation by dimethyl sulfoxide. Proc Natl Acad Sci 68:378–382
219. Leder A, Leder P (1975) Butyric acid, a potent inducer of erythroid differentiation in cultured erythroleukemic cells. Cell 5:319–322
220. Riggs MG, Whittaker RG, Neumann JR, Ingram VM (1977) n-Butyrate causes histone modification in HeLa and Friend erythroleukaemia cells. Nature 268:462–464
221. Candido EP, Reeves R, Davie JR (1978) Sodium butyrate inhibits histone deacetylation in cultured cells. Cell 14:105–113
222. Yoshida M, Nomura S, Beppu T (1987) Effects of trichostatins on differentiation of murine erythroleukemia cells. Cancer Res 47:3688–3691
223. Tsuji N, Kobayashi M, Nagashima K, Wakisaka Y, Koizumi K (1976) A new antifungal antibiotic, trichostatin. J Antibiot 29:1–6
224. Yoshida M, Kijima M, Akita M, Beppu T (1990) Potent and specific inhibition of mammalian histone deacetylase both *in vivo* and *in vitro* by trichostatin A. J Biol Chem 265: 17172–17179
225. Kim MS, Kwon HJ, Lee YM, Baek JH, Jang JE, Lee SW, Moon EJ et al (2001) Histone deacetylases induce angiogenesis by negative regulation of tumor suppressor genes. Nat Med 7:437–443
226. Kijima M, Yoshida M, Sugita K, Horinouchi S, Beppu T (1993) Trapoxin, an antitumor cyclic tetrapeptide, is an irreversible inhibitor of mammalian histone deacetylase. J Biol Chem 268:22429–22435
227. Nakajima H, Kim YB, Terano H, Yoshida M, Horinouchi S (1998) FR901228, a potent antitumor antibiotic, is a novel histone deacetylase inhibitor. Exp Cell Res 241:126–133
228. Piekarz RL, Frye R, Turner M, Wright JJ, Allen SL, Kirschbaum MH et al (2009) Phase II multi-institutional trial of the histone deacetylase inhibitor romidepsin as monotherapy for patients with cutaneous T-cell lymphoma. J Clin Oncol 27:5410–5417
229. Tanaka M, Levy J, Terada M, Breslow R, Rifkind RA, Marks PA (1975) Induction of erythroid differentiation in murine virus infected eythroleukemia cells by highly polar compounds. Proc Natl Acad Sci 72:1003–1006

230. Reuben RC, Wife RL, Breslow R, Rifkind RA, Marks PA (1976) A new group of potent inducers of differentiation in murine erythroleukemia cells. Proc Natl Acad Sci 73:862–866
231. Richon VM, Webb Y, Merger R, Sheppard T, Jursic B, Ngo L et al (1996) Second generation hybrid polar compounds are potent inducers of transformed cell differentiation. Proc Natl Acad Sci 93:5705–5708
232. Richon VM, Emiliani S, Verdin E, Webb Y, Breslow R, Rifkind RA, Marks PA (1998) A class of hybrid polar inducers of transformed cell differentiation inhibits histone deacetylases. Proc Natl Acad Sci 95:3003–3007
233. Duvic M, Talpur R, Ni X, Zhang C, Hazarika P, Kelly C et al (2007) Phase 2 trial of oral vorinostat (suberoylanilide hydroxamic acid, SAHA) for refractory cutaneous T-cell lymphoma (CTCL). Blood 109:31–39
234. Rock KL, Gramm C, Rothstein L, Clark K, Stein R, Dick L, Hwang D, Goldberg AL (1994) Inhibitors of the proteasome block the degradation of most cell proteins and the generation of peptides presented on MHC class I molecules. Cell 78:761–771
235. Adams J et al (1995) Boronic ester and acid compounds. US Patent 5780554
236. Teicher BA, Ara G, Herbst R, Palombella VJ, Adams J (1999) The proteasome inhibitor PS-341 in cancer therapy. Clin Cancer Res 5:2638–2645
237. Hideshima T, Richardson P, Chauhan D, Palombella VJ, Elliott PJ, Adams J, Anderson KC (2001) The proteasome inhibitor PS-341 inhibits growth, induces apoptosis and overcomes drug resistance in human multiple myeloma cells. Cancer Res 61:3071–3076
238. Richardson PG, Barlogie B, Berenson J, Singhal S, Jagannath S et al (2003) A Phase 2 study of bortezomib in relapsed, refractory myeloma. N Engl J Med 348:2609–2617
239. Meng L, Mohan R, Kwok BH, Elofsson M, Sin N, Crews CM (1999) Epoxomicin, a potent and selective proteasome inhibitor, exhibits *in vivo* antiinflammatory activity. Proc Natl Acad Sci 96:10403–10408
240. Kuhn DJ, Chen Q, Voorhees PM, Strader JS, Shenk KD, Sun CM et al (2007) Potent activity of carfilzomib, a novel, irreversible inhibitor of the ubiquitin-proteasome pathway, against preclinical models of multiple myeloma. Blood 110:3281–3290
241. Siegel DS, Martin T, Wang M, Vij R, Jakubowiak AJ, Lonial S, Trudel S et al (2012) A phase 2 study of single-agent carfilzomib (PX-171-003-A1) in patients with relapsed and refractory multiple myeloma. Blood 120:2817–2825
242. Lee ST, Welch KD, Panter KE, Gardner DR, Garrossian M, Chang CW (2014) Cyclopamine: from cyclops lambs to cancer treatment. J Agri Food Chem 62:7355–7362
243. Binns W, James LF, Keeler RF, Balls LD (1968) Effects of teratogenic agents in range plants. Cancer Res 28:2323–2326
244. Chiang C, Litingtung Y, Lee E, Young KE, Corden JL, Westphal H, Beachy PA (1996) Cyclopia and defective axial patterning in mice lacking Sonic hedgehog gene function. Nature 383:407–413
245. Johnson RL, Rothman AL, Xie J, Goodrich LV, Cox DR, Epstein EH Jr, Scott MP (1996) Human homolog of patched, a candidate gene for the basal cell nevus syndrome. Science 272:1668–1671
246. Xie J, Murone M, Luoh SM, Ryan A, Rosenthal A, Epstein EH Jr, de Sauvage FJ (1998) Activating Smoothened mutations in sporadic basal-cell carcinoma. Nature 391:90–92
247. Cooper MK, Porter JA, Young KE, Beachy PA (1998) Teratogen-mediated inhibition of target tissue response to Shh signaling. Science 280:1603–1607
248. Taipale J, Chen JK, Cooper MK, Wang B, Mann RK, Milenkovic L, Scott MP, Beachy PA (2000) Effects of oncogenic mutations in Smoothened and Patched can be reversed by cyclopamine. Nature 406:1005–1009
249. Robarge KD, Brunton SA, Sutherlin DP, Ubhayaker S, Wang S, Wong S, Xie M et al (2009) GDC-0449-a potent inhibitor of the hedgehog pathway. Bioorg Med Chem Lett 19:5576–5581
250. Sekulic A, Migden MR, Oro AE, Dirix L, Lewis KD, Hainsworth JD, Solomon JA et al (2012) Efficacy and safety of vismodegib in advanced basal-cell carcinoma. N Engl J Med 366:2171–2179

Chapter 10
Complications of Anticancer Drugs and Their Management

Anticancer therapy targets actively growing and dividing cells. Because of this characteristic, anticancer drugs assaults not only cancer cells but also normally proliferating cells such as blood cells, mucosal epithelial cells, and skin epithelial cells. Therefore, they inevitably have various side effects. Most of such side effects are mild and transient, but some can become severe and irreversible. To increase compliance with anticancer therapy and to maintain the quality of life of cancer patients, the complications of anticancer therapy must be well understood and properly managed.

10.1 Chemotherapy-Induced Nausea and Vomiting (CINV)

Chemotherapy-induced nausea and vomiting is one of the most-feared side effects by cancer patients. It imposes such an extreme physiological and psychological burden to many patients that it even drives some patients to refuse treatment. In the recent 20 years, effective anti-emetics have been developed to prevent and control the symptoms of nausea and vomiting, and they have dramatically improved the quality of life of patients receiving chemotherapy. The purpose of anti-emetic treatment is to block all three steps of nausea and vomiting. The first step is the anticipatory phase, in which nausea and vomiting is induced even before chemotherapy and the psychological reaction start. This is a type of conditioned reflex after stimulation with anticancer drugs. The second step is the acute phase, which is induced within the first 24 h of the anticancer drug administration. It usually starts within 1–2 h of the administration and peaks in 4–6 h. The third step is the delayed phase, which occurs after 24 h of anticancer drug administration, peaks in 2–3 days, and gradually improves over the next 2–3 days (Fig. 10.1).

Chemotherapy-induced nausea and vomiting has drug-related factors and patient-related factors. The drug-related factors include the type of the anticancer drug and its dosage, administration schedule, and administration method. The

K.-W. Kim et al., *Cancer Drug Discovery*, DOI 10.1007/978-94-024-0844-7_10

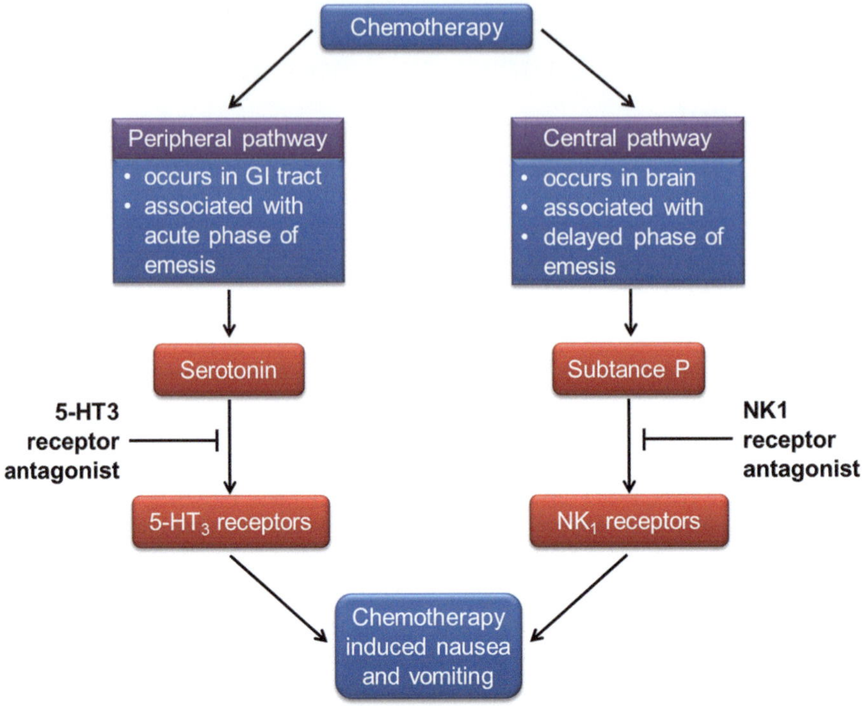

Fig. 10.1 Mechanism of Chemotherapy-induced nausea and vomiting (CINV)

patient-related factors include a history of nausea and vomiting as well as of alcoholism, a female gender, an age lower than 50 years, anxiety, and a history of motion sickness [1].

10.1.1 Emetogenic Risk of Anticancer Drugs

To effectively manage chemotherapy-induced nausea and vomiting, anticancer drugs must be grouped according to their emetogenic risk (Table 10.1). The emetogenic risk differs according to the administration dosage, route, and rate. In combination chemotherapy, in which several drugs are used concurrently, the anticancer drug with the highest vomiting risk must be confirmed and the risk of the co-administration of other anticancer drugs must be considered [1].

10.1.2 Types of Anti-emetics

Many effective anti-emetics have been developed in the past 20 years. Currently, the therapy that combines serotonin receptor antagonists, neurokinin-1 receptor antagonists, and corticosteroids shows the most significant prevention and treatment effects.

Table 10.1 Classification of chemotherapeutic drugs according to emetogenic risk

Minimal (<10 %)	Low risk (10–30 %)	Moderate risk (30–90 %)	High risk (>90 %)
Asparaginase	Paclitaxel	Carmustine	Carmustine
Bleomycin	Nab-paclitaxel	(≤250 mg/m^2)	(≥250 mg/m^2)
Bortezomib	Docetaxel	Cisplatin	Cisplatin
Busulfan	Pemetrexed	(≤50 mg/m^2)	(≥50 mg/m^2)
Cetuximab	Capecitabine	Methotrexate (250–	Cyclophosphamide
Chlorambucil	Cytarabine	1000 mg/m^2)	(≥1500 mg/m^2)
Decitabine	(100–200 mg/m^2)	Cyclophosphamide	Dacarbazine
Dasatinib	5-fluorouracil	(≤1500 mg/m^2)	Combination of
Dexrazoxane	Gemcitabine	Cytarabine	cyclophosphamide with
Erlotinib	Ixabepilone	(≥1 g/m^2)	Doxorubicin or Epirubicin
Fludarabine	Methotrexate	Carboplatin	Mechlorethamine
Gefitinib	(50–250 mg/m^2)	Oxaliplatin	Procarbazine
Hydroxyurea	Mitomicin	Ifosfamide	Streptozocin
Lapatinib	Mitoxantrone	Doxorubicin	
Lenalidomide	Nilotinib	Daunorubicin	
Melphalan	Topotecan	Epirubicin	
Methotrexate	Vorinostat	Idarubicin	
(≤50 mg/m^2)		Imatinib	
Panitumumab		Irinotecan	
Rituximab		Temozolomide	
Sorafenib		Azacitidine	
Sunitinib		Busulfan (>4 g/day)	
Temsirolimus			
Everolimus			
Thalidomide			
Trastuzumab			
Vinblastine			
Vincristine			
Vinorelbine			

10.1.2.1 Serotonin Receptor (5-HT3) Antagonists

Currently, various serotonin receptors antagonists are being widely used. Ondansetron (Zofran), granisetron (Kytril), dolasetron (Anzemet), and tropisetron (Navoban) are first-generation drugs, and palonosetron (Aloxi) is a second-generation drug. First-generation drugs show similar effects, and show no difference whether administered once or several times a day, intravenously or orally. However, these drugs have nearly no effect on the prevention of delayed vomiting caused by cisplatin. The second-generation drug palonosetron has a more than a dozen times higher binding affinity to 5-HT3 with a very long (40 h) half-life. When administered on its own, its prevention of acute and delayed vomiting caused by moderate emetogenic anticancer drugs is superior to that of ondansetron and dolasetron. When administered with dexamethasone, however, its prevention of acute and delayed vomiting caused by high emetogenic anticancer drugs is similar to when administered alone [1].

10.1.2.2 Neurokinin-1 (NK-1) Receptor Antagonists

The prevention of acute and delayed vomiting caused by high- or moderate emetogenic drugs was greatly improved by the introduction of aprepitant (Emend), a neurokinin-1 receptor antagonist. Several phase 3 clinical trials demonstrated that the combination therapy of aprepitant, ondansetron, and dexamethasone is superior to the previous combination of ondansetron and dexamethasone in preventing acute and delayed vomiting. Based on these results, the FDA approved its use in 2003. Fosaprepitant, an intravenous aprepritant formulation, is known to be converted to aprepitant within 30 minutes of intravenous administration. It received FDA approval in 2008 [1].

10.1.2.3 Corticosteroids

The anti-emetic mechanism of corticosteroids, such as dexamethasone, is not yet fully understood, but it has been traditionally very effective against chemotherapy-induced acute and delayed vomiting. Dexamethasone is used alone for low emetogenic drugs, and its combination with serotonin receptor antagonists and aprepitant is recommended for moderate or high emetogenic anticancer drugs. When combining aprepitant and dexamethasone, the dosage of dexamethasone should be reduced, because aprepitant acts as a CYP3A4 inhibitor [1].

10.1.2.4 Other Anti-emetics

Metoclopramide, lorazepam, prochloperazine, trimethobenzamide, etc. are anti-emetics with a low treatment efficacy. They can be used to treat low emetogenic groups or as salvage treatment for breakthrough vomiting. Metoclopramide has an anti-emetic effect as a dopamine receptor antagonist when used in the standard dose, and has an anti-emetic effect as a serotonin receptor antagonist when used in a high dose. However, metoclopramide should be used with caution because it can cause extrapyramidal symptoms such as akathisia and dystonia. Benzodiazepine drugs, such as lorazepam, have a weak anti-emetic effect but can help prevent and treat anticipatory vomiting due to its anxiolytic effect. It can also be used as a salvage treatment when the standard treatment fails [1].

10.1.3 Prevention and Treatment of Chemotherapy-Induced Nausea and Vomiting

10.1.3.1 High Emetogenic Anticancer Drugs

It is recommended that the triple regimen of a serotonin receptor antagonist, dexamethasone, and aprepitant be used shortly before administering the anticancer drug, then aprepitant be adminitered for following 2 days and dexamethasone for following 3 days.

10.1.3.2 Moderate Emetogenic Anticancer Drugs

The double regimen of a serontonin receptor antagonist and dexamethasone must be used shortly before administering the anticancer drug. Then after 2–3 days, a serontonin receptor antagonist or dexamethasone can be added.

10.1.3.3 Low Emetogenic Anticancer Drugs

It is recommended that dexamethasone be administered once before administering the anticancer drug, and that it can be used with prochloperazine.

10.2 Myelotoxicity (Bone Marrow Toxicity)

Myelotoxicity is very frequent in patients receiving cytotoxic chemotherapy, and is socioeconomically and clinically important. Even though targeted agents are widely used today, the existing cytotoxic anticancer drugs are still the key treatment, but the myelotoxicity of most anticancer drugs limits their dosage. The forms of myelotoxicity are neutropenia, anemia, and thrombocytopenia [2].

10.2.1 Neutropenia

Neutropenia is the most serious result of myelosuppression, and can progress to neutropenic fever and sepsis. Several studies have confirmed that the use of G-CSF (granulocyte colony-stimulating factor), such as filgrastim and pegfilgrastim, or GM-CSF (granulocyte-macrophage colony-stimulating factor), such as sagramstim, in neutropenia decreases the period of neutropenia and the incidence of neutropenic fever.

Currently, the preventive use of G-CSF is recommended for anticancer drug therapy with a 20 % or higher risk of neutropenic fever. It is not recommended, however, for a lower than 10 % risk of neutropenic fever. For a 10–20 % risk of anticancer therapy, the preventive use of G-CSF must be decided on while considering the overall risk if the patient has risk factors such as an age of over 65 years, progressive cancer, and a history of neutropenic fever (Fig. 10.2) [3].

10.2.2 Anemia

Chemotherapy-induced anemia is common. Its incidence differs according to the cancer type. A 50–60 % incidence is reported in lung cancer, ovarian cancer, and lymphoma, and a less than 20 % incidence is reported in breast cancer or colon cancer. Chemotherapy-induced anemia adversely affects the patient's quality of life by

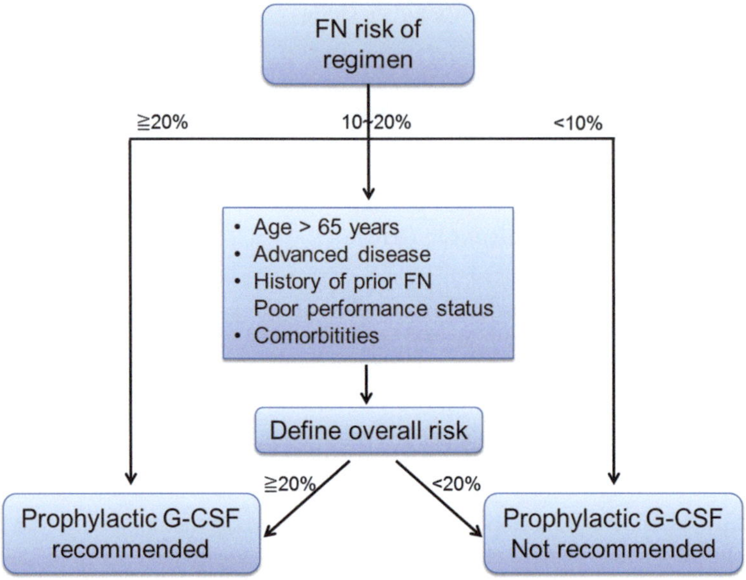

Fig. 10.2 Algorithm for prophylactic G-CSF treatment

causing fatigue, dyspnea, dizziness, etc. One-third of cancer patients experience transfusion due to anemia during their treatment. Transfusion rapidly and effectively relieves symptoms in patients with acute anemia, but a large amount of it is needed for long-term chemotherapy because its effect is temporary. Recombinant human erythropoietin (rhEPO) was developed to replace transfusion. In several randomized clinical studies in which recombinant erythropoietin, such as epoetin alfa (Epogen) or darbepoietin alfa (Aranesp), was administered to patients receiving chemotherapy, the use of epoetin alfa or darbepoietin alfa was shown to increase the average hemoglobin and decrease the transfusion demand in cancer patients. Based on these results, epoetin alfa was approved for use for chemotherapy-induced anemia in 1993. Darbepoietin alfa was also approved for use in 2001. However, the incidence of thromboembolism may increase when using epoetin alfa or darbepoietin alfa, so its use is recommended only when the hemoglobin level is less than 10 mg/dl [2].

10.2.3 Thrombocytopenia

Thrombocytopenia is a common side effect of anticancer therapy. Its incidence is increasing with the introduction of novel anticancer drugs, such as gemcitabine, and the development of new combination chemotherapies. Currently, platelet transfusion is the only treatment for thrombocytopenia, but repetitive platelet transfusion may cause infection or transfusion reaction. Thrombopoietin, an important factor of platelet growth, was discovered in 1994, based on which recombinant thrombopoietin was developed, but no such clinical drug is available yet [2].

10.3 Chemotherapy-Induced Diarrhea

10.3.1 Cause of Diarrhea

Chemotherapy-induced diarrhea decreases the patient's quality of life and disturbs effective anticancer treatment. Fluoropyrimidine drugs (especially 5-fluorouracil and capecitabine) and irinotecan are well known to induce diarrhea. Fluoropyrimidine induces acute damage and epithelial cell loss in the intestinal mucosa. Irinotecan can cause acute diarrhea within several hours of its administration, because its structure is similar to that of acetylcholine. This type of acute diarrhea can be mostly controlled with atropine which is a cholinergic antagonist. On the other hand, complex factors such as intestinal mucosa damage and motor abnormality affect the onset of late diarrhea. Tyrosine kinase inhibitors such as erlotinib and gefitinib often cause diarrhea but can be easily controlled [4].

10.3.2 Treatment

Mild (Grades 1–2) diarrhea with no accompanying symptoms or signs can be easily controlled through oral water intake and loperamide. For higher than Grades 3–4 diarrhea or for Grades 1–2 diarrhea with such symptoms as abdominal cramps, fever, neutropenia, and hemorrhage, active intravenous fluid therapy and antibiotics are needed. If severe diarrhea continues, the administration of octreotide, a somatostatin analogue, can be considered [4].

10.4 Chemotherapy-Induced Constipation

10.4.1 Cause of Constipation

The most common causes of constipation in patients receiving anticancer therapy are opioid analgesics and anti-emetics (serotonin receptor antagonists). All opioid analgesics cause constipation even after some time. Among anticancer drugs, vinca alkaloids commonly cause constipation, showing a neuropathic effect and decreasing the gastrointestinal passing time [4].

10.4.2 Treatment

A high-fiber diet, sufficient water intake, and increased physical activity are the most basic treatments. When they are not effective enough, laxatives can be helpful. Methylnatrexone is a pure opioid receptor antagonist that does not block the analgesic effect of opioid analgesics and is effective against the constipation caused by such analgesics. When there is no response to oral laxatives, enema or short-term use of a suppository can be effective [4].

10.5 Chemotherapy-Induced Urinary Toxicity

The major excretion route of many anticancer drugs and metabolites is the urinary system. Thus, patients receiving anticancer therapy may have kidney or urinary bladder complications. Chemotherapy-induced urinary toxicity has various clinical features, from asymptomatic proteinuria and renal function disorder to life-threatening renal failure. Hemodialysis must be conducted in an emergency condition, when body fluid and electrolyte control is fatal due to renal function disorder.

10.5.1 Cisplatin-Induced Nephrotoxicity

Cisplatin is the most widely known anticancer drug that causes nephrotoxicity. It is a strong cytotoxin that directly damages the proximal tubule and decreases the glomerular filtration rate. It also contributes to nephrotoxicity by decreasing the renal blood flow because it contracts the renal microvasculature and increases inflammatory cytokines such as TNF-α, IL-6, and IFN-γ. Cisplatin-induced nephrotoxicity becomes more severe according to the dosage and frequency of the cisplatin administration, and may become irreversible.

To prevent cisplatin-induced nephrotoxicity, the massive hydration with normal saline is recommended to maintain more than 100 ml of urine per hour. Mannitol or furosemide is sometimes used with cisplatin to induce forced diuresis, but this has no clear evidence. Carboplatin, a cisplatin analogue, can be used for patients with decreased renal function because it has low nephrotoxicity. It can be used instead of cisplatin in cancer patients, for which they are known to have similar treatment effects [5].

10.5.2 Hemorrhagic Cystitis

Hemorrhagic cystitis is commonly observed when using cyclophosphamide or ifosfamide. Acrolein, which is formed during the drug metabolism, damages urinary epithelial cells, causing hematuria, stimulant voiding syndrome, urinary bladder fibrosis, vesicoureteral reflux, etc. The incidence of hemorrhagic cystitis is 20–40 %, but up to 60–70 % has been reported after stem cell transplantation. Mesna is used as a preventive drug for hemorrhagic cystitis. It is a sulfhydryl compound that binds with acrolein in the urinary system and blocks epithelial damage due to acrolein. From several studies conducted in the early 1980s, it was reported that hemorrhagic cystitis can be prevented when mesna, including cyclophosphamide or ifosfamide, is added to chemotherapy.

Currently, when cyclophosphamide or ifosfamide is used in chemotherapy, it is recommended that mesna be administered right before (or simultaneously with) the anticancer drug with more than a 20 % dose, and that it be repeatedly administered every 4–8 h. Mesna can effectively detoxicate cyclophosphamide or ifosfamide, but does not influence the therapeutic efficacies of these drugs [6, 7].

10.5.3 Nephrotoxicity of Targeted Agents

Bevacizumab (Avastin), an antibody for VEGF (vascular endothelial growth factor), and sunitinib, sorafenib, pazopanib, and axitinib, which are small molecular tyrosine kinase inhibitors for the VEGF receptor, can cause proteinuria in 10–20 % of patients. The mechanism behind this is not fully understood, but it is assumed to be caused by vascular endothelial cell damage in the kidney. When the proteinuria induces clinical symptoms and is Grade 3 or 4, the drug administration must be suspended or reduced. These drugs have also been reported to cause thrombotic microangiopathy.

10.6 Chemotherapy-Induced Pulmonary Toxicity

10.6.1 Bleomycin-Induced Pulmonary Fibrosis

Pulmonary fibrosis appears in up to 10 % of patients using bleomycin. It is a serious complication that can be life-threatening. Bleomycin induces chromosomal damage through DNA cleavage. Bleomycin lyase is inactivated in the lung and skin, so the toxic effect of bleomycin is more severe in the lung, causing lung damage.

This pulmonary fibrosis symptom is more easily induced when a high dose of bleomycin is used, when the dose of combined bleomycin and cisplatin is high, when a high concentration of oxygen is inhaled, and when there is renal failure. Bleomycin-induced pulmonary fibrosis often progresses gradually 1–6 months after the initial drug administration, but some patients can experience acute chest pain syndrome. When bleomycin-induced pulmonary damage is strongly suspected, the drug administration should be suspended, and its re-administration is not recommended when the pulmonary fibrosis is confirmed. Corticosteroids are known to temporarily relieve the symptoms of pulmonary fibrosis, but their long-term effect has not been proven yet [8].

10.7 Chemotherapy-Induced Neurotoxicity

Neurotoxicity is a common side effect of anticancer drugs. Chemotherapy-induced neurotoxicity is increasing as patients are surviving longer due to the good treatment results of cancer patients [9, 10].

10.7.1 Platinum-Induced Neurotoxicity

Cisplatin is one of the drugs that commonly induce neurotoxicity. Cisplatin damages the peripheral nerves and induces numbness and pain in the fingers and toes, which progress to the arms and legs. When neurotoxicity occurs, the cisplatin dose must be reduced or delayed, because there is no effective treatment for this condition. Cisplatin also damages the cochlear epithelial cells, inducing a volume-dependent high incidence of sensorineural hearing loss.

Another platinum-based anticancer drug, oxaliplatin, induces acute neuropathy and cumulative neuropathy. Acute neuropathy is dysesthesia in the hands, feet, near the mouth, neck, etc., which worsens when exposed to the cold. Rarely can it cause seizure, voice change, ptosis, and visual field disorder. In such cases, the symptoms can be relieved by extending the oxaliplatin infusion time from 2 to 6 h. The cumulative neuropathy through oxaliplatin use is peripheral sensory neuropathy, accompanied by pain or function disorder. When symptoms of the condition occur, the oxaliplatin dose must be reduced or suspended [5, 9, 10].

10.7.2 Methotrexate-Induced Neurotoxicity

Aseptic meningitis is common in methotrexate-induced neurotoxicity, which can occur after intrathecal administration of methotrexate. This is accompanied by a headache or a neck stiffness, nausea and vomiting, and fever, usually occurs 2–4 h after the drug infusion, and can last up to 72 h. Most of the symptoms are self-limited and can be prevented through simultaneous intrathecal administration of steroids [9, 10].

10.7.3 Taxane-Induced Neurotoxicity

Taxanes, such as paclitaxel and docetaxel, induce sensory neuropathy accompanied by a burning sensation in the hands or feet or reflex loss, and may sometimes cause motor neuropathy in the proximal muscles. These symptoms depend on the cumulative drug dose or treatment schedule, and mostly improve by reducing the dose or delaying the treatment schedule [9–11].

10.8 Cardiotoxicity

10.8.1 Chemotherapy-Induced Cardiotoxicity

Long-term chemotherapy can cause cardiotoxicity. The resulting heart failure, myocardical infection, arrhythmia, etc. are serious complications that could affect the cancer patient's life expectancy. The incidence of cardiotoxicity is influenced by several factors, the more important of which are the type of anticancer drug, the dose used in each cycle, the cumulative dose, the administration route, and the combination with other drugs or radiotherapy. Also, cardiotoxicity can be affected if the patient has risk factors or a history of cardiovascular diseases or of radiotherapy [12].

10.8.2 Anthracycline-Induced Cardiotoxicity

The incidence of myocardial damage with the use of anthracycline is determined by the type of drug and its cumulative dose. Doxorubicin is well-known to increase the incidence of cardiotoxicity by as much as 4–36 % when its cumulative dose is higher than 500–550 mg/m^2 (Fig. 10.3), although epirubicin or idarubicin can also induce cardiotoxicity, albeit at a lower rate. Anthracycline-induced cardiotoxicity is caused by myocardial damage from the increase in oxygen radicals and oxidation stress. Myocardial damage induces lipid peroxidation and death of the cell membrane, which irreversibly damage the myocardial tissue [12, 13].

There are three types of anthracycline-induced cardiotoxicity. Acute toxicity (incidence: 1 %) occurs immediately after the drug administration. Early-onset chronic toxicity (incidence: 1.6–2.1 %) occurs within 1 year following the drug administration. Late-onset chronic toxicity occurs a year after the drug administration and progresses to dilated cardiomyopathy, but it can appear as late as 10–30 years after the initial administration of anthracycline. The severity of myocardial toxicity varies, from an asymptomatic decrease in the left ventricular ejection fraction to irreversible and fatal heart failure [13].

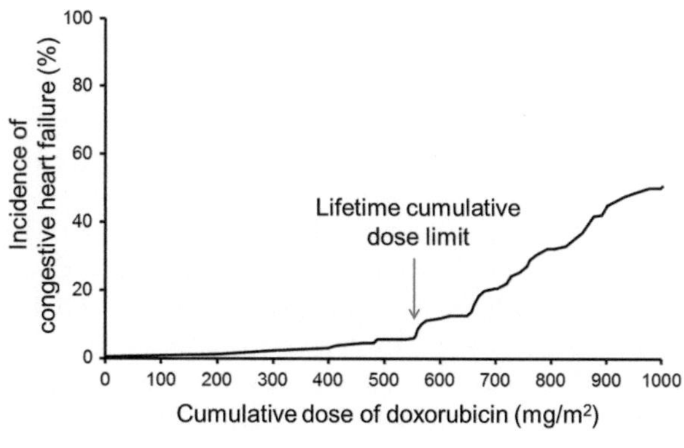

Fig. 10.3 Doxorubicin induced cardiotoxicity

To prevent and decrease the risk of anthracycline-induced cardiotoxicity, the total cumulative dose of anthracyclines must be kept below the recommended dose, and cardiac disorders must be detected in advance through regular heart function tests. In addition, there is a report that continuous infusion of antracycline rather than bolus injection can help prevent cardiotoxicity, but this is still controversial. Liposome forms of doxorubicin and daunorubicin have lower cardiotoxicity with the same efficacy, so an increase in their cumulative dose is possible [13].

Dexrazoxane (Cardioxane) is an EDTA derivative discovered by K. Hellimann in 1972. It was found to reduce the formation of oxygen radicals and protect the myocardium by chelating metal ions and block complex formation with anthracycline. Thus, its use to prevent the cardiotoxicity in cancer patients using doxorubicin was approved by the FDA in 1995. However, additional studies showed that dexrazoxane may be related to the incidence of secondary cancer in pediatric cancer patients; so in 2011, the FDA changed the drug indications to only adult breast cancer, and the drug dose to a cumulative dose of higher than 300 mg/m^2 of doxorubicin or higher than 540 mg/m^2 of epirubicin [12, 13].

10.9 Chemotherapy-Induced Oral Mucositis

Oral mucositis is a common complication of chemotherapy, especially of high-dose chemotherapy, in one-third to one-half of patients. It is experienced by almost all patients receiving radiotherapy in the head and neck [14].

10.9.1 Pathogenesis and Clinical Features

Chemotherapy or radiotherapy induces direct damage of the oral mucosal cell. Reactive oxygen species are important in this process. Early damage promotes inflammatory cytokine secretion, which damages the surrounding tissue, induces loss of the mucosal integrity, and forms a painful ulcerative lesion, thereby inducing secondary bacterial infection [14].

10.9.2 Prevention and Treatment

To prevent oral infection, the oral condition must be thoroughly inspected and appropriate dental treatment must be conducted before chemotherapy. Cryotherapy, by holding ice in the mouth 5 minutes before to 30 minutes after 5-fluorouracil bolus injection, is known to decrease the incidence and severity of stomatitis. Palifermin (Kepivance) is a recombinant keratinocyte growth factor that promotes the proliferation and differentiation of gastrointestinal epithelial cells. In the early

2000s, randomized clinical trials were conducted to confirm the effect of palifermin. It was shown to decrease the incidence and duration of severe stomatitis in patients with hematologic malignancies receiving high-dose chemotherapy and whole-body radiation before autologous hematopoietic stem cell transplantation. Based on these results, the FDA approved in 2004 the use of palifermin for patients with hematologic malignancies [14].

10.10 Anorexia

Anorexia and its resulting cachexia are common conditions experienced by more than 80 % of progressive cancer patients. The causes of anorexia are gastrointestinal obstruction and loss of appetite due to cancer, and systemic effects of chemotherapy. Malnutrition can directly affect cancer treatment outcome and increase the toxicity of chemotherapy. The 2-year survival rate of cancer patients with more than 4 % weight loss is 72 %, and the 3-year survival rate is less than 65 %.

In the 1970s, there was a clinical study in which the corticosteroid dexamethasone was used to improve the appetite of cancer patients. An improvement in the appetite was reported, but with significant weight gain. Enteral and tube feeding can increase the calorie supply of patients, but it is not cost- and time-effective. Besides, a randomized clinical study in the 1980s revealed that enteral and tube feeding did not improve the long-term nutritional state of patients [15].

Megestrol acetate is a progesterone derivative originally developed for hormone therapy of breast cancer patients. However, an unexpected side effect, weight gain, was reported from a clinical study in the 1980s. The mechanism of megestrol is not yet clearly known, but it is known to promote neuropeptide Y secretion from the hypothalamus, regulate calcium channels in the ventromedial hypothalamus, and suppress the secretion of cytokines that affect the appetite, such as IL-1a, IL-1b, IL-6, and TNF-α. In several randomized clinical studies conducted in the early 1990s, megestrol acetate was found to increase the appetite and cause weight gain in cancer patient with cachexia, which led to its FDA approval in 1994 and its current wide use [15].

10.11 Tumor Lysis Syndrome

Tumor lysis syndrome is a s metabolic disorder induced by massive lysis of tumor cells and subsequent release of intracellular molecules during chemotherapy. Tumor lysis syndrome usually occurs when proliferation rate of tumor is very fast, the tumor mass is bulky, and the response to anticancer drug is very good. Hexane, protein, phosphate, potassium, and calcium are the materials released when a cell dies, and they can cause hyperuricemia, hyperkalemia, hyperphosphatemia, hypercalcemia, and uremia. Especially, uric acid or calcium phosphate damages the renal tubule and causes renal failure, and may lead to death.

Table 10.2 Risk factor for Tumor lysis syndrome

	Risk factors
Tumor type	Burkitt's lymphoma Lymphoblastic lymphoma Diffuse large-cell lymphoma Acute lymphoblastic leukemia Solid tumors with high proliferation and rapid response to treatment
Extent of disease	High tumor burden (>10 cm) elevated LDH level (>twice the upper limit of normal) Leukocytosis (>25,000/μl)
Renal function	Pre-existing renal dysfunction, Dehydration
Uric acid	Elevated pre-treatment uric acid >7.5 ml/dL (450 μmol/L)

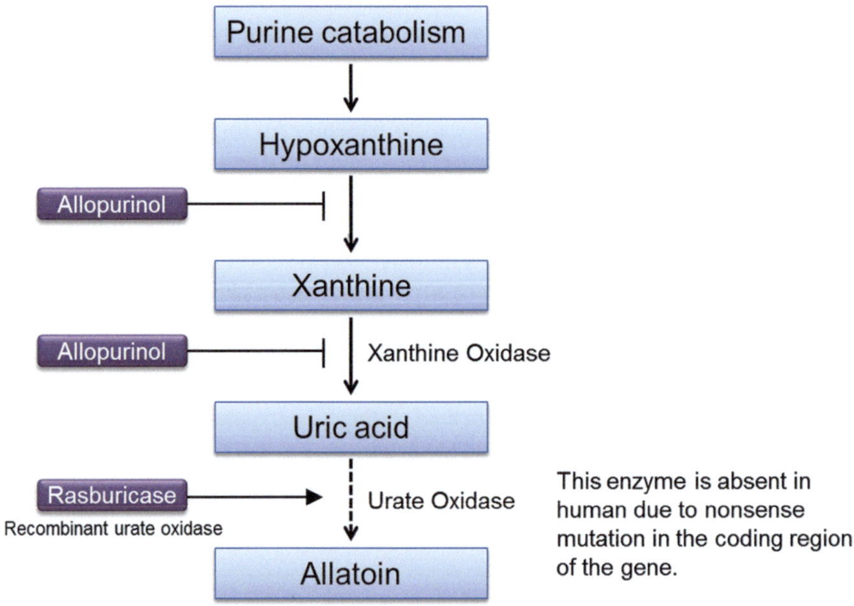

Fig. 10.4 Purine catabolism pathway and targeting durgs

Hematologic malignancies, such as Burkitt's lymphoma, solid tumors with a rapid proliferation rate, tumors larger than 10 cm, a high LDH level or white blood cell count, and underlying renal failure are some of the risk factors of this syndrome (Table 10.2) [16].

Management of hyperuricemia is the most important treatment of tumor lysis syndrome. Allopurinol has been used traditionally to prevent this disease. Cellular purine is catabolized to hypoxanthine and xanthine after its metabolism, and metabolized to uric acid by xanthine oxidase. Allopurinol suppresses this xanthine oxidase and blocks the synthesis of uric acid (Fig. 10.4). Therefore, allopurinol suppresses the synthesis of new uric acid but cannot degrade the pre-existing uric acid. In addition, a high accumulated concentration of hypoxanthine and xanthine can cause nephrotoxicity when allopurinol is given [16, 17].

Rasburicase (Elitek), a recombinant urico-oxidase, was formulated to catabolize uric acid in hyperuricemia. Many mammals, excluding humans, have urico-oxidase, which catabolize uric acid to allantoin. This enzyme is absent in humans because they have nonsense mutation in the coding region of this gene. Rasburicase is a recombinant protein obtained by expressing a cloned urico-oxidase from Aspergillus flavus in yeast. In a randomized clinical study reported in 2007, a dramatic decrease in uric acid was shown within 4 h after rasburicase administration. Based on this result, the FDA approved the use of rasburicase in 2009 for patients receiving chemotherapy with hyperuricemia or a high risk of hyperuricemia [17]. Currently, it is recommended that adequate hydration and allopurinol be given at the start of anticancer therapy for patients with a moderate risk of tumor lysis syndrome, and that rasburicase administration be considered when hyperuricemia occurs. For high-risk patients, rasburicase should be given together with the treatment [16, 17].

10.12 Extravasation of Anticancer Drugs

10.12.1 Skin Irritation from Extravasation of Anticancer Drugs

Extravasation is the leakage or penetration of anticancer drugs from blood vessels into the surrounding subcutaneous tissue. Irritant drugs induce pain or inflammation near the extravasation site, and vesicant drugs induce tissue necrosis and exuviation. Table 10.3 shows the drugs with side effects through extravasation [18].

10.12.2 Treatment of Extravasation

Several therapies have been attempted to block the necrosis in the extravasation site, but there has been no proper randomized clinical study including a control group. This is due to the small number of patients and the ethical issues of the placebo group during the conduct of a randomized trial.

Discovering the extravasation as soon as possible and holding the drug administration are most important in treating extravasation. The next step is to remove the remaining anticancer drug near the extravasation site as quickly as possible. Several institutions have presented various antidotes up to now, but most are ineffective, and reports show that they even increase the damage in the extravasation site. Application or local injection of corticosteroid in the extravasation site is not recommended, because it has shown many conflicting results. According to a study conducted in 1988, hypodermic injection of sodium thiosulfate is effective for the extravasation of

Table 10.3 Drugs with side effects through extravasation

Vesicants	Irritants
Alkylating agent Mechlorethamine Bendamustine	Alkylating agents Carmustine Ifosfamide Dacarbazine Melphalan
Anthracyclines Doxorubicin Daunorubicin Epirubicin Idarubicin	Anthracyclines Liposomal doxorubicin Liposomal daunorubicin
Antibiotics Dactinomycin Mitomycin C Mitoxantrone	Topoisomerase II inhibitor Etoposide Teniposide
Vinka alkaloids Vincristine Vinblastine Vinorelbine	Antimetabolites Fluorouracil
	Topoisomerase I inhibitor Irinotecan Topotecan
Taxanes Docetaxel Paclitaxel	Platinums Carboplatin Cisplatin Oxaliplatin

mechlorethamine. The application of DMSO to the extravasation site is a treatment option when there is extravasation of anthracycline, mitomycin C, or platinum. Dexrazoxane has the effect of reducing oxygen radicals, which substantially reduces the skin necrosis site through anthracycline extravasation in animal models, and also effectively prevented skin damage due to anthracycline in two prospective studies. Based on these results, the FDA approved the use of dexrazoxane for the extravasation of anthracycline. Surgical debridement is recommended if the necrosis through extravasation progresses and the pain cannot be controlled. Surgical treatment includes surgical removal of the extravasated skin, dressing, and skin graft. It has been reported that about one-third of patients with extravasation need surgical treatment [18].

10.13 Chemotherapy-Induced Skin Toxicity

10.13.1 Hyperpigmentation

Hyperpigmentation is a common complication of anticancer drugs. It is caused by many drugs, including fluoropyrimidine, doxorubicin, and platinum. It can be induced locally or systematically in the skin and mucosa. It often improves after suspending the drug administration [19].

10.13.2 Nail Change

Anticancer drugs can cause a nail change. Most prominently, paclitaxel or docetaxel causes inflammation of the nail base. This is also present in the use of fluoropyrimidine, doxorubicin, and cyclophosphamide [19].

10.13.3 Hand-Foot Syndrome (Palmar-Plantar Erythrodysesthesia)

Hand-foot syndrome can be caused by capecitabine, 5-fluorouracil, and doxorubicin. First, the patient's palms and soles become numb. This leads to erythema with tenderness, and in serious cases, there may be vesicles or desquamation. The application of moisturizing cream and the avoidance of friction or pressure on the palms and soles are needed to prevent hand-foot syndrome. When symptoms occur, it is also helpful to reduce the drug dosage or to increase the drug administration intervals. Most cases of hand-foot syndrome are treated within a month when the drug administration is suspended.

Hand-foot syndrome can also be caused by the targeting agents sunitinib or sorafenib, which show slightly different clinical features. Hand-foot syndrome caused by targeting agents may be accompanied by numbness, sensitivity to pain and heat, and paresthesia [20].

10.13.4 Acneiform Eruption

Acneiform eruption is common in patients using gefitinib (Iressa) and erlotinib (Tarceva), which are epidermal growth factor receptor tyrosine kinase inhibitors, and cetuximab (Erbitux), which is a monoclonal antibody for epidermal growth factors.

Papules and pustules that accompany a rash are the common symptoms, which form within one week of the drug administration and become most severe on the second week. They mostly develop on the face, scalp, and neck, and improve when the administration of the causative drug is hold.

The treatment of acneiform eruption is similar to that of acne or folliculitis: i.e., by taking doxycyclin or minocyclin and using isotretinoin [19].

References

1. Hesketh PJ (2008) Chemotherapy-induced nausea and vomiting. N Engl J Med 358: 2482–2494
2. Daniel D, Crawford J (2006) Myelotoxicity from chemotherapy. Semin Oncol 33:74–85, Elsevier

3. Aapro M, Bohlius J, Cameron D et al (2012) 2010 update of EORTC guidelines for the use of granulocyte-colony stimulating factor to reduce the incidence of chemotherapy-induced febrile neutropenia in adult patients with lymphoproliferative disorders and solid tumours. Eur J Cancer 47:8–32
4. Gibson RJ, Keefe DM (2006) Cancer chemotherapy-induced diarrhea and constipation: mechanisms of damage and prevention strategies. Support Care Cancer 14:890–900
5. Hartmann JT, Lipp HP (2003) Toxicity of platinum compounds. Expert Opin Pharmacother 4:889–901
6. Meisenberg B, Lassiter M, Hussein A et al (1994) Prevention of hemorrhagic cystitis after high-dose alkylating agent chemotherapy and autologous bone marrow support. Bone Marrow Transplant 14:287–291
7. Luce JK, Simons JA (1988) Efficacy of mesna in preventing further cyclophosphamide-Induced hemorrhagic cystitis. Med Pediatr Oncol 16:372–374
8. Catane R, Schwade JG, Turrisi AT III et al (1979) Pulmonary toxicity after radiation and bleomycin: a review. Int J Radiat Oncol Biol Phys 5:1513–1518
9. Park S, Krishnan A, Lin C et al (2008) Mechanisms underlying chemotherapy-induced neurotoxicity and the potential for neuroprotective strategies. Curr Med Chem 15:3081–3094
10. Argyriou AA, Bruna J, Marmiroli P et al (2012) Chemotherapy-induced peripheral neurotoxicity (CIPN): an update. Crit Rev Oncol Hematol 82:51–77
11. Lee JJ, Swain SM (2006) Peripheral neuropathy induced by microtubule-stabilizing agents. J Clin Oncol 24:1633–1642
12. Bovelli D, Plataniotis G, Roila F (2010) Cardiotoxicity of chemotherapeutic agents and radiotherapy-related heart disease: ESMO Clinical Practice Guidelines. Ann Oncol 21: 277–282
13. Shan K, Lincoff AM, Young JB (1996) Anthracycline-induced cardiotoxicity. Ann Intern Med 125:47–58
14. Keefe DM, Schubert MM, Elting LS et al (2007) Updated clinical practice guidelines for the prevention and treatment of mucositis. Cancer 109:820–831
15. Bruera E, Macmillan K, Kuehn N et al (1990) A controlled trial of megestrol acetate on appetite, caloric intake, nutritional status, and other symptoms in patients with advanced cancer. Cancer 66:1279–1282
16. Coiffier B, Altman A, Pui CH et al (2008) Guidelines for the management of pediatric and adult tumor lysis syndrome: an evidence-based review. J Clin Oncol 26:2767–2778
17. Cortes J, Moore JO, Maziarz RT et al (2010) Control of plasma uric acid in adults at risk for tumor lysis syndrome: efficacy and safety of rasburicase alone and rasburicase followed by allopurinol compared with allopurinol alone-results of a multicenter phase III study. J Clin Oncol 28:4207–4213
18. Fidalgo JP, Fabregat LG, Cervantes A et al (2012) Management of chemotherapy extravasation: ESMO-EONS Clinical Practice Guidelines. Ann Oncol 23:167–173
19. Huang V, Anadkat M (2011) Dermatologic manifestations of cytotoxic therapy. Dermatol Ther 24:401–410
20. Janusch M, Fischer M, Marsch W et al (2006) The hand-foot syndrome-a frequent secondary manifestation in antineoplastic chemotherapy. Eur J Dermatol 16:494–499, 382

Part III
A Paradigm Shift in Cancer Research

Chapter 11
Advancements in Bioscience and New Cancer Drugs

11.1 Development of Cancer Drugs According to Scientific Advancements

The parallel development of life science and cancer treatment after the introduction of the cell theory in 1838 can be briefly summarized as shown in Fig. 11.1. In the mid-1850s, cancer entered the field of science after being designated as neoplasm, which is defined as a new mass of cells created from the division of tumor cells.

Among the three representative modalities of cancer treatments, surgery has progressed as the primary treatment modality beginning from the radical mastectomy in 1889 for breast cancer to the supraradical mastectomy in the 1950s and the ultra-radical mastectomy in the 1960s. The second treatment modality is radiotherapy, which began in 1896 and has progressed to high-dose radiotherapy. The third mode, chemotherapy, has become a conventional treatment option since 1948, appearing as the universal treatment for all types of cancer under the hypothesis that cancer is an abnormal proliferation of cancer cells. Chemotherapy has also advanced to its maximum therapeutic efficacy as high-dose combination chemotherapy in the 1960s and ultra-high-dose combination chemotherapy in the 1980s. However, these concepts of maximum dose combination therapy ceased after clinical data showed that they were not superior compared to conventional dose chemotherapy in the treatment of metastatic solid tumors.

The limitations of cancer treatments are exemplified by the characteristic spread of cancer in the 1960s-1980s and the statistical data of studies referring to cancer prevention. Basic research at the molecular level of cancer cells, which is the basis of tumor heterogeneity, became extensive in 1980–2000 and identified the fundamental differences between cancer cells and normal cells. A molecular understanding of these differences, as shown in Fig. 11.2, resulted in the development of molecular-targeted treatments [1].

Because these molecular targets are mainly based on differences in genomic information among cancer patients, personalized cancer therapy is expected to be implemented in the near future owing to the technology which will enable rapid and

K.-W. Kim et al., *Cancer Drug Discovery*, DOI 10.1007/978-94-024-0844-7_11

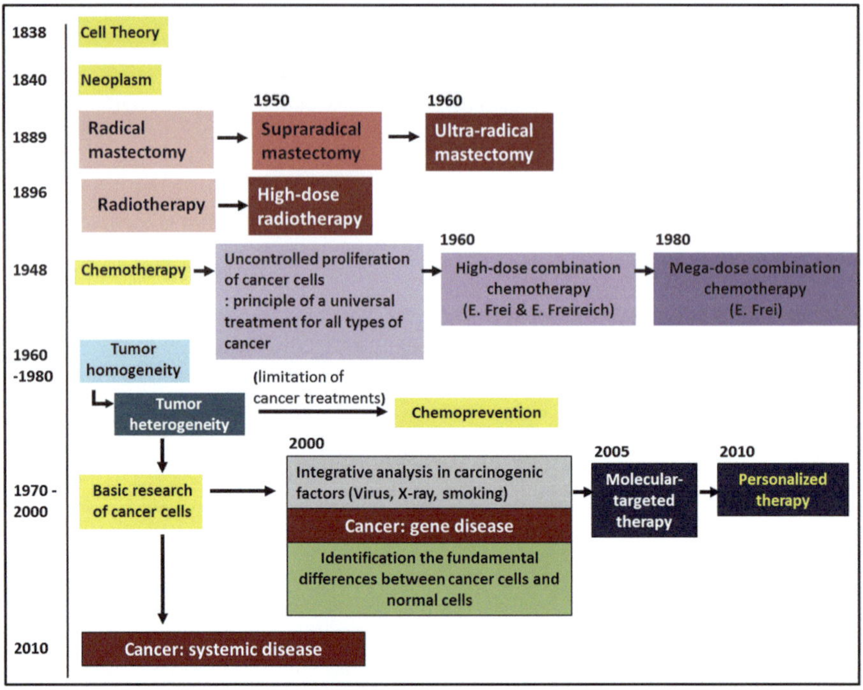

Fig. 11.1 Advancement of cancer therapy

Fig. 11.2 The differences between normal cells and the cancer cells

1980-2000, Understanding of the fundamental differences between cancer cells and normal cells

Normal cells	Cancer cells
Contact inhibition	No Contact inhibition
Controlled growth	Uncontrolled growth
Specialized cells	Nonspecialized cells
Normal chromosomes	Abnormal chromosomes
Undergo apoptosis	No apoptosis
Even appearance	Variable appearance
Stay in organ	Ability to metastasize
Undergo maturation and senescence	Immature/undifferentiated

accurate genomic analysis. In addition, molecular profiles of cancer patients will be precisely analyzed and will result in the revision of classical histology-based cancer classification, enabling precision oncology.

In addition, a new concept regarding cancer has been proposed: cancer is a systemic disease involving various normal cells within tumor microenvironments,

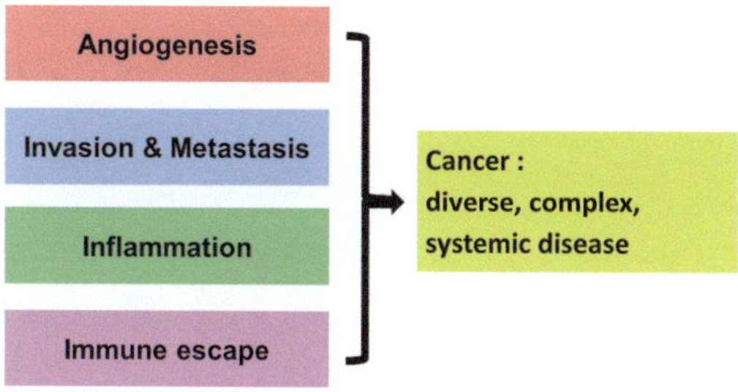

Fig. 11.3 Cancer is a diverse, complex, and systemic disease

such as the vascular system, lymphatic system, and immune system (Fig. 11.3). Thus, the development of cancer treatments based on this new concept will be pursued in the future.

11.2 New Anticancer Drugs

11.2.1 Development of Novel Targeted Agents

As previously described, most of the anticancer drugs currently used lead to inhibition of cell division. However, molecular targeted agents recently emerged and are based on extensive knowledge from the past 30 years of basic research on cancer cells as to how cellular metabolic pathways and signal transduction pathways differ between normal and cancer cells. Previous cytotoxic anticancer drugs suppressed the division of both cancer and normal cells by blocking the general mechanism of cell division, inducing various side effects. However, recent molecular targeted agents – for example, targeting signaling factors – differentiate normal cells by targeting signal transduction pathways related to cancer cell division and attempt to normalize its function. Such agents target the specific abnormal signaling factor in cancer cells rather than the general targeting associated with previous anticancer drugs and thus have been proposed to act more specifically on cancer cells. Among the target sites of the 160 anticancer drugs described in Chaps. 4–9, up to 80 % are focused on cancer cells, and most of the targets are metabolic pathways and signal transduction pathways related to cancer cell division, as shown in Fig. 11.4. The remaining 20 % of anticancer drugs target the other components, such as immune cells and endothelial cells. A detailed look at 80 % of anticancer drugs shows that alkylating agents act directly on DNA by suppressing cell proliferation, and antimetabolites act on the biosynthesis of nucleic acids, such as DNA and RNA. In addition, hormonal agents act on intracellular hormone receptors, such as estrogen or progesterone receptors, whereas plant alkaloids and antibiotics mainly act on microtubules and DNA topoisomerase. Many of the recently developed targeted agents block the aberrantly activated cell surface receptor tyrosine kinase (RTK), such as EGFR and HER2. The targeted anticancer drugs for these proteins were developed based on technologies such as monoclonal antibodies, DNA sequencing,

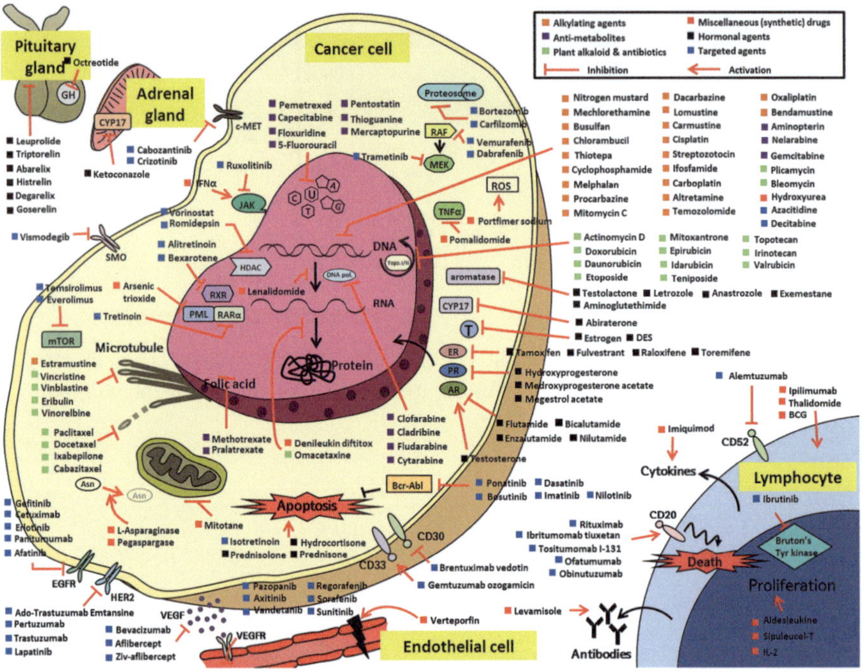

Fig. 11.4 Cancer drugs developed up to the present and their targets

and PCR, which were intensively developed in the 1970s to the 1980s. The following future studies will further develop targeted agents using these technologies (Fig. 11.5).

- More studies are expected to investigate how the approximately 500 mutations discovered via cancer genome analyses are involved in carcinogenesis. Some functions of these mutations are partially known, but the development and research of targeted agents that focus on tumors and carcinogenesis will be enhanced with research on the unknown functions of cancer mutations.
- In addition, more than 500 types of kinases are known to transduce proliferative signals of cancer cells; thus, there will be attempts to develop activity regulators of these kinases into anticancer drugs by determining how they contribute to carcinogenesis and studying their functions and molecular structures.
- Bioinformatics studies will continue in the future, which will provide an understanding of carcinogenesis at the molecular level by combining the vast amount of information gained from next generation sequencing. Potential therapeutic targets will also be discovered to identify novel classes of anticancer drugs that suppress carcinogenesis by blocking the essential mechanisms derived from such bioinformatic integrative studies.
- Research will be pursued on the mechanisms underlying cancer resistance to anticancer drugs and how to overcome such resistance. Drug resistance emerges

Future studies

1	**Research on unknown functions of cancer gene mutations**
2	**Analysis of newly identified oncogenic protein kinases**
3	**Integrative analysis in oncogenic signaling pathways**
4	**Research on the anticancer drug resistance**
5	**Molecular classification of cancers and development of personalized anticancer drugs**
6	**Research on the recovery of functional loss of tumor suppressor gene**
7	**Research on the microenvironment of cancer**
8	**Study of cancer stem cells (CSCs)**
9	**Improvement of the disease-free survival of cancer patients**
10	**Study of cancer prevention and development of early cancer diagnosis technologies**

Fig. 11.5 Future studies on cancer research

from the acquisition of new somatic mutations in target molecules or the activation of bypass signaling pathways, and thus, basic and clinical research on the combined use of anticancer drugs to overcome the resistance is necessary.

- In addition, cancer genomic studies reveal that cancer varies from patient to patient. Many more types of tumors will be identified using genomic analyses of cancer patients, and the adapted treatments and appropriate cancer drugs for the newly classified tumor will be developed. The number and location of mutations differ per patient according to the sequencing analysis of the cancer genome, such that anticancer drugs that target oncogenic genes will be personalized and designed optimally based on specific structures of the mutant protein. However, to develop such personalized anticancer drugs, technology that screens genomic mutations in cancer patients and manufacturing technology for different types of anticancer drugs must be developed with clinical validity, clinical utility, and cost-effectiveness. Thus, innovation is highly required in such technologies and much effort and time is required to establish a system for implanting these technologies in patient treatment.
- Currently, these targeted agents mostly suppress or block abnormally activated factors in cancer cells compared to normal cells. Thus, novel anticancer drugs

that restore the lost function of the tumor suppressor gene can be developed. However, recovery of the functional loss of the tumor suppressor protein is very difficult. Accordingly, the development of corresponding anticancer drugs may require a long time and many efforts. In addition, the cost of treatment per patient might rise considerably.

- The microenvironment of cancer includes various types of normal cells. Thus, research is required on cells that surround the cancer and constitute the microenvironment. The aforementioned diverse types of surrounding cells, such as fibroblasts, macrophages, endothelial cells, pericytes, and immune cells, will be studied in detail to understand how they are involved in carcinogenesis.
- In addition to the cancer-surrounding cells, recent studies have identified cancer stem cells (CSCs) in the cancer tissue. CSCs contribute to tumor progression and metastasis and confer drug resistance. Thus, investigations on how CSCs are formed and maintained and in-depth studies regarding CSC characteristics are required.
- From the perspective that cures for cancer are extremely difficult because of CSCs, treatments that improve the disease-free survival of cancer patients will be developed rather than focusing on complete eradication.
- To increase the survival rate of cancer patients, greater interest and effort in cancer prevention and the development of cancer prevention drugs are required, in addition to the innovation of cancer treatments. For example, drugs that can efficiently inhibit chronic inflammation involved in carcinogenesis may block the malignant transformation of precancerous lesions and may be used as cancer preventive agents. In addition, the activation of various chemicals in the 12 core pathways known in cancer genomic research can be used to test carcinogenicity. Moreover, the combination of molecular epidemiology with traditional epidemiology will help to identify such pathways, followed by studies on carcinogens according to differences in ethnicity, groups, social classes and regions. Furthermore, cancer screening analyses and early cancer diagnostic technologies based on individual gene mutations will become an important issue.

11.2.2 Future Research Prospects According to the Paradigm Shift

11.2.2.1 Necessity of Tissue-Specific Cell Network Research

"What is true for *E. coli* is also true for the elephant." This quote by J. Monod in 1954, when molecular biology studies began in earnest, is still valid today at the molecular level, but the expanded knowledge today indicates that multicellular organisms rely on biological phenomena that are non-existent in unicellular organisms. The multicellular life phenomena exist in tissues or organs that are aggregates of cells which constitute specialized systems, such as the circulatory system, nervous system, and immune system. Furthermore, defects and functional disorders of

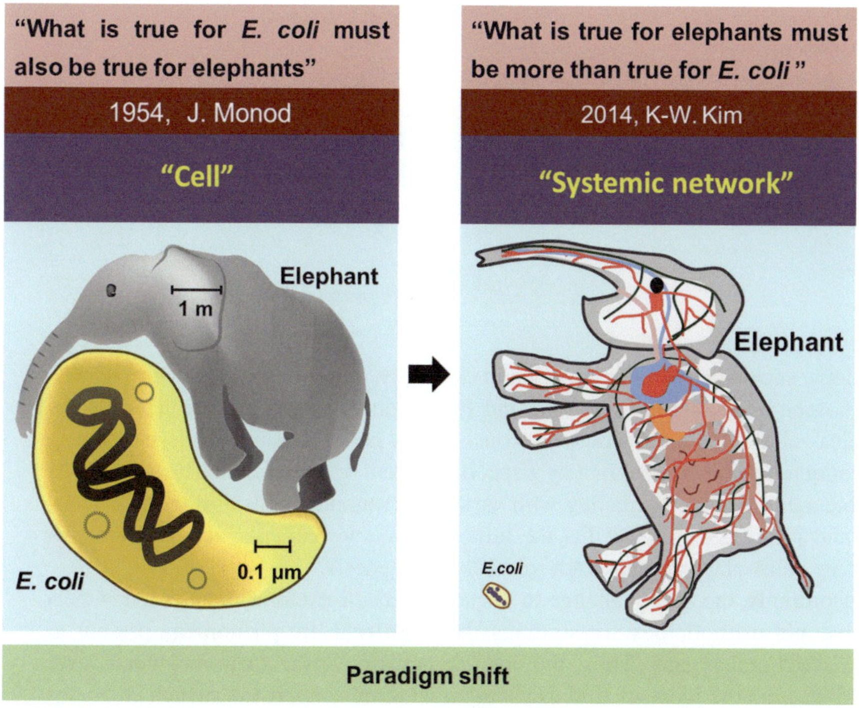

Fig. 11.6 Paradigm shift from studying cells to studying systemic cell network

these systems are closely related to the diseases of multicellular organism. Therefore, the understanding of life phenomena has changed over the last 60 years, as shown in Fig. 11.6. In this regard, cancer can be considered as a systemic disorder, because malignant cancer causes human death via metastasis through the vascular and lymphatic systems in its advanced stage, so that the fatal symptoms of cancer occur in association with the vascular and lymphatic systems.

Until recently, however, life science has focused on protein and gene functions at the molecular level of a single cell, based on the reductive approach of biochemistry and molecular biology. This method examines various functions of proteins and genes at the molecular or single-cell level without considering the cell-surrounding environment and the interaction between cells. However, this fragmented information cannot adequately explain the complex life phenomenon that occurs in the body with organic interactions between various cells. Multicellular organisms, such as humans, exhibit the emergence of new life phenomena at a superior level through hierarchical systematization (cell-tissue-organ-organism), unlike unicellular organisms. Vertebrates, including humans, strictly rely on the cooperative interaction between various tissues and organs that perform specialized functions to maintain their vital activities. Each tissue performs its unique function through the organic interaction of its various component cells, including specialized cells working in a specific tissue. For example, recent studies have shown that high-level brain

Fig. 11.7 Necessity of integrative approaches

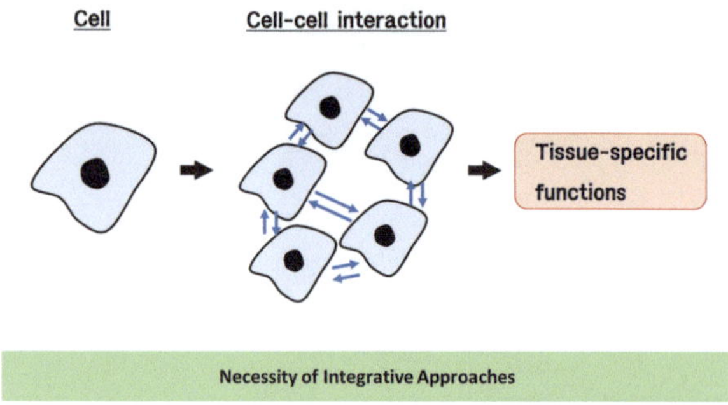

functions, such as learning, memory and creativity, as well as various cerebral disorders, such as Alzheimer's disease and Parkinson's disease, are mediated by the complex cellular interaction network consisting of nerve cells, glia cells, astrocytes, and endothelial cells rather than by a specific protein or gene. Similarly, tumor cells become malignant by interacting with various surrounding cells during tumorigenesis, and it has been shown that the tumor microenvironment, including the surrounding cells, plays an important role in tumorigenesis.

Accordingly, the new challenge to life science is the establishment of a new perspective and methodology for studying the high-level life phenomena present in such tissues and organs. Thus, the cellular network at the meta-molecular level should become the focus of studies using an integrative approach, which emanates from previous reductive approaches, and using changes in the paradigm to study tissue characteristics and functions from the superior level of cells. The cellular level shows a high specificity from the numerous activities accumulated at the molecular level, and thus an understanding of diseases drawn from previous research focused on only molecules is not sufficient to understand systemic diseases. Consequently, new alternatives to overcome these limitations could be provided by studying at the cell network level (Fig. 11.7).

From this point on, studies explaining the interaction network between tissue-specific cells in various tissues and the emergence of tissue specificity because of this cell network are required, as shown in Fig. 11.8.

The tissue-specific cell network plays an important role in integrating and expressing tissue characteristics and functions via unique interactions among various cells [2]. This function differs from division, differentiation, and migration of individual cells at the cellular level; rather, it involves synchronized coordination in the migration, division, and differentiation and the spatiality of various cellular functions of a group of cells. That is, a cell group constitutes a tissue-specific cell network and collectively and covalently shares the division and migration simultaneously at the entire tissue level. This aspect presents a new field of interest and study at the tissue-specific cell network level (Fig. 11.8). The types of tissue-specific cell networks in the body are poorly understood at present but can be classified as follows.

For cells to express their function as tissues in a normal state, they exist in a network that is connected to a single type or multiple types of cells, as shown in Fig. 11.9. Diverse functions are generated according to the type and constitution of

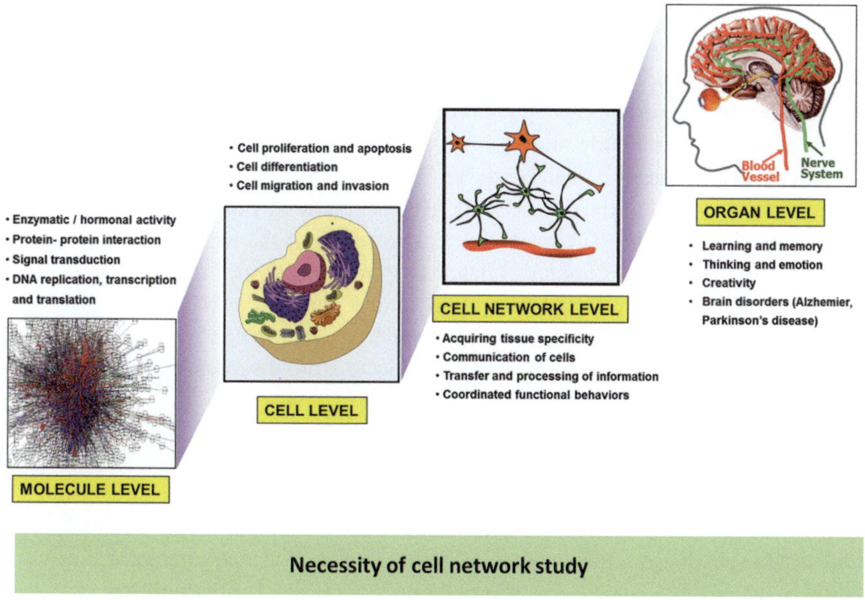

Fig. 11.8 Emergence of tissue specificity via cell-cell network

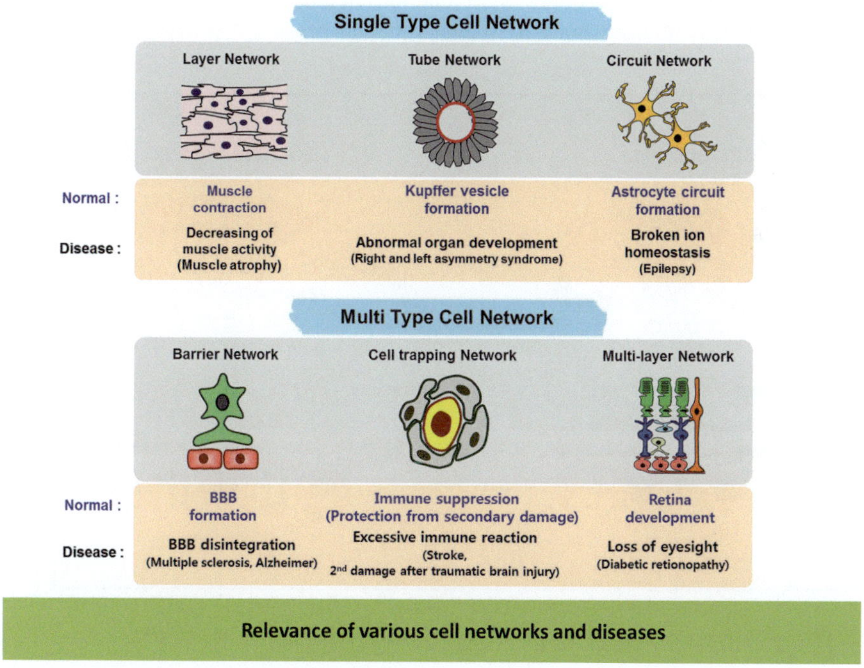

Fig. 11.9 Relevance of various cell networks and diseases

the connected cells. For example, in a single-type cell network, paraxial mesodermal cells, which are a component of a somite, induce myotome formation along the body axis via the overlapping layer. If there is a problem with the network formation because of abnormal overlapping of paraxial mesodermal cells, then disorder of muscle development and body movement results. Another example, Kupffer's Vesicle, which determines the bilateral tissue position of the heart and pancreas of zebrafish, creates a vesicle-type cell network after separation from the nearby ectoderm through cell migration. The asymmetrical secretion of the tissue localization factor from Kupffer's Vesicle induces bilateral asymmetric tissues through ciliary cell movement. Moreover, astrocytes in brain tissues form an astrocyte network, similar to the network observed in nerve cells, and regulate the activity of neural circuits. Cerebral disorders such as epilepsy may occur from disorders in this astrocyte network.

In addition to the single-type cell network, tissue functions are generated through a multi-type cell network (Fig. 11.9). A typical example of a tissue-specific cell network consisting of multi-type cells is the network of blood vessels. Each human blood vessel consists of endothelial cells (ECs), but the same ECs create a completely different tissue-specific vascular system in terms of function and characteristics, depending on which tissue-specific cells form the network (Fig. 11.10). Representative examples are the blood–brain barrier (BBB) in brain tissue and the sinusoid in liver tissues. The BBB can transfer nutrients, such as glucose and amino acids, from blood, but it strictly blocks toxic materials to protect the nervous system of the brain. Thus, cerebrovascular ECs have the strongest tight junctions in the human body and various transport systems [3]. During the BBB developmental process, astrocytes form a

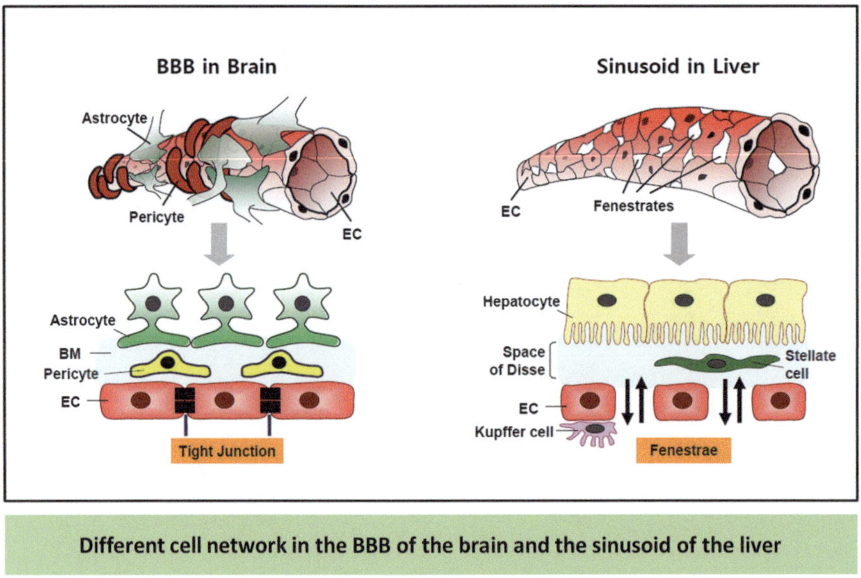

Fig. 11.10 Different cell network in the BBB of the brain and the sinusoid of the liver

network with ECs and induce strong tight junctions between ECs. However, liver tissues form fenestrae between ECs to loosen the cellular adhesion for the active exchange of materials between blood vessels and hepatocytes to supply nutrients to the body after detoxifying the materials at the Space of Disse in the hepatic plate. This creates a perforating vascular structure called a sinusoid, which allows the free exchange of materials. Perforating ECs can also be observed in the intestinal mucosa, endocrine gland, and glomerulus in the kidney and pancreas. A network with liver-specific surrounding cells is expected to be important in the development of perforating ECs, but detailed studies have not yet been performed. Furthermore, recent studies have reported a barrier network of meningeal cells that surrounds the brain in the wound healing process of the central nervous system. The meningeal cells suppress the inflammatory response and recover the meningeal barrier. To protect the brain during the wound healing process, meningeal cells form a specific cell network structure that captures the inflammatory cells derived from blood [4, 5]. In this case, the meningeal cells interact with various inflammatory cells and form a specific and transient cell network. These results indicate that multi-type cells express tissue-specific functions via interacting networks (Fig. 11.9).

Thus, new studies based on the cell network, unlike previous studies at the molecular level, can elucidate how cell networks specifically generate tissues and can determine the tissue-specific functions. These studies can be expanded to introduce a methodology for interpreting the pathogenesis of systemic disorders such as cancer in a novel manner. Currently, few cell networks are known to exist in various human tissues, and thus, various cell networks must be first investigated, and the emergence of new structures and functions at the tissue level via the cell network can then be studied in detail. Subsequently, damage and destruction of the cell network and its recovery during the pathogenesis of disorders such as cancer should be studied so that a new perspective can be proposed on the pathogenesis and treatment of systemic disorders.

11.2.2.2 Development of New Anticancer Drugs by Cell Network Studies

A paradigm shift is required in the study of cancer, particularly in the integrative cell network concept. As previously described, cell division inhibitors and targeted drugs comprise most of the current anticancer drugs, which were developed based on the intracellular characteristics of cancer cells. Since the cell theory was proposed in the nineteenth century, biochemical/molecular biology studies were actively conducted in the 1950s to 1960s, and further extensive studies on the characteristics of the cancer cell were performed in the 1970s to 2000s (Figs. 11.4 and 11.11).

However, these anticancer drugs were not as successful as expected for most solid tumors, and this was discussed at the World Oncology Forum held in Lugano, Switzerland in 2012 (Fig. 11.12) [6]. Current anticancer drugs, including targeted drugs, are not very effective for advanced malignant tumors, except hematological tumors [6]. To overcome the limitations of these current cancer drugs, we must rethink the current cancer research studies.

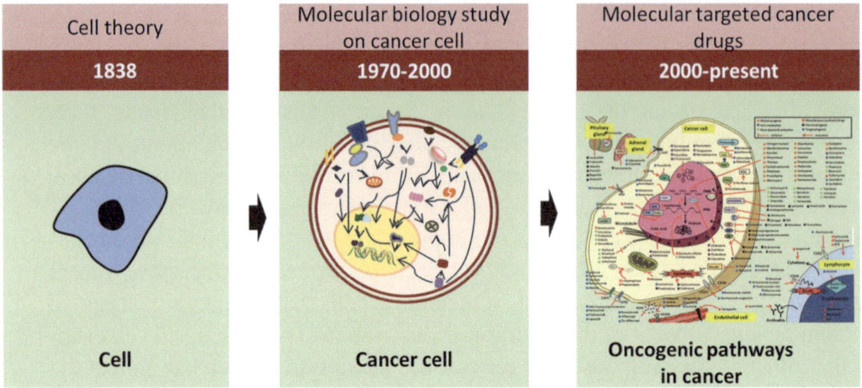

Fig. 11.11 Molecular targeted cancer drugs were developed based on cancer cell study

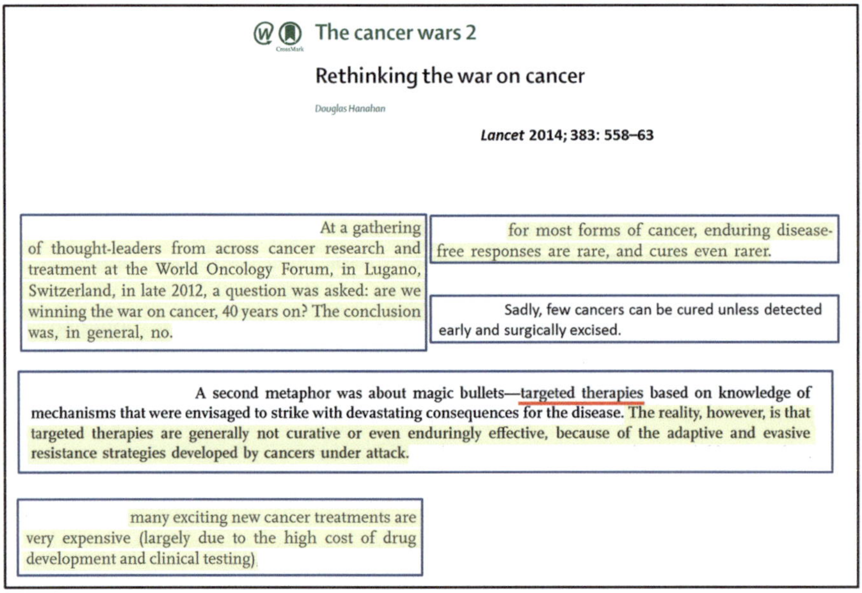
The cancer wars 2

Rethinking the war on cancer

Douglas Hanahan

Lancet 2014; 383: 558–63

At a gathering of thought-leaders from across cancer research and treatment at the World Oncology Forum, in Lugano, Switzerland, in late 2012, a question was asked: are we winning the war on cancer, 40 years on? The conclusion was, in general, no.

for most forms of cancer, enduring disease-free responses are rare, and cures even rarer.

Sadly, few cancers can be cured unless detected early and surgically excised.

A second metaphor was about magic bullets—targeted therapies based on knowledge of mechanisms that were envisaged to strike with devastating consequences for the disease. The reality, however, is that targeted therapies are generally not curative or even enduringly effective, because of the adaptive and evasive resistance strategies developed by cancers under attack.

many exciting new cancer treatments are very expensive (largely due to the high cost of drug development and clinical testing)

Fig. 11.12 Are the current cancer drugs successful?

Currently, cancer research studies are mostly centered on the cell biology and molecular biology of cancer cells. For example, R. A. Weinberg's "A perspective on cancer cell metastasis," published in 2011, focused on cancer cells by explaining that the cancer overcomes the six steps of metastasis via the capability gained by the cancer cell itself (Fig. 11.13) [7].

In Step 1, the cancer cells keep proliferating and acquire invasion capabilities. Step 2 involves the intravasation of the cancer cells, their disassembly of the surrounding extracellular matrix, and their entry into the blood vessel. In Step 3, the

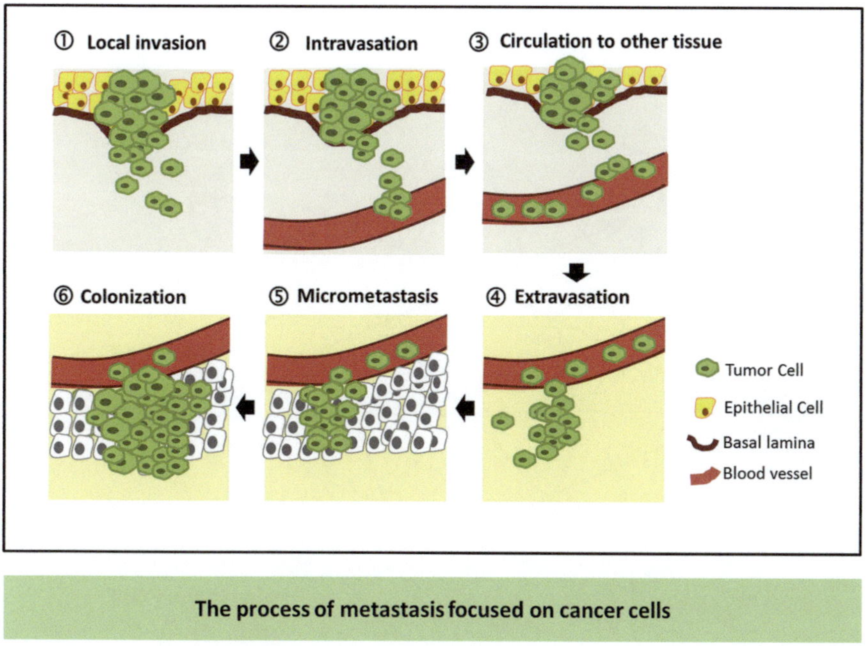

Fig. 11.13 The process of metastasis focused on cancer cells

cancer cells become CTCs in the blood vessel and are capable of surviving without attachment. Step 4 involves extravasation of the cancer cells, their breaking away from blood flow circulation, and their gaining the ability to invade the microenvironment of a new tissue. In Step 5, the cancer cells gain the ability to avoid an innate immune response in new tissues and also become capable of surviving as a single cell (or a small cancer cell mass). In the last step, Step 6, the cancer cells adjust to the new microenvironment and begin to proliferate. This superior ability of cancer cells creates a tumor mass in the new tissue and causes metastasis. This review clearly demonstrates that cancer cells perform the most important role in metastasis, and cancer cells are thought to accomplish metastasis by overcoming several difficulties with their acquired abilities. Thus, until now, many studies have focused on the various abilities acquired by cancer cells during the metastatic process.

However, as mentioned in Chap. 1, cancer characteristics can be divided into the characteristics of the cancer cells themselves and the characteristics from the interaction with the surrounding other cells and the microenvironment. The second type of tumor characteristics arises from the interaction between the cancer cells and their surrounding cells or the tumor environment, resulting in angiogenesis, invasion and metastasis, immune escape, and chronic inflammation. These characteristics are closely related to the systemic characteristics of multicellular organisms. As shown in many recent studies, not only cancer cells but also their tumor microenvironment, including ECs, pericytes, fibroblasts, macrophages, lymphocytes, and extracellular matrices, participate in cancer metastasis (Fig. 11.14). In

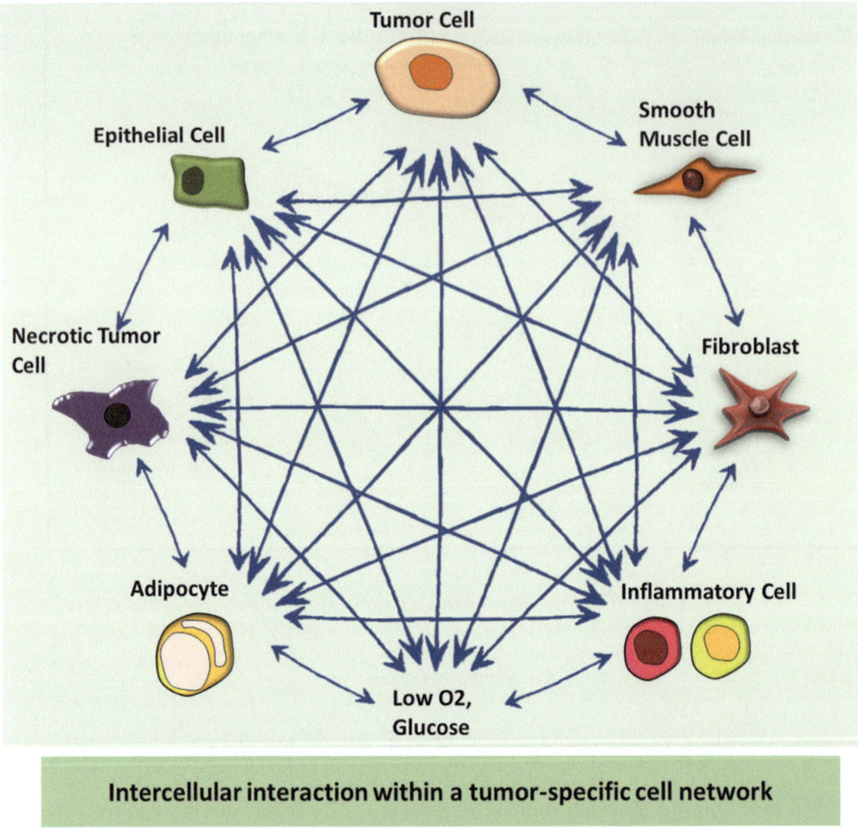

Fig. 11.14 Intercellular interaction within a tumor-specific cell network

addition, this microenvironment includes various factors, such as the oxygen concentration, ROS, blood perfusion, plasma components, cytokines, and growth factors, in addition to the cells. Thus, cancer cells are placed in a constant inflammatory environment caused by the nearby immune cells even during the metastatic process, and they gain not just the ability to escape the host immune system, but they also stimulate the vascular system to create new blood vessels and cause metastasis via the vascular and lymphatic systems.

On the basis of this recently gained knowledge, the tissue-specific cell network concept can be implemented in tumor research. The tumor research direction should be changed from an intracellular study of the cancer cell to a study on the cell network of cancer tissue and how they become malignant. To study this new cancer research concept, a corresponding methodology must be established. For example, the specific roles of the cells surrounding cancer cells in tumorigenesis and their relationship to various characteristics of cancer tissues must be investigated to truly understand the malignancy and variety of cancer. These studies are possible through a shift of focus from the cancer cells themselves to a cell network perspective that is

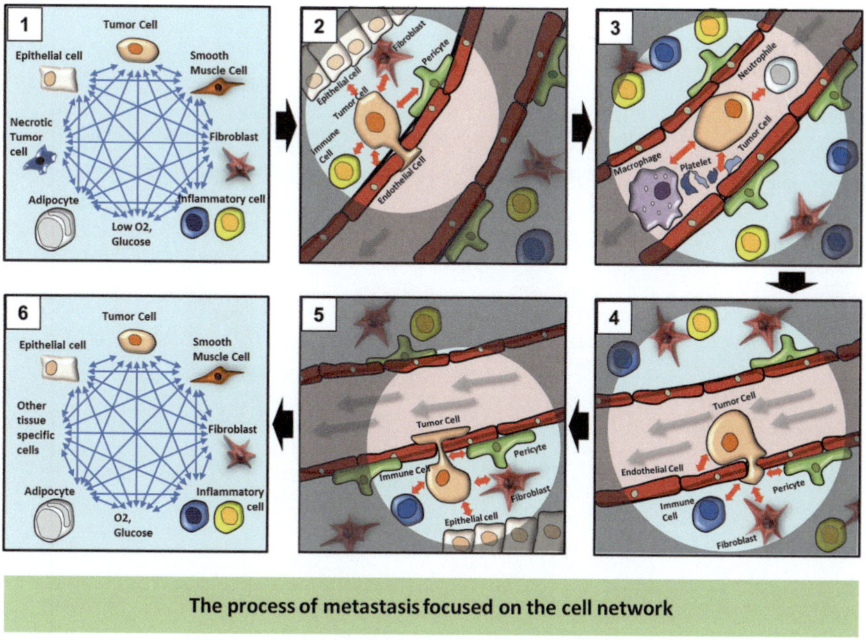

Fig. 11.15 The process of metastasis focused on the cell network

unique for cancer tissue. After an understanding and establishment of the cell network view of cancer, we can comprehend the true characteristics of metastasis and tumorigenesis. Consequently, new anticancer drugs or anticancer treatments can be developed on the basis of such an understanding of the fatal end-stage cancer that disrupts the system. From this perspective, the six steps of metastasis proposed by R. A. Weinberg in 2011 can be reconstituted into a dynamic tumor specific cell network, as follows (Fig. 11.15).

In Step 1, the cancer cells will constitute a network with the surrounding ECs, fibroblasts, necrotic cancer cells, inflammation-inducing cells, such as fat cells, lymphocytes (T-lymphocytes, B-lymphocytes, NK cells, and NKT cells), smooth muscle cells, and tissue-specific cells, along with hypoxia and a nutritionally deficient microenvironment state. In Step 2, the cancer cells will constitute an interactive network with the ECM, ECs, and pericytes. In Step 3, the cancer cells will constitute an interactive network with intravascular immune cells (macrophages, B cells, T cells, etc.), platelets, and rapid blood flow. Subsequently, in Step 4, the cancer cells will constitute an interactive network with ECs, pericytes, the basement membrane, etc.; and in Step 5, with the fibroblasts, ECs, inflammation-inducing cells, etc. of the new tissue. In the last step, Step 6, the interactive network forms with the cancer cells themselves, the lymphocytes (T-lymphocytes and B-lymphocytes), myeloid cells [tumor-associated macrophages (TAMs), myeloid-derived suppressor cells (MDSCs), tumor-associated neutrophils (TANs), and dendritic cells], NK cells, NKT cells, smooth muscle cells, fibroblasts, epithelial cells, endothelial cells, peri-

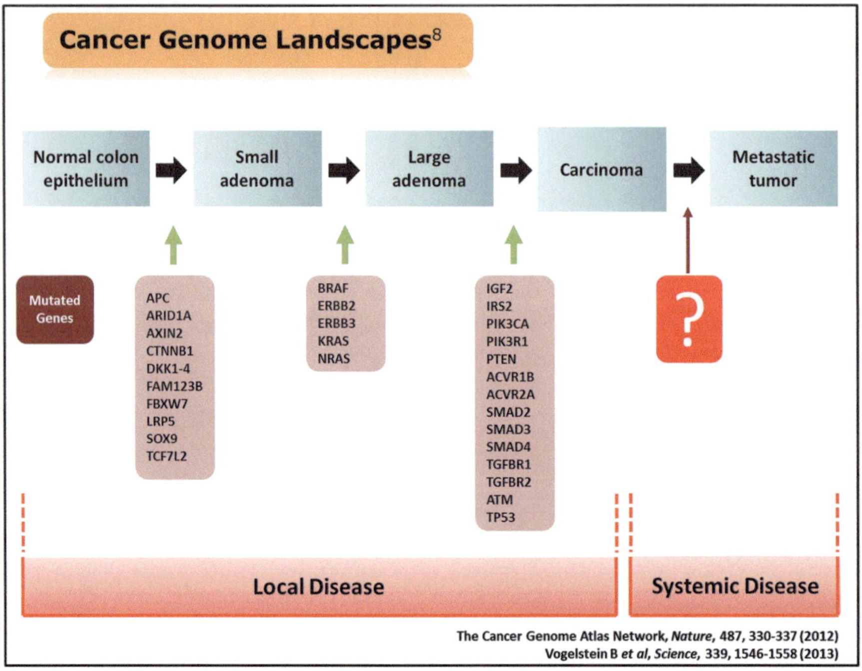

Fig. 11.16 Switch of disease characteristics from local disease to systemic disease during cancer progression

cytes, and new tissue-specific cells. During this process, the cancer cells exchange information with various surrounding cells to change and evolve constantly, eventually transforming into metastatic tumor cells or tumor stem cells.

Recent cancer genomic studies allow the large-scale screening of genetic mutations for various human cancers not in animal tissues or in cancer cell lines. The resulting genomic mutations are shown in Fig. 11.16 during the transformation of normal tissues to benign tumors and of benign tumors to malignant tumors [8]. However, the genetic mutations that are consistently common during the transformation of non-metastatic tumors to metastatic tumors have not yet been discovered. This result strongly suggests the importance of the interaction network between cancer cells and their surrounding cells in the advanced stage. Thus, in tumorigenesis, the step from normal epithelial tissue to adenoma, and then to carcinoma, can potentially be regarded as a local disease predominantly characterized by cell proliferation, whereas the final step from carcinoma to the metastatic tumor is presumed to involve a change to a systemic disease. Thus, the intercellular interaction network of cancer tissues is expected to play a critical role during this systemic change of cancer. Therefore, investigation of the tumor-specific cell network can propose a new breakthrough in explaining the metastatic stage.

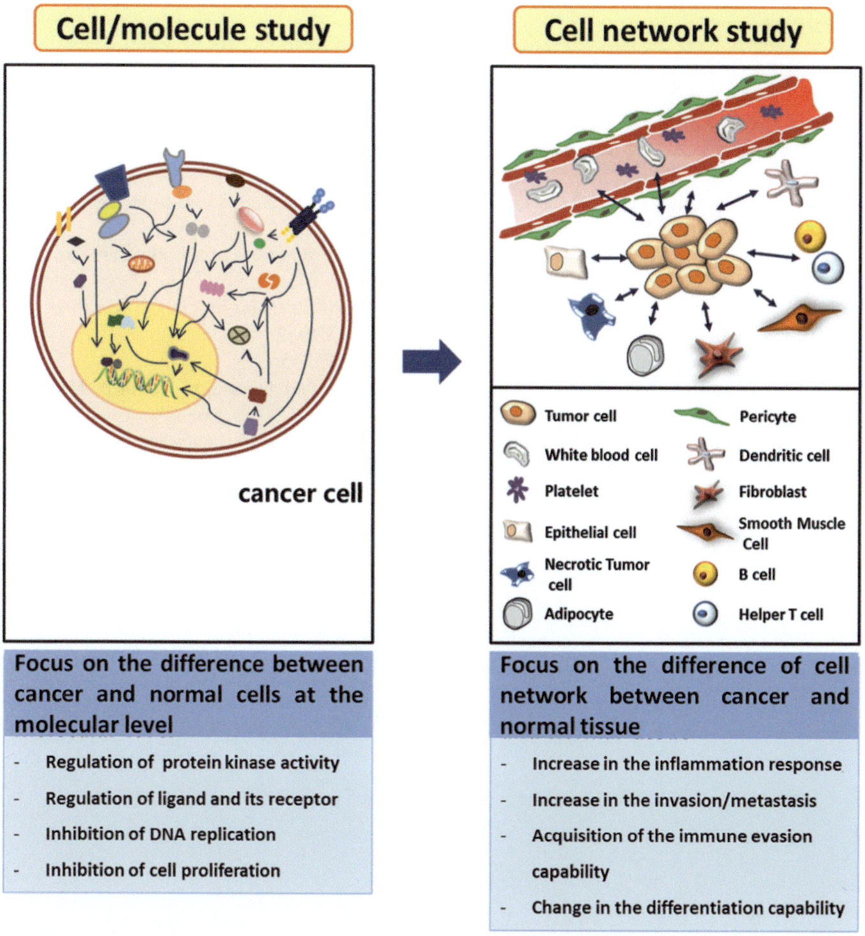

Fig. 11.17 Criteria of cellular and molecular level studies and cell network study

However, the cell network study of cancer tissue becomes enigmatic beyond imagination when the molecular changes in the interacting cells are the point of focus, which makes it difficult to identify a solution. Molecular level study will generate a huge amount of data and information, which will be too complex to solve the problems. Such complexity can be overcome by tissue level study instead of investigating it at the molecular level of the cells. Such tissue level study criteria shows that the cell network targets may include an increase in the inflammatory response, an increase in invasion/metastasis, acquisition of the immune evasion capability, a change in the differentiation capability, etc as shown in Fig. 11.17. Through these attempts, tumorigenesis can be newly understood and defined at the cell network level, which would enable the development of new-concept cancer drugs and treatments that can regulate or block malignant metastatic tumorigenesis.

References

1. Kleinsmith LJ (2005) Principles of cancer biology. Pearson, San Francisco
2. Park J, Choi KS, Kim SY et al (2003) Coordinated interaction of the vascular and nervous systems: from molecule- to cell-based approaches. Biochem Biophys Res Commun 311: 247–253
3. Lee SW, Kim WJ, Choi YK et al (2003) SSeCKs regulates angiogenesis and tight junction formation in blood–brain barrier. Nat Med 9:900–906
4. Cha JH, Wee HJ, Seo JH et al (2014) AKAP12 mediates barrier functions of fibrotic scars during repair. PLoS One 23:e94695
5. Cha JH, Wee HJ, Seo JH et al (2014) Prompt meningeal reconstruction by oxygen-sensitive AKAP12 scaffolding protein after CNS injury. Nat Commun 5:4952.
6. Hanahan D (2014) Rethinking the war on cancer. Lancet 383:558–563
7. Chaffer CL, Weinberg RA (2011) A perspective on cancer cell metastasis. Science 331: 1559–1564
8. Vogelstein B, Papadopoulos N, Velculescu VE et al (2013) Cancer genome landscapes. Science 339:1546–1558

MIX
Papier aus verantwortungsvollen Quellen
Paper from responsible sources
FSC® C105338

If you have any concerns about our products,
you can contact us on
ProductSafety@springernature.com

In case Publisher is established outside the EU,
the EU authorized representative is:
Springer Nature Customer Service Center GmbH
Europaplatz 3, 69115 Heidelberg, Germany

Printed by Libri Plureos GmbH
in Hamburg, Germany